The Biological Basis of Mental Health

This book explores the underlying biology associated with the pathology of mental health disorders and the related nervous system. Fully revised for this third edition, each chapter has been updated to include the latest research, ideas, and concepts in each field, and includes a new chapter on sleep.

Integrating up-to-date pharmacological and genetic knowledge with an understanding of environmental factors that impact on human biology, *The Biological Basis of Mental Health* covers topics including brain development, neural communication, neurotransmitters and receptors, hormones and behaviour, genetic disorders, pharmacology, drug abuse, anxiety, schizophrenia, depression, epilepsy, subcortical degenerative diseases of the brain, dementia, developmental disorders, and sleep.

Accessible and engaging, this is an essential text for mental health students, practitioners, and educators.

William T. Blows is a former Lecturer in the School of Health Sciences at City University London. His research centres on the biology of the brain, particularly in relation to mental health disorders.

The Biological Basis of Mental Health

Third edition

William T. Blows

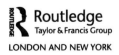 Routledge
Taylor & Francis Group

LONDON AND NEW YORK

First published 2016
by Routledge
2 Park Square, Milton Park, Abingdon, Oxon OX14 4RN

and by Routledge
711 Third Avenue, New York, NY 10017

Routledge is an imprint of the Taylor & Francis Group, an informa business

British Library Cataloguing-in-Publication Data
A catalogue record for this book is available from the British Library

Library of Congress Cataloging in Publication Data
Names: Blows, William T., 1947-, author.
Title: The biological basis of mental health nursing / William T. Blows.
Description: Edition 3. | Abingdon, Oxon; New York, NY : Routledge, 2016. |
    Includes bibliographical references and index.
Identifiers: LCCN 2015041661| ISBN 9781138900585 (hardback) |
    ISBN 9781138900615 (pbk.) | ISBN 9781315707167 (ebook)
Subjects: | MESH: Mental Disorders—physiopathology—Nurses'
    Instruction. | Psychiatric Nursing—methods—Nurses' Instruction.
Classification: LCC RC455.4.B5 | NLM WM 140 | DDC 616.89—dc23
LC record available at http://lccn.loc.gov/2015041661

ISBN: 978-1-138-90058-5 (hbk)
ISBN: 978-1-138-90061-5 (pbk)
ISBN: 978-1-315-70716-7 (ebk)

Typeset in Times New Roman
by Swales & Willis Ltd, Exeter, Devon, UK

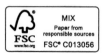

Printed and bound in Great Britain by
TJ International Ltd, Padstow, Cornwall

Contents

List of figures   vi
List of tables   x

1 Introduction to the brain   1

2 Brain development   22

3 Neural communication   39

4 Neurotransmitters and receptors   54

5 Hormones and behaviour   77

6 Genetic disorders affecting mental health   94

7 Pharmacology   119

8 Drug abuse   141

9 Stress, emotions, anxiety, and fear   168

10 Schizophrenia   200

11 Affective disorders   231

12 Epilepsy   264

13 Subcortical degenerative diseases of the brain   286

14 The ageing brain and dementia   306

15 Learning, behavioural, and developmental disorders   333

16 Sleep   355

Index   376

Figures

1.1	Exploded view of the brain	2
1.2	The meninges between the brain and the skull	3
1.3	A functional map of the left cerebral cortex	4
1.4	The components and location of the limbic system	8
1.5	Simplified connections of the amygdala	9
1.6	Coronal section through the brain	9
1.7	Areas of the basal ganglia	12
1.8	The basal ganglia motor loop	13
1.9	Sagittal section through the brain stem and cerebellum	15
1.10	Coronal section through the brain stem	16
1.11	Simplified scheme of the autonomic nervous system (ANS)	17
1.12	Sagittal section through the brain stem	19
2.1	Neurulation	23
2.2	The neuropores on days 26 and 28 of gestation	24
2.3	Schematic section through the neural tube	25
2.4	Lateral views of the folding brain	26
2.5	The reflexes at birth	27
2.6	Omega-3 and omega-6 fatty acids	36
3.1	The neuron	40
3.2	Axonal transportation	41
3.3	Resting potential in the neuronal membrane	42
3.4	The action potential	44
3.5	Sodium-potassium pumps	45
3.6	An unmyelinated axon	45
3.7	A section of myelinated axon	46
3.8	A synapse	47
3.9	Events at a synapse	47
3.10	Two types of postsynaptic receptor	48
3.11	Astrocytes	50
3.12	Astrocytes near a GABA synapse	51
4.1	The structure of three compounds: (a) an amine; (b) an amino acid; (c) the catechol group	55
4.2	An excitatory metabotropic receptor	56
4.3	An inhibitory metabotropic receptor	57
4.4	The formation of dopamine, noradrenaline, and adrenaline	58

4.5	The main dopamine pathways	59
4.6	The main noradrenaline pathways	60
4.7	The main serotonin pathways	61
4.8	The formation of serotonin	62
4.9	The synthesis of glutamate and gamma-aminobutyric acid	63
4.10	The main glutamate pathways	64
4.11	The main gamma-aminobutyric acid pathways	65
4.12	The NMDA glutamate receptor	66
4.13	The gamma-aminobutyric acid inhibitory receptor	67
4.14	The main aspartate pathways	68
4.15	The main somatostatin pathways	70
4.16	The main enkephalin pathways	71
4.17	The synthesis of acetylcholine	73
4.18	The main acetylcholine pathways	74
4.19	The main histamine pathways	75
5.1	Hormones and receptors	78
5.2	The complex of hormone and receptor	78
5.3	The hypothalamo–pituitary–adrenal axis	79
5.4	The production of various steroidal hormones	81
5.5	Adrenogenital syndrome	82
5.6	Adrenogenitalism	82
5.7	The control of production of catecholamines from the adrenal medulla	83
5.8	Aggression	88
6.1	The normal human karyotype	95
6.2	Dominant gene inheritance	96
6.3	Recessive gene inheritance	96
6.4	The genetic code for alanine	97
6.5	The gene locus	98
6.6	Genetic mutations	100
6.7	The human karyotype showing monosomy and trisomy	102
6.8	Down syndrome karyotype	103
6.9	The male Y chromosome	106
6.10	Inheritance patterns of sex determination	107
6.11	Sperm meets ovum	108
6.12	The X chromosome	109
6.13	Fragile X syndrome	111
6.14	Normal imprinting and imprinting errors in Angelman and Prader–Willi syndromes	113
7.1	Drugs binding to albumin	122
7.2	Illustration of a drug half-life	124
7.3	The enterohepatic cycle	125
7.4	Agonist drugs	126
7.5	An antagonist drug	127
7.6	Pharmacokinetic interaction	135
7.7	Drug interaction in the liver	136
7.8	Pharmacodynamic interactions at a receptor	137
8.1	The mesotelencephalic doperminergic system	142

8.2	The main pathways from the substantia nigra to the nucleus accumbens, and from the ventral tegmental area to the septal area	143
8.3	The mu receptor	145
8.4	Pathways of the extended amygdala	146
8.5	Opiate binding to the mu receptor	147
8.6	The action of amphetamines and cocaine at the dopaminergic synapse	150
8.7	Ecstasy intake and the events that follow	152
8.8	The chemical structure of cannabidiol	154
8.9	Cannabis causes dopamine release	154
8.10	POMC neurons and appetite	156
8.11	Molecular structure of serotonin, LSD, and psilocin	163
9.1	The main components of the limbic system	169
9.2	Inputs and outputs of the amygdala	170
9.3	The brain stem nuclei emotional responses	172
9.4	The neuroendocrine response to stress	173
9.5	The general adaptation syndrome (GAS)	175
9.6	The brain areas of love	179
9.7	The brain areas involved in music	181
9.8	The brain areas involved in General Anxiety Disorder	185
9.9	The mechanism of *Glo 1* and MG in anxiety-related behaviour	186
9.10	The genetic basis of fear	187
9.11	Adipose feedback to the brain	191
9.12	The liver control of hunger	192
10.1	The *DISC1* gene pathway	206
10.2	Views of the cerebral cortex to show the cingulate gyrus	207
10.3	Schematic view of the hippocampal complex	208
10.4	The hippocampal complex shown within the brain	209
10.5	The 'trisynaptic pathway' in the hippocampus	210
10.6	The four main types of dopaminergic pathway	215
10.7	The factors affecting the cause of schizophrenia	218
10.8	The chemical structures of some important antipsychotic drugs	220
10.9	The receptor antagonistic properties of the major atypical antipsychotic drugs	223
10.10	The atypical antipsychotic effects on the mesocortical and mesolimbic systems	225
10.11	The 'hit and run' theory of atypical antipsychotic activity	226
11.1	The PKC enzyme system in mania	235
11.2	The areas of the world with a high suicide rate	237
11.3	Areas of the brain involved in depression	239
11.4	The diffuse modulatory systems	241
11.5	The hypothalamo–pituitary–adrenal axis and the hypothalamo–pituitary–thyroid axis	244
11.6	The effect of blood cortisol concentration on adrenocorticotropic hormone	245
11.7	The relationship between cortisol concentrations and cytokine production	247
11.8	Location of the pineal gland	251

11.9	Structure of some important antidepressants	252
11.10	The short-term and long-term effects of SSRI drugs on the serotonin neurons	254
11.11	The action of lithium	261
12.1	The normal electroencephalogram (EEG) tracing	267
12.2	The EEG seen in absences	267
12.3	The EEG seen in simple partial seizures	268
12.4	The EEG seen in complex partial seizures	268
12.5	The EEG seen in general tonic–clonic seizures	269
12.6	The mitochondrial DNA loop	271
12.7	Changes at the epileptogenic focus neuron	273
12.8	The primary focus	273
12.9	The action of anticonvulsant drugs	281
13.1	The motor loop	287
13.2	Normal basal ganglia pathways	287
13.3	Parkinson's disease	290
13.4	The pathway in which MPTP causes neuronal damage and losses	292
13.5	Huntington's disease	296
13.6	Chromosome 4 with the huntingtin gene at 4p16.3	298
13.7	Huntingtin protein in normal brain tissue and Huntington's disease	300
13.8	Wilson's disease	302
14.1	Connections of the hippocampus important in memory	309
14.2	The brain gets old	310
14.3	Chromosome 21	317
14.4	Normal amyloid protein production and amyloid plaque formation	318
14.5	Normal tau synthesis and abnormal tau tangles	320
14.6	The *ApoEε-4* and cyclophilin A pathway in Alzheimer's disease	322
14.7	The inflammatory response in Alzheimer's disease	325
14.8	Ampakine drug action	330
15.1	The magnocellular layer in dyslexia	335
15.2	The planum temporale	336
15.3	The cerebellum showing the vermis	343
15.4	Phenylalanine hydroxylase action	346
15.5	Fetal alcohol syndrome (FAS)	348
15.6	Effect of smoking during pregnancy	348
15.7	The loop extending from the orbitofrontal cortex to the cingulate gyrus	350
16.1	Synaptic homeostasis hypothesis (SHY)	357
16.2	The 8-hour sleep cycle	358
16.3	Atonia during REM sleep	359
16.4	Brain waves	360
16.5	Peribrachial area, REM-on, REM-off	363
16.6	The ventrolateral preoptic nucleus	364
16.7	SCN and blue light impulses from retina in light and dark	365
16.8	Dreams and nightmares	367

Tables

1.1	Functions of the autonomic nervous system	18
1.2	Brain pathways involved in mental health	19
2.1	Comparison of prefrontal cortex development	30
2.2	Types of memory	31
2.3	The vitamins involved in brain development and function	34
2.4	Minerals involved in brain development and function	34
4.1	Classes of serotonin receptors and their intracellular actions	62
4.2	The affinity of endogenous opiates for opiate receptors	72
5.1	Sex differences in the brain in terms of task performance	85
6.1	Proportions of genes in common between relatives of different degrees	101
6.2	Changes in the incidence of Down syndrome with maternal age	103
6.3	X-linked syndromes involving intellectual disability	110
7.1	Routes of drug administration	121
7.2	Different types of dry oral medication	128
7.3	Different types of liquid medication	129
8.1	Drug interactions with opiates	148
8.2	Drug interactions with methadone	148
8.3	Drug interactions with cocaine	151
8.4	Drug interactions with amphetamines	153
8.5	Drug interactions with cannabinoids	157
8.6	Drug interactions with alcohol	160
8.7	The effects of inhaling nicotine on nonsmokers and smokers	161
8.8	Drug interactions with nicotine	161
10.1	The symptoms of schizophrenia	201
10.2	Genetic risk of developing schizophrenia	202
10.3	The major genes examined in schizophrenia research	203
10.4	The effects and side effects of the phenothiazine antipsychotic drugs	221
10.5	Receptor affinity for the major antipsychotic drugs	224
11.1	Previous and current classifications of depression	232
11.2	The symptoms of depression	232
11.3	The psychoimmunological changes reported in depression	246
11.4	Selective serotonin and noradrenaline inhibitors	255
11.5	Some atypical antidepressants	255
11.6	MAOI antidepressants	257
12.1	The known causes of seizures	269

12.2	Some genetic epileptic disorders	270
12.3	Stages of a tonic–clonic fit	274
12.4	Immediate first aid required at each stage of the fit	274
12.5	The classification of the antiepileptic drugs	279
12.6	Drugs used in specific epileptic categories	282
13.1	The genetic involvement in Parkinson's disease	291
13.2	The polyglutamine (PolyQ) diseases	297
14.1	The distinction between Alzheimer's disease (AD) and dementia with cortical Lewy bodies (DCLB)	327
16.1	Sleep and the risk of catching the common cold	368
16.2	Teenage sleep loss in America, UK, Korea, and Japan	368
16.3	Some common causes of insomnia	372

1 Introduction to the brain

- Introduction
- The meninges and cerebrospinal fluid
- The cerebrum
- The limbic system
- The thalamus, hypothalamus, and pituitary gland
- The basal ganglia and the cerebellum
- The brain stem
- The autonomic nervous system
- The main pathways involved in mental health
- The principal brain pathologies affecting mental health
- Key points

Introduction

The human brain is one of Nature's greatest achievements. It is the development of the brain that has allowed humans to progress from their humble origins to putting a man on the moon. This chapter consists of an overview of the brain and contains many references to other pages of this book where the area of the brain in question is explored in more detail, usually in relation to a particular mental health pathology. At the simplest level the brain works something like a computer, but this is a computer like no other. It has been said that to build a computer to do everything the human brain does, the computer would have to be the size of Europe. Like a computer, the brain has an input (called a **sensory nervous system**) and an output (called a **motor nervous system**). Between these two systems, the brain carries out **cognitive functions**, i.e. mental processing such as thought, language, intellect, memory, and interpretation of the world about us.

As with a computer, things can go wrong with the brain, and when they do, symptoms occur, just as with any other organ. The pathological conditions associated with the brain may be either **neurological** or **psychiatric**, depending on the degree of physical disturbance (neurological) or mental health disturbance (psychiatric) identified. These two types of brain dysfunction increasingly overlap, with the distinction between them becoming blurred. This is because we are learning that neurological conditions often involve disturbance of the mind and that mental health disturbance has some degree of physical (or biological) basis.

The brain can be divided into several anatomical, developmental, and functional areas as we move downwards from the top towards the base (Figure 1.1). The **cerebrum**, at the top, is the largest and most advanced region of the brain, carrying out all our cognitive and conscious processes. Beneath this is the **limbic cortex** (*cortex* means 'surface layer'), the area concerned with preservation of both the individual and the species. This is the area involved in emotions, such as fear, and behavioural patterns, such as eating, which are designed to keep us alive. Beneath this are the **basal ganglia** and the **cerebellum**, areas involved in control of movement at a subconscious (automatic) level. Finally, at the very base of the brain, the **brain stem** is involved in keeping the individual alive at the physiological level, controlling the heart, the blood pressure, and the lungs, among other functions.

At tissue level, the areas of the brain are either **grey matter**, made from the cell bodies of **neurons** (brain cells), or **white matter**, made from the **axons** of neurons. Grey matter

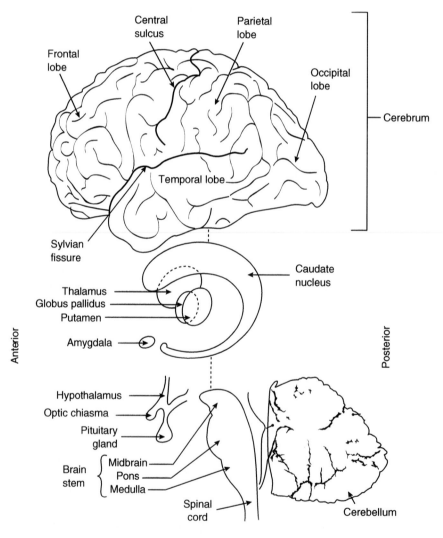

Figure 1.1 Exploded view of the brain seen from the left, showing the main components.

dominates the outer surfaces of the brain, known as the **cortex**, with white matter inside. The surfaces, or cortex, are folded into **gyri** (singular **gyrus**, i.e. the top of a fold), and **sulci** (singular **sulcus**, i.e. the bottom of a fold) in order to increase the surface area for the purpose of packing in more neurons. Cell bodies that are separate from the main outer surface, i.e. patches of grey matter deeper inside the white matter, are called **ganglia** (e.g. the basal ganglia). **Nuclei** are patches of grey matter that have a specific controlling function (e.g. the cranial nerve nuclei of the brain stem). Several areas of the brain, such as the **thalamus** and **hypothalamus**, are actually discrete collections of distinct nuclei, which are linked together by one name because they are anatomically positioned together and have similar, related functions.

The meninges and cerebrospinal fluid

The brain and the cord are covered by membranes called the **meninges**, which form three layers (Figure 1.2). The innermost layer is the **pia mater** ('gentle mother'), the middle layer is the **arachnoid mater** ('spider mother'), and the outermost layer is the **dura mater** ('tough mother'). Between the arachnoid mater and pia mater is the **subarachnoid space**, containing a watery fluid called **cerebrospinal fluid (CSF)**. This is formed from blood plasma inside the **ventricles** of the brain, i.e. the cavities within the brain substance (Marieb and Hoehn 2014). CSF fills the two **lateral ventricles**, the **third ventricle**, and the **fourth ventricle** before it flows out into the subarachnoid space. From here it circulates over the brain and cord surface before being absorbed back into blood via small projections of the arachnoid mater called **villi**. CSF also flows from the fourth ventricle through the **central canal** of the cord. CSF has several important functions.

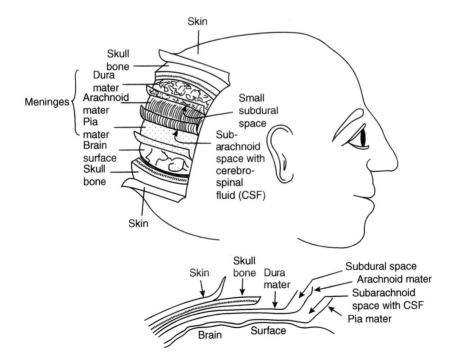

Figure 1.2 The meninges between the brain and the skull.

1   It protects the central nervous system by acting as a water jacket, giving a cushioning effect to the central nervous system. This is a very important function, helping to reduce brain injury in accidents involving the head.
2   It provides support and flotation for the brain, which would otherwise weigh 30 times heavier without it!
3   It delivers nutrition to some parts of the nervous system, since the CSF contains not just water but also some minerals and glucose.
4   It acts as part of an excretory pathway for the end products of neurotransmitter metabolism (known as **metabolites**) and some psychoactive drugs. These wastes pass from the brain into the CSF, then into the blood, which then goes on to the kidneys for filtering and the excretion of wastes in the urine.

CSF is often very important in mental health because of its role as an excretory pathway. One investigation, called **lumbar puncture**, is a method of collecting a sample of CSF in which the excretory products from brain chemicals or drugs can be measured (Blows 2002). A needle is put into the spinal subarachnoid space below the level of lumbar vertebra 2 (L2) so as not to hit the solid spinal cord. The quantity of metabolite found in the CSF sample gives an indication of the amount of neurotransmitter that is active in the brain.

The cerebrum

The largest and uppermost area of the brain, the cerebrum (Figure 1.1), is divided into two **hemispheres**, left and right, which are linked by the **corpus callosum**, a connection that allows the two halves to communicate with each other. Each hemisphere is further divided into four **lobes**: the frontal, parietal, temporal, and occipital lobes. **Brodmann numbers** form an internationally agreed numbering system to identify and map the major areas of the cerebral cortex (outer surface) according to their functions (Figure 1.3).

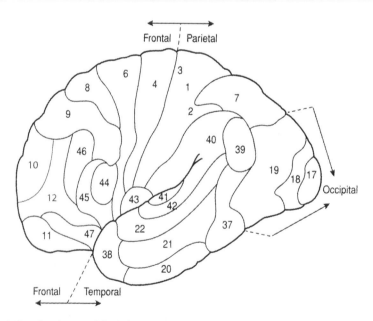

Figure 1.3 A functional map of the left cerebral cortex showing important Brodmann numbers.

Frontal lobe

The **frontal lobes** contain the main **motor cortex** (motor = movement) (Brodmann 4) for each side of the body. Each cortex, left and right, controls skeletal muscles via long pathways descending into the spinal cord, then out to the muscles; these motor pathways are called the **pyramidal tracts** (Marieb and Hoehn 2014). In addition, the **premotor cortex** (Brodmann 6), just anterior to the motor cortex, is involved in **motor planning**, a process that is vital for the swift and accurate execution of complex motor tasks. Speech motor areas (Brodmann 44 and 45), also known as **Broca's area**, control the muscles of speech.

The frontal lobe also has areas concerned with the following range of important higher intellectual activities:

- achieving and sustaining attention and concentration;
- carrying out language activities, both spoken and in thought;
- maintaining memory;
- forming part of the pathways involved in emotions;
- carrying out complex skills involving visual space (i.e. **visuospatial tasks**), which require, for example, sequence planning or detailed copying of figures;
- performing **executive functions** such as monitoring one's own performance and making corrections as required, formulating and achieving goals, planning, judgement and reasoning.

The frontal lobes are the last part of the brain to mature, sometime after puberty, so teenagers function with reduced levels of emotional control and reasoning.

The frontal lobes are the main centres of consciousness, particularly of self (i.e. self-awareness). Many of our **thought processes**, particularly **planning** (which requires forward thinking towards the future), reasoning, and deduction, are carried out by the frontal lobe, and in particular the prefrontal cortex. It has the most neural connections, it makes the most complex integrations with other systems, and it requires more than twice the energy requirements of other brain areas such as the limbic system. Thought processes, unlike other brain functions, do not rely on sensory input directly; they are an 'internal' mental function. However, thought does require processed information on the environment supplied via the sensory areas of the brain and influenced by the hippocampus, combined with previously stored information and knowledge, in particular knowledge of language. Because thought content and processing is strongly influenced by the hippocampus, any disruption of the hippocampus, as in **schizophrenia**, causes symptoms such as thought disorder.

Many components of what we regard as our **personality** are caused by the activities of the frontal lobes. It should therefore not be surprising to learn that many psychiatric disorders and some specific mental health symptoms either manifest within or involve the frontal lobes of the brain. No wonder then that one of the very few psychosurgical operations carried out in the past for mental health reasons was a **prefrontal leucotomy**, which involved severing pathways leading from the frontal lobe to the other parts of the brain.

Parietal lobe

The **parietal lobe** involves the main **somatic** (*soma* = 'body', thus *somatic* = 'from the body') sensory cortex (Brodmann 1, 2 and 3), and the somatic sensory association area (Brodmann 5 and 7). **Association areas** are essential for the interpretation and memory of senses, and therefore the understanding of sensory stimuli. This is important because the brain is itself shut away from the world inside the skull. The only way the brain is going to know what is happening outside the skull is via the sensory nervous system, and by its ability to interpret the signals brought in by that system. Association areas are therefore critical in the brain's understanding of the world around us. A language area, also known as **Wernicke's area**, occurs partly within the parietal (Brodmann 39) and the temporal lobes (Brodmann 22), and is the main site for understanding and formulation of spoken sentences.

Temporal lobe

The **temporal lobe** houses the auditory area for the conscious sensation of hearing (Brodmann 41 and 42) and the auditory association area (Brodmann 22, part of Wernicke's area). What we actually hear is generated in the temporal lobe auditory area and not in the ears. Ears are organs necessary to convert sound waves into nerve impulses. The temporal lobe makes sense of these impulses as conscious sound. This lobe is also involved in the creation of personality and is involved in emotional responses to sensory stimuli.

Occipital lobe

The **occipital lobe** has the main visual cortex (Brodmann 17) and the visual association areas (Brodmann 18 and 19) (Blows 2000a). This is therefore the conscious area for vision; i.e. as with the temporal lobe and hearing, we actually 'see' the world with the back of the brain. The eyes only convert light energy into nerve impulses; it is the occipital lobe that makes sense of these impulses as a conscious visual picture.

The cingulate cortex (or limbic cortex) and the insular cortex

The **cingulate cortex** is situated in the medial aspect of the cerebral cortex and is part of the **limbic association area**. It overlies the upper surface of the corpus callosum, from front to back, and tucks beneath the corpus callosum anteriorly (Chapter 9, Figure 9.1). Part of the cingulate cortex is the **cingulate gyrus**. The cingulate cortex is usually divided into an anterior part (Brodmann 24, 32 and 33) and a posterior part (Brodmann 23 and 31). The anterior cingulate cortex is closely linked with the limbic system (see below) and is therefore involved in processing emotions. The posterior cingulate is involved with learning and memory. It is implicated as part of the pathology of schizophrenia (Chapter 10, Figure 10.2), depression (Chapter 11, Figure 11.3) and obsessive compulsive disorder (Chapter 15, Figure 15.7).

The **insular cortex** is that part of the cerebral cortex that lies within the **lateral sulcus**, i.e. the deep fissure between the temporal lobe below and the parietal/frontal lobes above. The insular cortex cannot be seen from the outside unless parts of the temporal lobe and some of the frontal or parietal lobes are removed. It is involved with consciousness, regulation of homeostasis, perception, cognitive processing, and emotions (Chapter 9, Figures 9.6 and 9.7).

Functions of the cerebrum

One of the most important functions of the cerebrum is the government of three important aspects of **consciousness**: awareness (sensory); cognition (e.g. thought); and response (motor). The entire cortex plays a role in consciousness, although for the most part the parietal, temporal, and occipital lobes are involved in conscious interpretation of sensory stimuli, whereas the frontal lobe is concerned with cognition and consciousness of the 'self'. A discussion of consciousness can be found in Blows (2012, Chapter 10; see also Blows 2000b).

The left hemisphere of the cerebrum is dominant for several functions, notably fine motor control, logic, analytical work, language, and verbal tasks. Fine motor control means digital and hand movements, an essential part of many activities. Since most of the motor (i.e. pyramidal) fibres cross in the medulla, the dominance of motor control in the left hemisphere makes most people right handed. However, we know that it is entirely normal for left-handed people to be an exception to this, although left-handed dominance has not always been accepted by society. The right hemisphere is dominant for non-language skills, spatial perception, and artistic and musical endeavours. People who have a general dominance of left hemisphere function are sometimes called 'thinkers', whereas those with right hemisphere function dominance are sometimes referred to as 'creators'. This is an oversimplification, and gives the impression that the two hemispheres work in isolation. This is not true; they work together, communicating with each other through the corpus callosum, which joins the left hemisphere to the right hemisphere (Marieb and Hoehn 2014).

Sleep is a vital function for the brain and is discussed in detail in Chapter 16. During waking hours, the brain is able to concentrate on the specific task at hand, but there are times when the brain is allowed to wander, and not concentrate on anything. During this time, it would be easy to suspect that the brain is inactive, but this is far from the truth. The brain appears to be active on 'internal matters' rather than 'external matters', but these internal matters remain unknown to us, and have therefore been called *dark energy*. The **default mode network (DMN)** is the system in the brain responsible for dark energy; it is a system that keeps active even when the brain is not doing anything. This is rather similar to a car engine 'ticking over' or 'running idle' when not involved in moving the car. The DMN is probably involved in establishing and maintaining consciousness, and it keeps the brain in a state of instant readiness for when focus on a specific activity is necessary. Before the discovery of the DMN, neurologists thought that the brain was cycling between moments of no activity and moderate activity; but now the new concept is that the brain is cycling between moderate activity and high activity. This, plus the notion that the brain is active during sleep, suggests that, from birth to death, the brain *never* rests. The main areas of the brain that make up the DMN are the **ventral** and **dorsal medial prefrontal cortex**, the **inferior** and **medial parietal cortex**, the **lateral temporal cortex**, the **hippocampus**, and the **posterior cingulate cortex**. Other areas are also involved, but these regions appear to control the activity levels of the brain's idle state. This new discovery may be important for mental health because there is growing evidence that altered connections in the DMN are possibly linked to disorders such as autism, depression, Alzheimer's disease (AD), and even schizophrenia. In fact, some researchers are suggesting that one day AD may be classified as a disorder of the DMN (Raichle 2010).

The **salience network** is another network of brain connections, consisting of two main areas: the **anterior insula** and the **dorsal anterior cingulate cortex**. As with the DMN, the salience network also involves other brain areas, including the **amygdala**, the **ventral tegmental area (VTA)**, and the **ventral striatum** (i.e. the ventral **corpus striatum**; see below for discussion of these brain areas). The salience network monitors and filters the constant stream of incoming sensory stimuli to select which is the most salient (or relevant) to pass onto the rest of the brain. Only the most important sensory stimuli become salient, e.g. aspects currently under our attention, surprise stimuli and potential threats to our well-being. Without this process, the brain would be constantly overwhelmed and swamped with irrelevant sensory data.

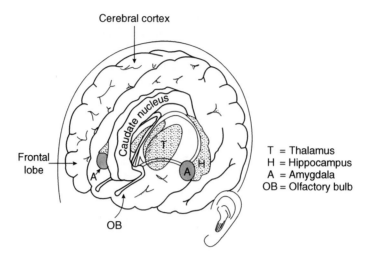

Figure 1.4 The components and location of the limbic system.

Learning and **memory** are also two vital functions for the brain. Learning is the process by which long-term memory is formed. These are covered in more detail in Chapters 2 and 15.

The limbic system

The limbic system is the brain's emotional centre, and it is also important for learning and for maintaining the brain's role in relation to a sense of human needs and safety. The system consists of a ring of structures, notably the amygdala, the **hippocampus**, the **cingulate gyrus**, the **mammillary bodies of the hypothalamus**, and the **orbitofrontal cortex** (Figure 1.4 and Chapter 9, Figure 9.1).

The amygdala

The amygdala is a small pea-sized collection of nuclei situated at the tail end of the caudate nucleus (Figure 1.4). This tiny area is the emotional centre of the brain. It receives sensory input from several sources, particularly the cerebral cortex, the thalamus, and the hippocampus (Figure 1.5) (Blows 2000c). All kinds of stimuli from the external environment, or from the internal environment of the body, pass through the amygdala. The amygdala may respond to these stimuli by initiating specific emotional responses. Any adverse stimuli are known as **stressors** – i.e. potential threats to which the brain must respond with either an emotional or physical change. Output from the amygdala, in response to either good stimuli or stressors, passes to the brain stem (for emotional responses) and to the hypothalamus (for any physical response) (Figure 1.5). The amygdala is described in more detail in Chapter 9 in relation to emotions and phobic states.

The hippocampus

The hippocampus is tucked up underneath the temporal lobe (Figure 1.6). The main function of this area is that of short-term memory conversion to long-term memory, i.e. memory of

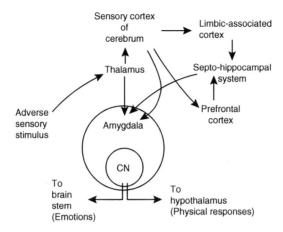

Figure 1.5 Simplified connections of the amygdala. CN = central nucleus.

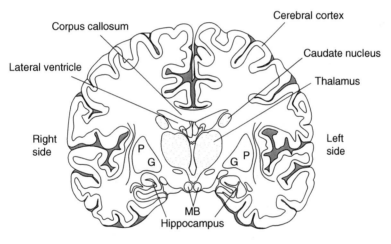

Figure 1.6 Coronal section through the brain showing the location of the cerebral cortex, the corpus callosum, the thalamus, the hippocampus, the mammillary bodies (MB) of the hypothalamus, and parts of the basal ganglia. P = putamen, G = globus pallidus.

very recent events (within the last few hours) is held temporarily until it is either committed to long-term memory or forgotten (Blows 2000c). The conversion of short-term memory to long-term memory is a component of learning (Chapter 15). Emotional behaviour and thinking are both influenced by hippocampal activity, notably during aggression. The hippocampus is described in more detail in relation to schizophrenia (Chapter 10).

The orbitofrontal cortex

Although strictly part of the cerebrum, the orbitofrontal cortex has strong links with the limbic system and is sometimes considered to be part of the limbic associated cortex.

This part of the frontal lobe lies ventral to the prefrontal cortex, i.e. it is the brain area found immediately above the eyes. It is one of the most complex parts of the brain, and its functions are only just coming to light. All sensory stimuli (vision, hearing, etc.), is first processed by the relevant sensory areas, then passes into the posterior orbitofrontal cortex. The main function of the orbitofrontal cortex is to use this sensory input to guide behaviour, learning, memory, and pleasure-seeking activity.

The thalamus, hypothalamus, and pituitary gland

The thalamus

The thalamus is a collection of more than 30 nuclei situated underneath the cerebrum, close to the midline of the brain on each side (Figure 1.6) (Blows 2000c). The nuclei are set in four main groups: anterior, medial, midline, and lateral. The thalamus is the sensory relay station; i.e. sensory impulses originating in the body (somatic) or the special senses (e.g. vision and hearing) pass into the thalamus, from where they are relayed to the appropriate part of the cerebrum. Visual nerve impulses from the retina must be relayed by the thalamus to the visual cortex of the occipital lobe (Brodmann 17, Figure 1.3), and nerve impulses generated from sound by the ear are relayed by the thalamus to the auditory cortex in the temporal lobe (Brodmann 41 and 42, Figure 1.3). Even somatic sensations from the body, e.g. touch or pain, are relayed by the thalamus to the appropriate part of the sensory cortex in the parietal lobe (Brodmann 1, 2, and 3, Figure 1.3). The sensory cortex has a cellular layout rather like a body plan, with cells in specific sites on the cortex accepting sensations from particular parts of the body. Impulses arising from the toes, for example, would be directed by the thalamus to the cortex occurring down the midline division, while impulses destined for the cells that accept sensations from the face would be directed to the lateral aspect of the cortex (Blows 2000b). Pain is the only sensation that is 'conscious' at both thalamic and cerebral levels, whereas all other sensations must arrive at the cerebrum before we become aware of them.

The thalamus also focuses attention to specific sensations by making certain sensory areas of the cerebrum more receptive to sensory stimuli and other areas less receptive. Integration of some different sensory stimuli takes place inside the thalamus, a process essential for full appreciation of the information received by the sense organs.

The thalamus has a motor function as well. One particular thalamic nucleus links with the premotor cortex (Brodmann 6) of the frontal lobe, influencing motor function by increasing the focus of attention on the motor activity in progress. This influence is normally deactivated by the **basal ganglia motor loop** when no movement is happening, or activated when movement begins.

The hypothalamus

The hypothalamus occurs as a collection of nuclei at the base of the brain (Figure 1.6) (Blows 2000c). These nuclei are arranged in anterior, posterior, ventromedial, dorsomedial, and lateral groups. The **mammillary body**, a bulbous part of the hypothalamus, is a member of the posterior group of nuclei and a useful landmark on the undersurface of the brain. The hypothalamus is connected to the **pituitary gland** by a narrow stalk, the **pituitary stalk** (or **infundibulum**) (Marieb and Hoehn 2014).

The hypothalamus has a wide range of functions and controlling centres:

1   It is part of the **reticular formation** (see brain stem on page 15) that controls the **sleep–wake cycle** (Chapter 16); the role of the hypothalamus is that of the **alerting centre**. It wakes the brain from sleep by sending impulses out to the cerebrum.
2   It controls the body's temperature via the **temperature regulation centre**, keeping the body at 37°C. By monitoring blood temperature and acting as a thermostat it corrects the temperature if it goes too high or too low. The *anterior* part of the hypothalamus controls heat loss if the body gets too hot (e.g. by promoting sweating) and the *posterior* part controls heat conservation if the body gets too cold.
3   It regulates eating by giving a feeling of fullness (**satiation**), which prevents further food intake. This is the function of the **satiety centre** within the ventromedial part of the hypothalamus. Hunger and the seeking of both food and drink, however, are controlled by the lateral part of the hypothalamus (Chapter 9, Figures 9.11 and 9.12).
4   It controls the functions of both the **sympathetic** and **parasympathetic** components of the **autonomic nervous system (ANS)**.
5   It influences sexual activity in combination with other regions of the brain.
6   It plays a role in emotions.
7   It controls the hormonal output of the pituitary gland, both anterior and posterior lobes.

Anterior pituitary lobe

Releasing hormones (RH) or **inhibiting hormones (IH)** (sometimes called releasing or inhibiting factors) pass down from the hypothalamus into the anterior lobe and either release or inhibit the release of the anterior lobe hormones. Anterior pituitary lobe hormones are:

- **growth hormone** – as the name suggests, it is important for growth;
- **adrenocorticotropic hormone (ACTH)**, which acts on the adrenal cortex to stimulate the production of cortisol (Chapter 5, Figure 5.3);
- **thyroid-stimulating hormone (TSH)**, which acts on the thyroid gland and causes release of the thyroid hormones **T3** and **T4** (Chapter 5, Figure 5.3);
- **prolactin**, which promotes breast milk production during breastfeeding;
- **follicle-stimulating hormone (FSH)**, which stimulates the ovarian follicles to mature the ova (egg cells) in females and stimulates cells in the male testes to produce sperm;
- **luteinzing hormone (LH)**, which promotes ovulation in females and stimulates the production of testosterone from the male testes.

Posterior pituitary lobe

The hormones that are released from the posterior lobe are produced in the hypothalamus. They pass down into the pituitary gland, where they are stored and released by hypothalamic control. These hypothalamic hormones are:

- **Antidiuretic hormone (ADH)**, from the **supraoptic nucleus** of the hypothalamus, is a hormone that is released into the blood and acts on the renal nephron to conserve water.

- **Oxytocin**, from the **paraventricular nucleus** of the hypothalamus, is a hormone that is released into the blood and causes smooth-muscle contraction (for example, it contracts the uterus during labour), and also contraction of special breast cells which push milk toward the nipple during breastfeeding. It also appears to drive maternal behaviour and social attachment; a so-called 'bonding molecule'. Research is underway to see if this hormone may have benefits for autistic children, in combination with other therapies (see autism, Chapter 15).

The basal ganglia and the cerebellum

These areas are part of what is called the **extrapyramidal tract** system; that is, they control the finer details of skeletal muscle movement at a subconscious level (Blows 2000c; Blows 2012). The extrapyramidal tract side effects of drugs such as the antipsychotics are caused by disturbance to this system, particularly the basal ganglia.

The basal ganglia

The basal ganglia are made up of five main nuclei: the **putamen**, the **caudate nucleus**, the **globus pallidus**, the **substantia nigra**, and the **subthalamus** (it is important not to muddle the thalamus with the hypothalamus and the subthalamus) (Figure 1.7). Several terms are used

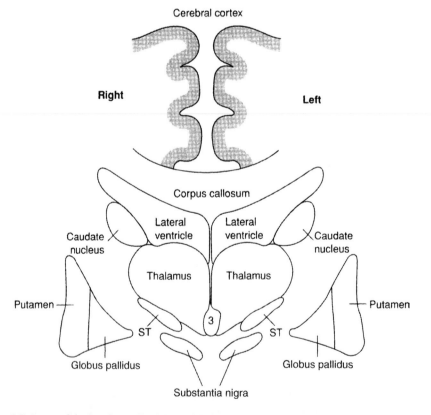

Figure 1.7 Areas of the basal ganglia. ST = subthalamus, 3 = third ventricle.

to describe the different ways in which some of these nuclei are grouped. The corpus striatum is the area involving the putamen and the caudate nucleus combined, with the main pyramidal motor pathways, called the **internal capsule**, passing between them. But the putamen is also part of the lentiform nucleus, which also includes the globus pallidus (Figure 1.7).

Collectively, the function of the basal ganglia is the fine control of muscle contraction (Marieb and Hoehn 2014). The corpus striatum receives input from the main motor and sensory areas of the cerebrum, as well as inputs from the thalamus, subthalamus, and the brain stem (particularly the substantia nigra). Degeneration of the caudate nucleus is seen in Huntington's disease, in which excessive uncontrollable movement is a major symptom (Chapter 13). Output from the corpus striatum passes via the globus pallidus to the motor areas of the frontal lobe. The globus pallidus has several vital functions, notably the control of trunk and limb movements, including the positioning of limbs just prior to the movements of the digits, a function of the main motor cortex.

The globus pallidus and the putamen are also involved in the **basal ganglia motor loop** (Figure 1.8; Blows 2012). When the body is not moving, the globus pallidus inhibits a particular thalamic nucleus which, when active, influences movement. As movement starts, stimulation of the putamen causes a blocking of the globus pallidus, removing the inhibition on the thalamus. The thalamus then becomes free to influence the main motor areas of the frontal lobe.

The substantia nigra is particularly important as the area that controls decreasing **muscle tone**, the state of tension within a muscle, which is essential for the muscle to achieve full contraction. The axonal tracts coming from the substantia nigra to go to the corpus

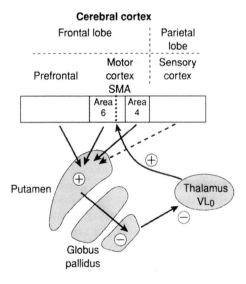

Figure 1.8 The basal ganglia motor loop. Input to the putamen comes from the frontal cortex, with less input coming from the parietal sensory cortex. This activates (+) neurons running from the putamen to the globus pallidus, which, in turn, then deactivates (–) neurons linking the globus pallidus with the ventral lateral nucleus of the thalamus (VLo). These globus pallidus neurons were preventing (i.e. inhibiting, shown as –) any feedback from the VLo to the cerebral cortex. However, deactivation from the putamen has removed this inhibition, and the VLo then is free to feed back to the cortex (+): more precisely, the supplementary motor area (SMA) of area 6 of the motor cortex.

striatum are the **nigrostriatal pathway**, and these neurons use the neurotransmitter dopamine. Degeneration of the substantia nigra causes Parkinson's disease, and parkinsonian-like symptoms are a feature of some drug side effects.

The subthalamus has the role of inhibiting excessive motor activity from the cerebral motor cortex (i.e. acting as a breaking system for the pyramidal tracts). Disturbance of this function can result in excessive pyramidal activity, affecting skeletal muscle contraction.

Apart from Huntington's disease and Parkinson's disease, disturbance of basal ganglia function includes several other different movement disorders, which are described in relation to psychotropic drug side effects in Chapter 10.

The cerebellum

The cerebellum (Figure 1.9) is another part of the extrapyramidal tract system, controlling muscle function at a subconscious level (Blows 2000d). There are two hemispheres, as in the cerebrum, but just three main lobes: the **anterior**, **posterior**, and **flocculonodular** lobes. Each lobe is further subdivided into smaller regions of surface area. This surface is made of grey matter, which is folded to increase the area to about 75% of the surface area of the cerebrum. There is white matter below the surface and at the core of this white matter are further patches of grey matter, the **cerebellar nuclei**. The routes for impulses to pass into and out from the cerebellum are through the brain stem via the **cerebellar peduncles**, foot-like connections between the cerebellum and the brain stem (Marieb and Hoehn 2014).

The functions of the cerebellum are as follows:

1   To maintain the balance of the body: the cerebellum makes fine adjustments to muscle tensions to stabilise body position, especially when upright, to prevent falling over. Sensory feedback on balance, to the cerebellum, is from somatic **proprioception** (sensory information on body position from muscles, tendons, and joints) and **vestibular** information from the semicircular canals of the inner ear. The proprioception impulses enter the anterior lobe of the cerebellum, whereas the vestibular impulses pass into the flocculonodular lobe.
2   To smooth out muscle movement, preventing erratic movements and facilitating fine, well-controlled movements.
3   To increase muscle tone in opposition to the substantia nigra.
4   To effect *synergy*, i.e. a collection of different muscle movements made simultaneously to achieve a particular objective. The cerebellum creates a motor plan, whereby multiple muscles function together in one activity. A good example is the coordination required to catch a ball that is moving toward you. Visual information on the nature of the object, its speed, and its direction, is flashed to the cerebellum. The entire muscle sequence needed to catch the ball is planned, slightly ahead of time (to allow for movement of the ball while planning and muscle movement takes place), and the activity is then executed.

These skills are not present in the newborn infant. The cerebellum has to learn, by trial and error, to balance the body, smooth and coordinate muscle activity, and to interact with moving objects (Chapter 2). Parents can often identify the moments in the development of a child when the cerebellum achieves a new skill, such as the first moment the infant stands unsupported, balancing on both legs. Repeated attempts at a skill, along with sensory feedback, improve the cerebellum's ability to learn and perfect that skill. *Practice makes perfect* could be rewritten to read *Practice makes better cerebellar function.*

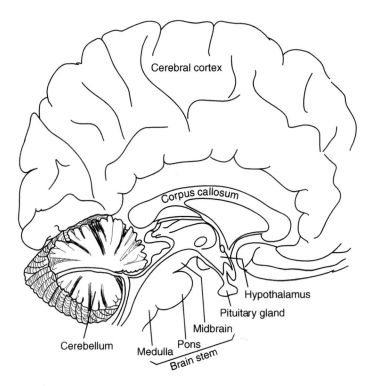

Figure 1.9 Sagittal section through the brain stem and cerebellum.

The brain stem

This part of the brain is the most primitive in that it carries out the basic functions of living (Blows 2000d). It is the lowest area of the brain (Figure 1.9) and is continuous with the spinal cord. The distinction between brain stem above and cord below is approximately at the level of the **foramen magnum**, the 'large window' at the base of the skull.

The brain stem is divided into three parts, the uppermost part being the **midbrain**. Below this and bulging anteriorly is the **pons**, and the lowest part is the **medulla** (Figure 1.9). The pons is often described as *bulbar*, meaning that it is swollen like a bulb. The brain stem houses many nuclei, a number of which control the functions of most of the 12 pairs of **cranial nerves** (numbers **III** to **XII** arise from the brain stem). Cranial nerves are the nerves that come directly from the brain. Cranial nerves **I** (olfactory) and **II** (optic) come from the brain at a higher level than the brain stem.

The midbrain is the smallest part of the brain stem, just above the pons. Here cranial nerve nuclei numbers III (oculomotor) and IV (trochlear) are found. These nerves and their nuclei are concerned with eye movements.

The pons has cranial nerve nuclei numbers V (trigeminal), VI (abducent), VII (facial), and VIII (vestibulocochlear). Two other nuclei are part of the respiratory control centres shared with the medulla.

The medulla is the lowest part of the brain stem. The remaining cranial nerve nuclei are found here with their associated nerves: IX (glossopharyngeal), X (vagus), XI (accessory),

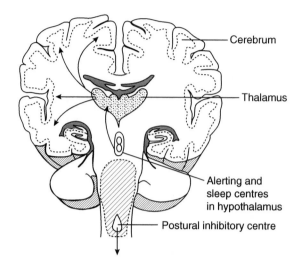

- Cerebrum
- Thalamus
- Alerting and sleep centres in hypothalamus
- Postural inhibitory centre

Figure 1.10 Coronal section through the brain stem showing area of the reticular formation (cross hatched) and the main centres of the sleep–wake cycle, the sleep and alerting centres in the hypothalamus (Chapter 16). Impulses from these centres are distributed either to the cortex via the thalamus or to the body via the spinal cord (Chapter 16, Figure 16.3), as shown by the arrows.

and XII (hypoglossal). The medulla also contains the vital centres that keep the body alive: the **cardiac centre** essential for heart function, the **respiratory centres** (shared with the pons), which together maintain breathing, and the **vasomotor centre (VMC)**, a diffuse set of nuclei that collectively influence peripheral vascular resistance, part of the mechanism for maintaining blood pressure. The medulla is also the location for a number of reflexes that, again, are primitive responses to stimuli designed to protect the body against harm or even death. Such reflexes include the **gag reflex** (which prevents unwanted substances from entering the throat), the **corneal reflex** (which prevents injury to the front of the eye by shutting the lids if something touches the eye), and the **pupillary reflex** (which shuts down the pupil in bright light, preventing light-induced retinal injury). Some of these reflexes are used in neurological investigations to assess brain stem function.

Parts of the medulla, the pons, the midbrain, and the upper cord contain discrete patches of small nuclei, referred to as the **reticular formation (RF)** (Figure 1.10) (Blows 2000d). These nuclei have connections with many parts of the brain. The reticular formation has the role of inhibiting those sensory stimuli entering the brain that can be considered as repetitive, weak, or unnecessary, allowing only strong, significant, or unusual impulses to pass. Other mechanisms such as vomiting, swallowing, coughing, and sneezing are brain-stem RF-mediated functions, and are all linked to the function of respiration in some way. Part of the RF is the **reticular activating system (RAS)**, i.e. those RF components that are responsible for the **sleep–wake cycle** (Figure 1.10, see also Chapter 16).

The autonomic nervous system

The autonomic nervous system (ANS) is that part of the peripheral nervous system that functions automatically, i.e. without conscious control. The two parts of the ANS are the **sympathetic**

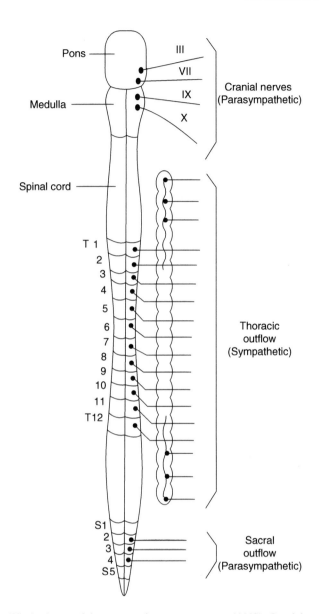

Figure 1.11 Simplified scheme of the autonomic nervous system (ANS). Cranial nerves (III, VII, IX, and X) are shown in roman numerals. T = thoracic, S = sacral.

and **parasympathetic** systems (Figure 1.11). They act between them to stabilise many physiological parameters (e.g. heart rate is stabilised at an average of 72 beats per minute), but the two parts allow the parameters to change when it becomes appropriate (e.g. the heart rate can increase or decrease depending on the circumstances). The sympathetic component serves to increase those parameters, and this is useful for reactions to adverse stimuli, such as fear. Sympathetic responses to stimuli like fear result in, among other things, fast pulse rates, sweating, and increased respiration, all of which are important in speeding up oxygen delivery to the

Table 1.1 Functions of the autonomic nervous system

Target organ (or system)	Sympathetic function	Parasympathetic function
Mental alertness	Increases	No effect
Eye (pupil)	Dilates	Constricts
Heart muscle	Increased heart rate and force of contraction	Decreased heart rate
Coronary arteries	Dilated	Constricted
Blood pressure	Raised	Lowered
Bronchi	Dilated	Constricted
Digestive tract	Reduced peristalsis and increased sphincter tone	Increased peristalsis and decreased sphincter tone
Stomach	Reduces digestion	Increases hydrochloric acid
Liver/blood glucose	Glucose released from glycogen into blood	No effect
Kidney	Decreased urine produced	No effect
Bladder	Allowed to fill, internal sphincter closed	Emptied, sphincter opened
Adrenal medulla	Releases adrenaline	No effect
Metabolism	Increased	No effect
Skin	Increased sweating	No effect

tissues for a physical response to the cause of the fear. The parasympathetic component causes an opposite effect by reducing the physical parameters, e.g. slower heart and breathing rates, at times of rest. The range of functions for each system can be seen in Table 1.1.

Excessive sympathetic activity is seen in anxiety and phobic states when patients come into contact with their fears. Some parameters do not have an opposing parasympathetic activity.

The main pathways involved in mental health

Table 1.2 shows the major pathways of the brain that are chiefly involved in mental health disorders, **psychotropic** (affecting the mind) drug activity, and drug side effects. Figure 1.12 illustrates some of these important pathways. Further discussion of these pathways (or tracts) is given under the relevant neurotransmitter (Chapter 4), under the appropriate disorder, and under the pharmacology involved.

The basic principles of brain pathologies affecting mental health

Pathology is the study of the nature and causation of disease. Disease is either congenital ('born with', i.e. the condition is present from birth, and therefore occurred before birth), or acquired (occurs at a later date after birth). Of the congenital causes, some may be hereditary (i.e. passed to the infant from the parent through gene errors, called mutations), or teratogenic (i.e. caused by a harmful chemical or viral agent passing through the placenta from mother to fetus – either a microorganism, a drug, or a toxin – causing harm or malformation of the fetus).

Of the acquired causes, there are a number of different categories that can involve the brain and therefore cause symptoms of mental health disorder, as follows:

- **Inflammatory**: inflammation produces redness (rubor), swelling (tumor), pain (dolor) and heat (calor), with a corresponding loss of function. It may be due to an immune reaction to microorganisms (infection) or other antigens, such as cancer cells (sterile reaction) (Blows 2005). Inflammation involving the brain could be meningitis (inflammation of the meninges covering the brain) or encephalitis (inflammation of the brain itself).

Table 1.2 Brain pathways involved in mental health

Pathway	Pathway		Importance to mental health
	From	To	
Mesolimbic pathway	Brain stem	Limbic system	Probably involved in positive symptoms in schizophrenia
Mesocortical pathway	Brain stem	Cerebral cortex	Probably involved in negative symptoms in schizophrenia
Nigrostriatal pathway	Substantia nigra	Corpus striatum	Site of extrapyramidal side effects of drugs and of Parkinson's disease
Diffuse modulatory systems	Brain stem	Many parts of limbic area and cerebral cortex	Appears to be involved in depression and possibly eating disorders
Median forebrain bundle	Brain stem	Frontal lobe of cerebrum	Involved in the brain reward pathways, which are implicated in drug addiction
Dorsolateral prefrontal circuit	Frontal lobe (Brodmann 9 and 10)	Head of caudate nucleus (basal ganglia)	Involved in deficits of frontal lobe executive functions
Lateral orbitofrontal circuit	Prefrontal cortex (Brodmann 10)	Caudate nucleus	Involved in mood and personality changes
Anterior cingulate circuit	Anterior cingulate gyrus (Brodmann 24) of the frontal lobe	Several areas of brain stem and basal ganglia	Involved in speech and emotional loss, and apathy

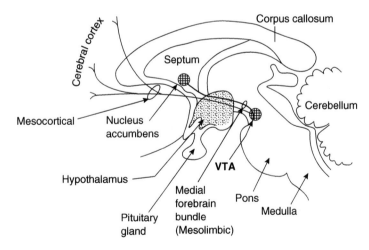

Figure 1.12 Sagittal section through the brain stem showing the ventral tegmental area (VTA) and the main dopaminergic pathways; the mesolimbic pathways (through the medial forebrain bundle) and the mesocortical pathways.

- **Traumatic**: physical injury, for example, damage to the brain from a blow to the head (Blows 2012). Long-term complications of brain injury include epilepsy and depression.

- **Neoplastic**: new growths of the brain, either benign or malignant, such as meningioma, a new growth of the meninges. Many malignant new growths in the brain are known as secondaries because they are formed from metastases, i.e. cells broken free from a primary growth elsewhere (Blows 2005). New growths of the brain can cause confusion, personality changes, and fits.
- **Nutritional**: deficiency or excess of a dietary nutrient, e.g. a vitamin or mineral, can cause a brain malformation or reduced level of neurotransmitter. An absence of adequate protein in the diet would reduce the amount of neurotransmitters in the brain that relied on a supply of amines, since amines are derived from protein.
- **Allergic**: the adverse reaction of the immune system to a foreign substance (called an antigen) (Blows 2005). An antigen is any foreign substance – often a protein that enters the body and provokes an immune reaction. Such reactions can affect the brain to cause fits, confusion, or loss of consciousness.
- **Metabolic**: abnormal changes in cellular metabolism that often produce toxic wastes, which can cause confusion, fits, or reduced level of consciousness. An example of this is an excess production of urea, which then enters the blood and causes uremia.
- **Degenerative**: deterioration and the ultimate death of cells due to age-related and other pathological changes. Degeneration of brain cells causes disorders such as dementia and Parkinson's disease. Age-related degeneration of the arterial walls supplying blood to the brain can cause strokes (also known as cerebrovascular accidents, or CVA), which can cause confusion, fits, and loss of consciousness (Blows 2012).
- **Psychological**: disorders caused by environmental stress and mental trauma, often over a long period, e.g. anxiety states and depression.
- **Iatrogenic**: health-related 'injuries' caused by the medical and nursing profession. Examples are: drug side effects, caused when a drug is prescribed by the doctor; a puncture wound caused by the nurse during the administration of an injection; or a pressure sore caused by a patient being immobilised in one position for too long. Some are inevitable (e.g. wounds and other trauma caused during surgery), but others are preventable, and the medical and nursing staff should be working to minimise the harmful effects of their actions as much as possible.
- **Idiopathic**: 'of unknown cause'. Research has done much to reduce the number of disorders that fall into this category, and much progress has been achieved in finding the cause of many psychiatric disorders. However, there is still much more research to be done in order to remove some very important brain disorders from this category.

Key points

The meninges and cerebrospinal fluid

- The brain and the cord are covered by the meninges in three layers: the pia mater, the arachnoid mater, and the dura mater.
- Between the arachnoid mater and pia mater is the subarachnoid space, containing cerebrospinal fluid (CSF).
- Two lateral ventricles, the third ventricle and the fourth ventricle inside the brain are filled with CSF.
- Lumbar puncture is a method of collecting a sample of CSF from the subarachnoid space below the lumbar vertebra 2 (L2) level.

The cerebrum

- The cerebrum is the largest part of the brain, carrying out our cognitive and conscious processes.
- The frontal lobe is a major part of the brain involved in many mental health functions; in particular it is the site of consciousness of the 'self' and thinking.

The limbic system

- The limbic system below the cerebrum is involved in preservation of the individual and the species, and involves emotions and controlling behavioural patterns.
- The amygdala is the emotional centre of the brain.
- The functions of the hippocampus are: short-term memory, learning, emotional behaviour, and influencing thought.

The thalamus and hypothalamus

- The thalamus is the sensory relay station, passing sensations to the cerebrum.
- The hypothalamus has a wide range of functions, notably temperature control, regulation of eating, alerting the brain after sleep, and controlling both the pituitary gland's hormones and the autonomic nervous system.

The basal ganglia and the cerebellum

- Below the limbic area are the basal ganglia and the cerebellum, areas involved in control of movement at a subconscious level (i.e. part of the extrapyramidal tract system).
- The function of the substantia nigra is the reduction of muscle tone.
- The functions of the cerebellum are fine control of balance, smoothing out muscle movement, and synergy.

The brain stem

- The brain stem contains the nuclei that control the cranial nerve functions and the vital centres, such as respiration, cardiac function, and blood pressure.
- The brain stem houses the reticular formation and the reticular activating system that is involved in the sleep–wake cycle.

References

Blows, W. T. (2000a) The nervous system, part 1. *Nursing Times*, **96** (35): 41–44.
Blows, W. T. (2000b) The nervous system, part 2. *Nursing Times*, **96** (40): 45–48.
Blows, W. T. (2000c) The nervous system, part 3. *Nursing Times*, **96** (44): 45–48.
Blows, W. T. (2000d) The nervous system, part 4. *Nursing Times*, **96** (48): 47–50.
Blows, W. T. (2002) Lumbar puncture. *Nursing Times*, **98** (36): 25–26.
Blows, W. T. (2005) *The Biological Basis of Nursing: Cancer*. Routledge, London.
Blows, W. T. (2012) *The Biological Basis of Clinical Observations* (2nd edition). Routledge, Abingdon, Oxon.
Marieb, E. N. and Hoehn, K. N. (2014) *Human Anatomy and Physiology* (9th edition). Pearson Education Limited, Harlow, UK.
Raichle, M. E. (2010) The brain's dark energy. *Scientific American*, **302** (3): 28–33.

2　Brain development

- Introduction
- The nervous system up to birth
- The debate: when does consciousness start?
- The brain at birth
- Infant and child brain development
- Learning and memory
- The teenage brain
- Hormone influences on brain development
- Nutritional influences on brain development

Introduction

The human brain is a remarkable structure, with functions that go beyond anything other organisms can achieve. However, although the human brain is fully in place at birth, with many of its functions already working, it still has a lot more development to do, and will not be completely mature until about 23 years of age. Being locked up inside a bony box (the **skull**) the brain relies entirely for much of that development on the sensory nervous system. It is through the senses that the brain keeps in contact with the outside world, and it is the outside world that has the biggest influence on the brain (Blows 2003). Therefore the brain can only make progress in development if the sensory systems are fully functioning. Fortunately, the sensory systems are always the most advanced at all stages of development.

The nervous system up to birth

The human nervous system starts as a groove forming along what will become the back of the early embryo. This groove deepens and closes over to form a tube, the neural tube. Forming this groove and the neural tube is a process called **neurulation** (Figure 2.1). The enclosed lumen within the tube is destined to become the **ventricular system** of the brain and the central canal down the cord, and will eventually contain a watery fluid called **cerebrospinal fluid (CSF)**. The head (**rostral**) end of the tube and the tail (**caudal**) end initially remain open to the **amniotic fluid** that bathes the entire embryo. These tubal openings (called **neuropores**) will close between 26 and 28 days, the days counted from the start of

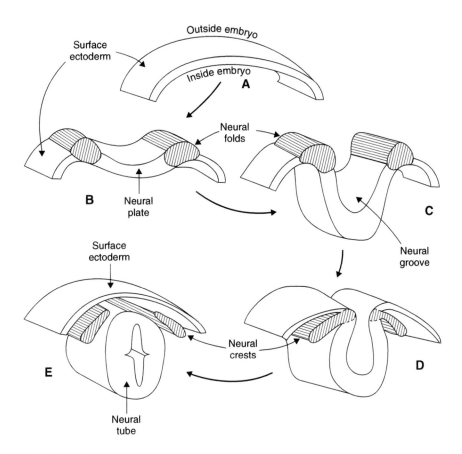

Figure 2.1 Neurulation.

pregnancy, i.e. conception (Figure 2.2). While the tube itself becomes the **central nervous system** (**CNS**, i.e. the brain and spinal cord), cells that originate from the tube form a crest (the **neural crest**) (Figure 2.1) between the tube and the embryonic surface, and this crest will develop into the **peripheral nervous system** (**PNS**, i.e. peripheral nerves).

Deep within the neural tube wall, in a cell layer next to the lumen called the **ventricular zone** (**VZ**), many millions of new cells are formed from **mitosis** (cell division), and these will eventually become mostly **neurons** (Figure 2.3). In the next zone out, the **subventricular zone** (**SZ**), more cells are dividing and these will become mostly **glia cells** (known as **neuroglia**), i.e. the support cells of the CNS.

At first, these layers contain early **stem cells**, meaning that the cells are not yet designated to become any particular cell type (i.e. they are **undifferentiated**). Cells of the VZ then pass through three stages of development to become neurons: (1) **neural epithelial cells**, (2) **radial progenitor cells**, and (3) **intermediate neural precursors**. One key gene, called **glycogen synthase kinase 3** (*GSK-3*) has a major influence over radial progenitor cells, being responsible for the product that causes these cells to move on to neuronal status. Failure of this gene has been shown to prevent these cells from further development, and they simply

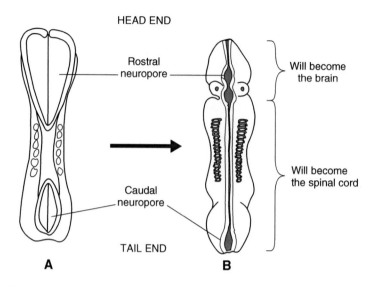

HEAD END

Rostral neuropore

Will become the brain

Caudal neuropore

Will become the spinal cord

TAIL END

A   B

Figure 2.2 The neuropores on days (A) 26 and (B) 28 of gestation.

continue to divide. The normal progress from intermediate neural precursors is to go on to become neuronal cell bodies. They are still in a very primitive state at this point; for example, these neurons are cell bodies only, and have no **axon**, **myelin**, or **synaptic** connections.

Three waves of **neuronal migration** occur during the **second trimester** of pregnancy (i.e. the third to the sixth month of pregnancy). Migration involves the movement of millions of cells from the VZ inner layer of the tube to the surface. How they find their correct finishing point on the tube surface is not fully understood, but it involves a framework of glial projections extending from the lumen to the surface, and a critical protein coded by a gene called *srGAP2*. The protein produced from this gene has an active part called the **F-BAR domain**, which causes temporary finger-like extensions of the neuronal cell body, called **filopodia**, which then drag the cell to its new position on the tube surface. Once in their final destinations these primitive neuronal cell bodies form three cellular layers (Figure 2.3). The innermost layer is the product of the first wave, and the outermost layer is the product of the third wave. The position of these cells within these layers is both critical and irreversible, and once placed, cells are ready to begin axon development and synapse formation. On completion, these neuronal migrations will never happen again. If cells are misplaced during migration, nothing can be done to correct this, and the brain will have some errors in synaptic connection. Mutations of *srGAP2* and the incorrect positions and connections of misplaced neurons are now considered to be part of the problem in schizophrenia and autism. Correct axonal growth, guidance to the final destination, and synaptic connections are due to the production of a large number of specific proteins; examples include the **Notch** cell signalling proteins and the **Netrin** and **Semaphorin** axonal guidance proteins.

The rostral end of the tube thickens and folds to form three primary brain vesicles, the **forebrain, midbrain,** and **hindbrain** (Figure 2.4). The primitive brain also begins to fold: the start of the process of packing as much brain matter into the skull as possible. These folds consist of two folds forward (the **midbrain** and **cervical flexures**), which are then

NEURAL TUBE

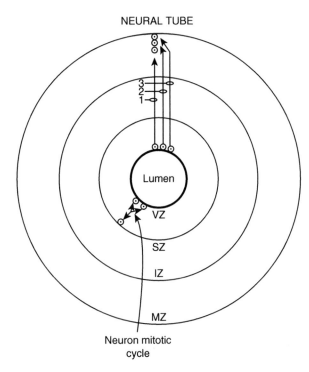

Figure 2.3 Schematic section through the neural tube during the early development of the nervous system. VZ is the ventricular zone near the tube lumen. The other zones are SZ (subventricular zone), IZ (intermediate zone), and MZ (marginal zone). Cell mitosis (division) takes place in the VZ, with the cell alternating from close to the lumen (where it divides) to close to the SZ. At specific times, three waves of cell migration out of the VZ into the MZ take place (labelled 1, 2, and 3). The first migration places cells short of the outer layer, but successive migrations place cells closer to the surface.

separated by a fold backwards (the **pontine flexure**) (Figure 2.4). The forebrain vesicle enlarges and expands in all directions to form the cerebrum. This begins to engulf the parts behind (notably the **thalamus**, **hypothalamus**, and **basal ganglia**), which will ultimately take up a position surrounded by the rapidly developing cerebrum (Figure 2.4). The midbrain and hindbrain have also grown, although not to the same extent, and between them these will form the **brain stem** and **cerebellum**.

The debate: when does consciousness start?

When do we first develop consciousness? This is a question that is often asked, and is important when we have to consider what sensations an unborn fetus can experience. The question is linked to another problem in biology: How does the brain create consciousness? Trying to understand this is known as *the hard problem* because it is just that, virtually unsolvable (see Chapter 10 in Blows 2012).

Part of the answer may be determined by establishing at what point in gestation the pathways in the brain that are involved in consciousness are in place and functioning.

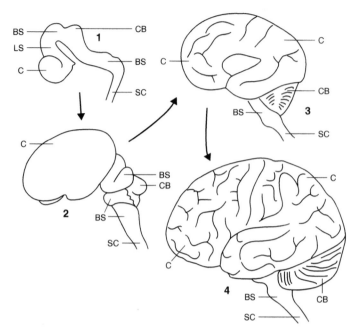

Figure 2.4 Lateral views of the folding brain during development. 1. At 5 weeks' gestation, the upper (head, or rostral) end of the neural tube is folding forwards and backwards, and expanding, especially the cerebrum (C). 2. At 13 weeks' gestation the cerebrum is the largest component and is expanding backwards to encompass the limbic system (LS). 3. At 26 weeks' gestation the cerebrum is still expanding backwards and has encompassed the limbic system and part of the cerebellum (CB) and brain stem (BS). 4. At birth the brain has completed its formation but has a lot or maturation to go. The remaining tube has developed into the spinal cord (SC).

Many areas of the brain, especially the cerebral cortex, are important with regards to consciousness, and these are anatomically formed by between weeks 24 and 28 of gestation (Koch 2009). This is followed a few weeks later by evidence that both cerebral hemispheres are in communication with most parts of the brain. The groundwork for consciousness is therefore set up ready for the third and final trimester of pregnancy. However, it appears from multiple studies that the unborn fetus is alternating between two different sleep modes (called active and quiet sleep) throughout 95% of this final trimester. The fetus is kept sedated and asleep by a mixture of chemicals secreted by the placenta. So, it would appear that the unborn child is not conscious enough to be aware of very much until the day of its birth, when it becomes detached from the placenta and is released into an environment rich in sensory stimuli.

The brain at birth

The major anatomical structures of the brain are all in place at birth, and a number of functions essential for keeping the baby alive are working. These functions are mainly those of the brain stem where the vital centres are located. The brain stem is the most developmentally advanced

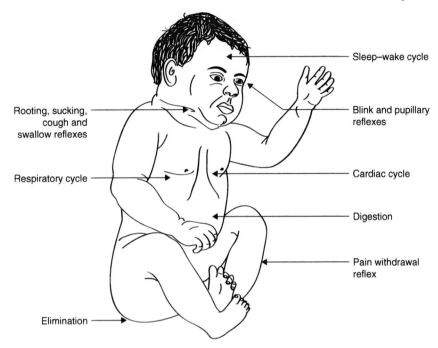

Sleep–wake cycle

Rooting, sucking, cough and swallow reflexes

Blink and pupillary reflexes

Respiratory cycle

Cardiac cycle

Digestion

Pain withdrawal reflex

Elimination

Figure 2.5 The reflexes at birth.

brain area at birth, and houses the **cardiac centre** (regulating heart function), the **respiratory centre** (controlling breathing), and the **vasomotor centre** (stabilising blood pressure). The brain stem is also the centre for controlling reflexes, and again these are functioning from birth. There are two types of reflexes: the **avoidance reflexes** and **approach reflexes**. Avoidance reflexes are there to protect the baby against harm, and they include the **blink reflex**, which protects against eye injury, the **pupillary reflex**, which protects against bright light, and the **vomit, cough,** and **sneeze** reflexes. The approach reflexes help the child obtain food, e.g. the **sucking** and **swallow reflexes** (Figure 2.5). Other than these brain stem functions, the brain at birth is also quite advanced in sensory perception.

The newborn can see, hear, and feel pain and touch, as well as other senses, and these first started to happen before birth. However, the child at birth is lacking the motor skills we see in older children and adults. The motor system is well behind in terms of development at birth, and remains behind at all stages until near full maturity. The reason for this is threefold. First, the motor system is behind in physical development, i.e. it is slower in creating synaptic connections and forming myelin sheaths. Second, many of the motor skills involve **learning**, and this not only takes time but can only start to happen after birth. How much time learning takes depends on the skill in question, but it can typically be months or years. This is linked to the first reason because learning involves forming and strengthening synaptic connections. Third, motor development is heavily dependent on sensory feedback, and there is a distinct lack of sensory **feedback** before birth. Only after birth can sensory feedback really begin to make a difference to the formation of motor skills. So the newborn can breath, cry and move their limbs a little, but not much else. It's going to take years for the motor system to catch up with the rest of the brain.

The human brain at birth contains around 100,000,000,000 (100 billion) neurons, virtually the full complement of brain cells it is going to have, but is just 25% of the weight of the adult brain. However, it is already in the middle of a brain **growth spurt**. This started before birth and continues until about 2 years of age, i.e. the age when the brain weighs about 75% of the adult brain weight. By the age of 6 years, the brain is about 90% of the adult size. Brain growth spurts do not generally involve the addition of new neurons. The child at birth will add very few new neurons after birth. A brain growth spurt involves the addition of new neuroglia cells, an increase in synaptic connections and myelination, and an increase in the protein content of the brain.

Infant and child brain development

Infancy has a number of definitions, depending on different interpretations, but a good approach is to define infancy as the period from birth to the development of a language (i.e. the first few years of life, given there is considerable normal variation in the age of language development). During this time, three main processes are involved in brain growth: synaptogenesis, myelination, and plasticity.

- **Synaptogenesis** is the formation of new synapses – the connections between neurons. Each neuron is capable of having hundreds of synaptic connections with other cells, and these are forming daily from the time neuronal migration is complete (the second trimester of pregnancy). Some of the unused synapses may be removed by a process called **synaptic pruning**, the purpose of which is to make the brain more efficient. Many unused synapses still remain, however, to allow for future new learning and adaptation to changes in circumstances.
- **Myelination** is the process of laying down a fat-based layer called myelin around the axons of neurons in order to provide some degree of insulation and to speed up transmission of nerve impulses. Some neurons are fully myelinated (called '**A**' **fibres**), and they have a speed of transmission about 120 metres per second; others are unmyelinated (called '**C**' **fibres**), and their speed is 2.3 metres per second. Because myelination speeds everything up, this process improves brain efficiency, but is not fully complete until the early twenties.
- **Plasticity** is defined as the brain's ability to adapt to new environments and new experiences. We are encountering new environments throughout our lives; new homes, new schools, even new countries, and with these new environments come new experiences. Childhood is no different, with new experiences each day. Plasticity is achieved by creating many more synapses (**synaptogenesis**) than we actually use now, and not pruning them all away. This leaves us with considerable spare capacity that we can adopt for new environments, new events, and new experiences. Plasticity also involves synaptic remodeling, improvements in dendritic function, axon development, and even the creation of new neurons (**neurogenesis**) in specific brain areas, notably the hippocampus. Plasticity is also linked to learning, and since everything new in our lives involves a degree of learning, plasticity allows for this. In this way the changing environment moulds the mind, making childhood a time when brains are set up for the future. After full brain maturity, plasticity is probably better than previously recognised. This is because neuronal differentiation (i.e. neurons becoming specialised in a particular function), axonal guidance (i.e. processes that ensure axons arrive where they should), and axonal branching continues on beyond full maturity. Certain proteins (notably **Notch**, **Mash**, **Netrin**, and **Semaphorins**) control these neuronal developments, and these molecules are known to be produced well beyond the maturity of the brain.

Although behind in development, the motor system progresses rapidly through childhood, that progress being made possible by synaptogenesis, myelination, and sensory feedback. The motor system is able to gradually adopt more functions, such as lifting the head, rolling over, crawling, and eventually walking. These are all learnt motor skills with the emphasis on sensory feedback through trial and error. You can witness this process when you see a child pull themselves up to stand for the first time. They quickly fall, but eventually they learn to balance through many attempts, until they can stand properly. Once learnt, a motor skill will be stored as a motor memory in the brain for life, so that skill will never be lost unless that part of the brain is damaged.

Speech is partly a motor skill, since it involves muscular movements of the voice box (the larynx), the tongue, jaw, and lips. It is also another good example of sensory feedback and learning, since in order to say words they must be heard first, then learnt (Hartshorne 2009). The first words usually appear between 8 and 18 months of age, but it should be noted that there is a considerable normal variation between individual children in the ages at which speech develops. After the first words, development is slow at first; for example, only about 10 words are mastered over the next 3 months or so. As soon as the child has a vocabulary of about 50 words, speech development increases. By about 3 years of age, the child should have a vocabulary of about a thousand words, and is adding to this at the rate of about two new words per day. The first sentences appear at about 2 years of age and consist of two words (e.g. 'I do'). Prior to this they make themselves understood by **holophrasing**, i.e. by combining one word with a hand gesture (e.g. pointing at a biscuit and saying 'me'). **Telegraphic speech** is the first attempt to form true sentences, i.e. leaving out non-essential words. The ability of babies to learn speech eventually to adult levels of fluency appears not to be dependent entirely on brain maturity but is more to do with achieving a number of linguistic milestones, such as acquiring a certain number of words in the vocabulary. This is known as the **'stages of language hypothesis'** and is independent to brain maturity in all children (Hartshorne 2009). Two main areas of the brain involved in speech are **Broca's area** (the speech motor area; i.e. it controls the muscles of speech) and **Wernicke's area** (the language centre, or area of word processing).

Cerebral **lateralisation** is well underway by birth, and continues throughout life. This is the process by which new information, skills, and experiences are assigned for storage in one side of the brain or the other. The cerebral hemispheres, left and right, are the sites of most long-term memory, and a learnt skill must be stored either on the left, or the right, or both. Males tend to lateralise more than females, who usually assign skills to both sides. In practice, this makes no difference to carrying out the skill, but it helps to have stored the skill on both sides when trying to recover brain function after injury or disease to the brain. This helps us to explain why females tend to recover normal brain function better than males after disruption by disease or trauma.

Learning and memory

Childhood is all about learning, and memory is a major component of the learning process. Humans have the longest childhood, longer than any other species, and this length of time is as much about brain growth, learning, and memory as it is about body development. Evidence is growing that higher intellectual abilities come with time, i.e. the longer the period before brain maturity the greater the intellect (see Table 2.1).

Children with different levels of intelligence, measured by **intelligence quotation (IQ)** tests, were shown to have variations in the thickness of the cerebral cortex, especially the

Table 2.1 Comparison of prefrontal cortex development, as determined by magnetic resonance imaging (MRI) studies, between children of different IQ test scores. Prolonged thickening of the cortex in Child A (from age 8 to 12) is possibly essential for development of higher intellectual cognitive circuits. Thinning of the cortex is happening in all teenage brains and is a mark of increased brain efficiency

Child and IQ tests results	Brain at age 7 to 8 years	Brain at age 11 to 12 years
Child A High IQ test scores	This child has a thin prefrontal cortex, which starts to thicken rapidly.	The cortex thickens rapidly to peak at 12 years old, then thins out slowly through teens.
Child B Average IQ test scores	This child has a thick prefrontal cortex peaking at aged 8 years.	At 11 years old the cortex has already been thinning slowly for 3 years and continues through teens.

prefrontal cortex. Table 2.1 suggests that the variations in the thickness and activity of the prefrontal cortex at different ages profoundly influence intelligence levels.

Learning and memory are products of strong synapses. Initially these synapses are formed from temporary proteins, but these are ultimately replaced by permanent proteins provided that the synapse has been used enough. Usage of synapses therefore strengthens them, and they can then become permanent. This process will be improved by stimulating the brain, and by **rehearsal**, i.e. repeating the same learning multiple times, as actors do when learning their parts, and as students do before an examination. Synapses are also strengthened by excitement, a good reason why we tend to remember the exciting events in our lives. Strengthening synapses in this way is known as creating **long-term potentials (LTPs)**; and therefore LTPs are the basis of the learning process. LTPs require activity through two types of **glutamate receptors** on the **post-synaptic membrane**, and these receptors are explained further in Chapter 4. Of the synapses not strengthened in this way, many (but not all by a long way) may be subject to synaptic pruning in order to improve brain efficiency.

There are a number of ways to classify memories (see Table 2.2), but the simplest is to consider two forms of memory: **long-term memory** and **short-term memory**. Temporarily holding short-term memory, and sometimes converting it to long-term memory, is one of the functions of the **hippocampus**. Within the hippocampus, a limited number of information bits can be held for a short period. To convert these to long-term memory requires rehearsal in order to establish LTPs. Long-term memory is held in many parts of the brain, the location depending on what is being memorised. For example, visual memory is stored in the **visual cortex** of the occipital lobe, whereas **motor memory** is held in the **motor association cortex** of the frontal lobe, and so on.

Memories are usually missing from the first 3 years of life, and remain poor before the age of 6 years. This is due to immaturity of the brain memory circuits at this early age, partly because of the immaturity of language skills that are necessary for all memory development, and partly because there is a poor sense of identity at such a young age (Weir 2015). The best years for acquiring and storing memory are between 13 and 25 years of age, i.e. before final completion of the front lobe myelination process (see the section on the teenage brain, page 31). After this period memory begins to deteriorate slowly. These years of best memory are known as the **reminiscence bump**, and are a good reason for using these years for serious learning. Myelination of the language area occurs mostly before the age of 13, which makes learning a language before this relatively easy, but after 13 it becomes harder.

Table 2.2 Types of memory

Type of memory	Explanation
Long-term	Permanently stored memory in various sites across the cerebrum, depending on the nature of the memory to be stored.
Short-term	Limited number of facts stored temporarily in the hippocampus. Conversion to long-term memory requires rehearsal.
Explicit	Memory involving conscious thought, e.g. remembering a relative's telephone number.
Implicit	Subconscious memory, such as knowing the route to the kitchen at home.
Declarative	Memory for facts and events. Divided into **semantic** memory for basic facts and figures, e.g. 9 is a number and fish have gills; and **episodic** memory of the context in which these facts exist, e.g. 9 is the ninth number in a sequence of numbers starting with number 1; and gills are part of a system by which vertebrates extract oxygen from the environment.

The teenage brain

The teenage years, from 12 years to around 23 years old, mark the final stages of brain development, with increasing skills far in advanced over anything seen in the first decade of life. There is an improvement in attention span, due largely to increased myelination and synaptic changes in the brain, which happen in a slow wave from back to front, and from bottom to top during the teenage years, the frontal lobe being the last to become fully myelinated (Dobbs 2011).

Among the most important changes are those that occur in the **prefrontal cortex**, the anterior part of the frontal lobe above the eyes. This is involved in decision-making and other higher executive functions. By the early twenties, information is processed faster by the teenager, using more logic and reasoning powers, and with a capability of abstract thought. The frontal lobe also shows changes in its organisation and function, eventually using less energy to do more work, i.e. it becomes energy efficient. However, these brain changes, in particular the frontal lobe changes, come at a cost. During these changes, if the brain is faced with a task to perform, the prefrontal cortex must work much harder in teenagers than the same brain area in adults in a similar situation. It seems that the adolescent prefrontal cortex tries to solve the task single-handed, unlike adults where they can call upon other brain areas for help. The teenage prefrontal cortex can, in some extreme circumstances, become overloaded, an unlikely scenario in the mature adult brain, and this overload will impair the frontal lobe's abilities to carry out its executive functions. The dorsolateral prefrontal cortex undergoes synaptic pruning, and during this process its function of controlling impulses is reduced and impulsive behaviour increases, especially when influenced by alcohol or drugs. Two types of behavioural control are recognised: **exogenous control**, where the brain responds to external stimuli and uses reflexes to control behaviour, thus not allowing for much involvement of rational thought, and **endogenous control**, where control is based on a predetermined, thus logically thought-through, voluntary plan. Endogenous behaviour can quite easily override exogenous control in the adult, but the adolescent finds this hard, and responds to situations more with exogenous control. Teenage behavioural patterns then seem more spontaneous and illogical, and the addition of stress, drugs, or alcohol will make matters worse (Sabbagh 2006). In addition, working memory (Chapter 15) is not fully developed during the teenage years and therefore this also cannot be fully recruited to help guide behaviour.

In the adult brain the frontal and temporal lobes, i.e. the **limbic association cortex,** have a major influence over the brain's emotional centres, i.e. the limbic system, but during teenage years the frontal and temporal lobes show a marked reduction in this influence. Emotions then become controlled largely by the amygdala, the main limbic centre for emotions. This reduction in the sobering influence of the conscious cerebrum over emotions allows the subconscious limbic system a greater free reign over emotions. This is far from the ideal situation, but it ultimately has a good outcome. Starting at about 12 years of age, the frontal lobe loses some of its ability to read the social situation correctly. The teenager then finds it difficult to identify other people's emotions (about 20% slower in doing this than during earlier years), and they become petulant, ill-tempered, sulky, and have confused emotions. However, during late teenage years, the shift back to the much improved frontal lobe for rational emotional influence occurs. Ultimately, during the early twenties, the brain will complete its myelination and synaptic changes, reaching full maturity at about 23 to 25 years of age (Sabbagh 2006).

Synapses that are frequently used are strengthened, whereas those that are never used may be lost by synaptic pruning (an example of synaptic pruning is the thinning of the prefrontal cortex identified in Table 2.1) while others are retained for plasticity. These changes show how important the environment is, in providing the stimuli to strengthen synapses. It is true to say that, just as in early childhood, the environment moulds the teenage mind, and these changes offer a second opportunity for families and society to influence development of the brains of its children. Providing positive stimuli (e.g. happiness, emotional support, education, freedom from want, music, etc.) will strengthen the brain in a positive manner, whereas providing negative stimuli (e.g. pain, fear, alcoholism, drug abuse, sexual abuse, crime, poverty) will strengthen the brain in a negative manner. The effects of strengthened brain pathways during early childhood, and during the teenage years, either in a positive or negative way, are generally for life, and negative pathways, once established, are very hard to change or eliminate. The lifelong outcome of environmental influences on the brain is the responsibility of those who deliver that experience: the child carers. They provide the environment the child is exposed to. Every child should be provided with a positive, loving, caring, happy, and stimulating environment from birth in order to guide brain development in the direction which will allow the resulting adult the best chances of a happy life, and success in meeting all the challenges life has in store. If the brains of children are moulded by exposure from an early age to crime, abuse, neglect, and other physical, social, and psychological hardships, these children find it very difficult, even impossible, to turn away from these negative effects later in life and lead a happy, fruitful life. Children with brains moulded in this negative manner may ultimately become parents who also provide a negative environment for their children, therefore perpetuating the problem (see Chapter 8, Drug abuse).

Apart from the frontal lobe, changes also occur in the corpus callosum (which increases in size), the **hippocampus** (which forms stronger links with the frontal lobes), the parietal lobe (which decreases in volume), the occipital lobe (which increases in volume), and the temporal lobe (which reaches maximum volume at 16 to 17 years of age).

Chemical changes in the brain also occur during the teenage years. Sensitivity to **dopamine**, a neurotransmitter (Chapter 4), increases during adolescence. This improves learning ability and decision-making, but also excites the reward pathways of the brain (Chapter 8). The effects of the hormone **oxytocin** (Chapter 1) is also enhanced in the brain, and this makes social connections with other teens more rewarding than at any time previously or after the teenage years (Dobbs 2011).

Hormone influences on brain development

The subject of hormonal and nutritional influences on the development of the brain has received much interest, as there is growing evidence that disorders such as autism and schizophrenia may be affected by such influences. During all the stages of brain development, from early embryo to full maturity, hormones are a key factor in the process, and abnormal hormonal production has a profound adverse influence on the brain. Hormones act on brain cells by first binding to receptors; therefore cells that are influenced by hormones must have these receptors present on the cell-surface membrane.

Testosterone, a hormone usually attributed to males, is produced in both sexes from an early stage of growth in relatively small quantities compared with during puberty. The source of the hormones during fetal development is the **adrenal cortex**, the outer part of the **adrenal glands**, which are found above the kidneys. These glands are formed and function long before the testes or ovaries. Both testosterone and oestrogen are produced from **cholesterol**. Boys produce surprisingly high levels of testosterone during fetal development, and for a short while after birth, but this level then drops until puberty, when it rises again. Girls produce much smaller quantities of testosterone before and after birth. The sex difference in testosterone concentrations causes different synaptic changes in the male brain from those in the female brain. Testosterone (and its derivatives) changes the synaptic connections to form a male-orientated brain.

Oestrogen is produced from testosterone, and therefore also originally comes from cholesterol. It also occurs in both sexes from the adrenal cortex. Oestrogen improves cell survival (known as a **neuroprotective** function) by altering gene expression that in turn changes the proteins in favour of cell survival. In addition, it has some control over the formation and maintenance of neural networks by promoting synaptic connections.

Thyroid hormone is produced by the thyroid gland in the neck. The function of thyroid hormone is to stimulate and regulate cellular **metabolism**, the chemistry essential for cell function. Brain cells are busy metabolic factories, consuming glucose and oxygen to produce energy that will be used in many cellular functions, including the production of **action potentials** (nerve impulses). The principal hormonal activity appears to be by **triiodothyronine** (T_3) since most brain cells have T_3 receptors. Its counterpart **tetraiodothyronine** (T_4) appears to be less important. Thyroid hormone changes gene expression inside the nucleus, and that in turn changes the way cells grow and develop.

Growth hormone, produced by the **pituitary gland**, works in conjunction with thyroid hormone in regulating growth in the brain's neural networks. A cascade of other hormones, including **insulin**, is involved in brain development, but their roles are not fully established. Most are likely to work through gene activation and regulation.

Nutritional influences on brain development

Nutriments have a part to play in brain development, so an adequate nutritious diet for the mother throughout pregnancy and for the child up to adulthood is essential. From birth to 2 years of age is a critical period for adequate nutrition, since the nervous system is particularly vulnerable to deficiencies during this time. Much has been said and written about the role of vitamins, minerals, and fatty acids in childhood intelligence. Vitamins are summarised in Table 2.3, and minerals in Table 2.4.

Table 2.3 The vitamins involved in brain development and function (see also Ramakrishna 1999)

Vitamin	Notes
Vitamin A (retinoids, e.g. retinol)	Essential for cell differentiation, proliferation, and migration, gene expression, and cell death. Excess and deficiency in the maternal diet during pregnancy can cause malformation of the fetal brain.
Vitamin B_1 (thiamine)	Thiamine is required for the activity of thiamine-dependent enzymes in the brain. These enzymes are involved in cerebral energy metabolism and myelin synthesis. Deficiency during critical stages in brain development results in permanent abnormal brain changes.
Vitamin B_2 (riboflavin)	Has a role in fatty acid metabolism, and a deficiency disrupts myelin synthesis.
Vitamin B_3 (niacin, nicotinic acid)	Deficiency during fetal development causes irregularities in cell replication and differentiation, and cerebellar structure becomes particularly abnormal.
Vitamin B_5 (pantothenic acid)	A coenzyme required for energy production. Deficiency in humans is rare and evidence for involvement in brain development is hard to obtain. It is involved in neurotransmitter production, DNA replication, and cell division, and therefore is important in brain development.
Vitamin B_6 (pyridoxine)	Deficiency causes inadequate myelination, disruption of synaptogenesis, and reduced brain cell organisation.
Vitamin B_7 (biotin)	Being widely distributed in food, and because the body can manufacture it, a deficiency of biotin is rare. A lack of biotin during in pregnancy could be a possibility. Biotin is essential for carbohydrate and fat metabolism and a deficiency could disturb metabolism in the brain.
Vitamin B_9 (folic acid)	Prevents neural tube defects during very early fetal development.
Vitamin B_{12} (cyanocobalamin)	Deficiency appears to affect basal ganglia function, causing limb spasticity and involuntary movements. At least one brain enzyme, essential for brain development, is dependent on vitamin B_{12}. Low B_{12} therefore causes infants to have poor brain development, and to be anorexic, irritable, and to fail to thrive.
Vitamin C (abscorbic acid)	Highly concentrated in brain cells throughout human development. Its role in brain development is not clear, but it may influence cell division. A deficiency during pregnancy may cause fetal brain cell losses, notably in the hippocampus.
Vitamin D (cholecalciferol)	There is a wide distribution of vitamin D receptors in the brain. It influences proteins involved in learning, memory, motor control, and possibly social behaviour. Metabolites of vitamin D are required for normal cerebellar development.
Vitamin E (tocopherols)	Important antioxidant but also essential for many aspects of nervous system development and function.

Table 2.4 Some of the important minerals involved in brain development and function

Mineral	Notes
Iodine (I) (a component of thyroid hormone)	Low levels associated with **hypothyroidism**, and causes infantile **cretinism**. This is associated with cerebral palsy, deafness, and mutism. The critical stage of brain development affected by low iodine is after 14 weeks' gestation. Both neuron and dendrite formation is affected, causing brain developmental failure.

Calcium (Ca)	Calcium ions play a central role in neuronal cell development, including cellular proliferation, differentiation, migration, and maturation. Calcium is also essential for neurotransmission, and therefore critical for brain development.
Copper (Cu)	Copper facilitates iron absorption; therefore low copper leads to poor iron uptake from the gut. Wilson's disease (Chapter 13) is a disturbance of copper metabolism.
Iron (Fe)	Maternal iron deficiency during pregnancy is not uncommon, and can seriously affect the fetal brain. Various regions of the fetal brain becomes dependent on iron at specific points in development, and deficiency at that time causes irreversible changes in myelination, neurotransmitters (especially dopamine), and neuronal networks. Iron deficiency slows the transmission of nerve impulses and has been linked with child and adult cognitive deficits.
Sodium (Na)	An essential component of nerve conduction, sodium is normally concentrated outside the neuronal cell body. Deficiency of sodium during pregnancy prevents normal neuronal function.
Potassium (K)	Potassium ions are an essential component of nerve conduction. Potassium is concentrated inside the neurons, all potassium outside the cell is controlled by **astrocytes**. Deficiency of potassium during pregnancy prevents normal neuronal function.
Zinc (Zn)	Zinc plays a role in neuronal replication and migration, brain growth, synaptogenesis, and gene expression. Zinc is concentrated in glutamatergic neurons in the brain. Impaired memory and learning skills are evident in children born to mothers with low zinc. Deficiency in zinc is now linked with depression, and prescribed zinc supplements may help to improve depressive symptoms.
Magnesium (Mg)	Magnesium is critical in activating over 300 enzymes, many of which are vital for brain function. It is also involved in the myelination of neurons, and so is vital to brain development. Low magnesium is linked to depression and anxiety, and the link involves changes in gut microbes (called **intestinal flora**).
Manganese (Mn)	Manganese is necessary for normal development and metabolism. However, in excess it is a neurotoxin, and high levels are now linked to dementia.

Fatty acids

Omega-3 and **omega-6** are terms used to describe certain forms of fatty acid, one of the components of fat (Figure 2.6).

The 'essential' form of omega-3 is **alpha-linolenic acid (ALA)** ('essential' meaning the only source is the diet because the body cannot produce it), and the 'non-essential' forms are **docosahexaenoic acid (DHA)** and **eicosapentaenoic acid (EPA)** ('non-essential' meaning the body can manufacture these from other forms). The 'essential' form of omega-6 is **linolenic acid (LA)**, and the 'non-essential' forms are **gamma-linolenic acid (GLA)** and **arachidonic acid (AA)**. As components of fats (or **lipids**), fatty acids in the brain are a part of fat-based structural elements, such as cell membranes and the myelin sheath around axons. DHA, for example, is widely found in these structures. Many claims are made for the improvement of mental health with the addition of essential fatty acids in the diet. For example, ALA in the diet improves the mood, promotes a sense of calm, increases learning ability

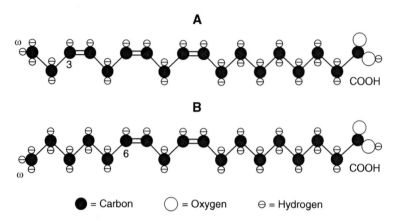

Figure 2.6 (A) Omega-3 and (B) omega-6 fatty acids.

and intellect, and allows for the brain to cope with stress better. There is substance to these claims, since many trials and clinical observations have strongly indicated links between the fatty acids and mental health. And DHA is a key player, since evidence now indicates that DHA is critical to optimum brain development at all stages of growth. Breast milk can have quite good levels of DHA (depending on the mother's diet), and long periods of breastfeeding, in some cases up to 2 years after birth, has resulted in children with fewer mental health problems. Infant milk formulas, until recently, have had very low levels of DHA, but this is now being corrected. Low DHA blood levels in children has been linked to **attention deficit hyperactivity disorder (ADHD**, Chapter 15).

Trans fats are chemical and physical distortions of unsaturated fatty acids. They can be caused by exposure to excessive heat, as in high temperature cooking for long periods, but this actually produces only small quantities. The biggest quantities are produced artificially by manufacturers when normal fatty acids are changed under extreme high pressure. Producing trans fat in this way converts liquid oils to solid fats at room temperature, and this is considered useful for long-term storage of fats and repeated use in cooking. However, consumption of trans fats can result in disturbance of blood cholesterol, causing an increase in heart disease. Recently, evidence is growing that trans fats in the diet are getting incorporated into neuronal cell membranes, possibly during infant brain development. Cell membranes are critical in neuronal function because everything the cell needs must pass through the membrane by one means or another. Membranes incorporating the abnormally shaped trans fats may not function properly, and distort what is passing into and out of the cell.

Key points

The nervous system up to birth

- The brain and cord is formed initially from a neural tube.
- Three waves of neuronal migration occur within the tube wall.
- Three primary brain vesicles, the forebrain, midbrain, and hindbrain, form at the head end of the tube, and these become the complete brain.
- The sensory systems are always the most advanced at all stages of development.

The debate: when does consciousness start?

- The most important areas of the brain for consciousness are anatomically formed by between weeks 24 and 28 of gestation.
- The unborn fetus is alternating between two different sleep modes, active and quiet sleep.
- Although conscious before birth, the child is not aware of very much until the day of its birth.

The brain at birth

- The brain stem is the most advanced brain area at birth, and houses the vital centres and reflexes necessary for life.
- The newborn has all the senses functioning, but is lacking motor skills, mostly because the motor system is less well developed at birth.
- The brain is in a growth spurt at birth, which started before birth and continues until about 2 years of age, when the brain weighs about 75% of the adult brain weight.

Infant and child brain development

- The environment has the biggest influence over brain development.
- Synaptogenesis is the formation of new synapses.
- Unwanted synapses may be removed by a process called synaptic pruning to improve brain efficiency.
- Myelination is the process of laying down myelin around the axons of neurons.
- Plasticity is the brain's ability to adapt to new environments.
- Cerebral lateralisation, the assignment of new skills to one side of the brain, is well underway by birth, and continues throughout life.

Learning and memory

- Learning is a product of strong synapses.
- Using synapses strengthens them and they can become permanent.
- Stronger synapses mean long-term potentials (LTPs), which are the basis of learning and memory.
- This process will be improved by rehearsal.
- Two main forms of memory are long-term memory and short-term memory.
- One of the functions of the hippocampus is the conversion of short-term memory to long-term memory.

The teenage brain

- During teenage years the frontal lobe shows a reduction in its influence over emotions, which then become controlled largely by the amygdala.
- A partial shutdown of frontal lobe function is to improve myelination, synaptic pruning, and energy efficiency.
- Between the years 11 to 18 the teenager finds it harder to identify other people's emotions.
- During late teenage, a shift occurs away from the amygdala to the much improved frontal lobes for rational emotional influence.

Hormone influences on brain development

- Hormones are a key factor in brain development, and abnormal hormonal production has a profound adverse influence on the brain.
- Hormones act by binding to cell-surface receptors and influencing gene activity.

Nutritional influences on brain development

- From birth to 2 years of age is a critical period for adequate nutrition.
- The nervous system is particularly vulnerable to deficiencies during this time.
- There are strong indications that fatty acids in the diet are important in mental health.
- DHA is vital for optimum brain development at all stages of growth.
- Brain cell membranes incorporating the abnormally shaped trans fats may not function properly.

References

Blows, W. T. (2003) Child brain development. *Nursing Times*, **99** (17): 28–31.

Blows, W. T. (2012) *The Biological Basis of Clinical Observations* (2nd edition). Routledge, Abingdon, Oxon.

Dobbs, D. (2011) Beautiful brains. *National Geographic*, **220** (4): 36–59.

Hartshorne, J. (2009) Why don't babies talk like adults? *Scientific American Mind*, **20** (5): 58–61.

Koch, C. (2009) Consciousness redux, when does consciousness arise? *Scientific American Mind*, **20** (5): 20–21.

Ramakrishna, T. (1999) Vitamins and brain development. *Physiology Research*, **48**: 175–187.

Sabbagh, L. (2006) The teen brain, hard at work. *Scientific American Mind*, **17** (4): 20–25.

Weir, K. (2015) A likely story, *in* The human brain, *New Scientist The Collection*, **2** (1): 108–109.

3   Neural communication

- The neuron
- Neurotransmission
- Synapses
- Neuroglia
- Key points

The neuron

The functional unit of the nervous system is a cell called the neuron. All nerve impulses, or **action potentials**, originate in neurons. They travel along the neuron's extended cytoplasm, called the **axon**, to the point inside or outside the brain where the impulse is required. The impulse then initiates one of three possible actions, e.g. triggering another action potential within a second neuron, or causing a muscle contraction to occur (in motor neurons), or possibly causing a glandular secretion to be released (in neurons of the autonomic nervous system). Action potentials make things happen, and therefore the cell generating the impulse has some control over that action. Strong or rapidly repeated impulses along a neuron result in powerful activities, such as muscle contraction.

We are born with 100 billion neurons, an amazing number by any standards, yet this vast mass of cells constitutes only about 10% of the entire nervous system. The remaining 90% is made up of 900 billion glial cells (also known as **neuroglia**), which have very different functions from neurons. There is a grand total of 1000 billion cells in the nervous system, all derived from the same single fertilised ovum as the rest of the body. A very high rate of cell mitosis is required *before birth* to produce this vast number of neurons, i.e. about 250,000 new neurons *per minute* at the peak of cell mitosis! Although recent evidence indicates that some neuronal division can occur after birth in the hippocampus, the neuron cell mass in the brain is essentially complete at the time of birth. However, many *neuroglia* retain the power to replicate after birth and continue to do so throughout life.

The neuronal connections, called **synapses**, are not complete at birth. They continue forming throughout childhood until the brain becomes fully mature in the early twenties (Chapter 2). Synaptic development in childhood is promoted by stimulation of the senses and by education, and involves the creation of memory.

The neuron (Figure 3.1) has a relatively standard cell body, with a surrounding cell membrane, a cytoplasm with **organelles** such as **mitochondria** (for cellular energy) and

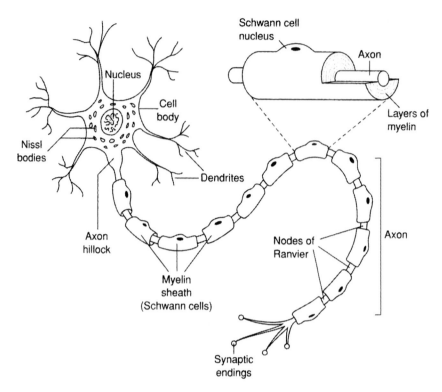

Figure 3.1 The neuron. The cell body shows a nucleus surrounded by Nissl bodies. The axon starts at the axon hillock and terminates at the synapse. Myelin covers the axon in segments with gaps between called the nodes of Ranvier. A myelin segment is shown enlarged. Each segment is laid down by a Schwann cell.

ribosomes (for producing proteins), and a nucleus with its own nuclear membrane. It is distinguished from other cells by the presence of cell body extensions, called dendrites and axons, and by the presence of **Nissl granules** (or **Nissl bodies**) within the cytoplasm (see below). **Dendrites** are mostly *afferent* pathways; that is, they convey impulses *towards* the cell body. There are usually many such dendrites, branching in a number of different directions, each branch covered by short processes called **spines**. The more dendrites or dendritic spines a neuron has, the greater the surface area available for forming synaptic connections. Dendrites are the sites of many synapses, which are formed from the local connections they have with other neighbouring neurons. **Axons** are *efferent* pathways, carrying impulses *away from* the cell body. Most neurons have only one axon, but there are examples of neurons with more than one. They can be long, and some are nearly the length of the body, and they have few branches, most of the branches occurring at the terminal end. The majority of neurons are myelinated and they make distant connections with other neurons, muscle cells, or glandular cells (Blows 2000).

Nissl bodies are patches of intracellular **rough endoplasmic reticulum (rough ER)** and are the site of protein synthesis carried out by **ribosomes** (protein factories) in the ER membrane. Nissl bodies are especially concentrated close to the nucleus, in the region of the

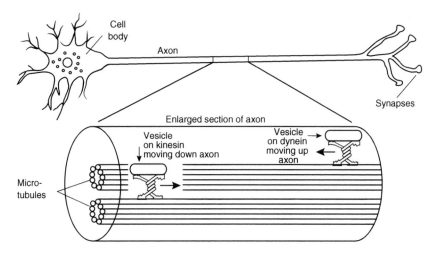

Figure 3.2 Axonal transportation. The protein kinesin transports vesicles filled with other proteins along microtubules towards the synapse. Another protein called dynein does the same in the opposite direction.

cytoplasm known as the **endoplasm**. Proteins produced in Nissl bodies are used within the cell to create membranes or organelles.

Axoplasmic transportation

Proteins are also required at the synapse, the terminal end of the axon, but because ribosomes are not found in the axon the proteins must be transported there from their source within the cell body. This **axoplasmic transport** (Figure 3.2) of proteins is a function of part of the cell's **cytoskeleton**; the protein support framework of the cell. Three structures are involved in this framework: **microtubules** (20 nm in diameter), hollow tubules made from the protein **tubulin** (see also Chapter 14); **microfilaments** (5 nm in diameter), cable-like structures made from two twisted proteins; and **neurofilaments** (10 nm in diameter), strong structures branching out in many directions. Like the bony skeleton inside the body, this protein framework of the cell provides shape, support, and some movement to the neuron, as well as allowing the mechanism of axoplasmic transport.

Axoplasmic transport first involves the packaging of essential proteins into vesicles that are destined for the synapse. These vesicles are then attached to another protein called **kinesin**. Using cellular energy in the form of **adenosine triphosphate (ATP)**, produced by another organelle, the **mitochondrion** (Blows 2012, Chapter 1), the kinesin moves down the axon. Kinesin acts like legs to 'walk' the vesicle along the microtubules, which extend in bundles along the full length of the axon. In the long journey to the synapse, two speeds of axonal transportation have been observed. **Slow transportation** moves the vesicles up to 8 mm per day, while **fast transportation** moves them anything from 50 to 400 mm per day. This is **anterograde** movement, i.e. from cell to synapse, involving the transportation of some neurotransmitters. However, **retrograde** movement also occurs, from synapse to cell body, using the protein **dynein** in place of kinesin.

Retrograde axoplasmic transport may be involved in feedback to the cell body related to the protein needs of the synapse (Figure 3.2). The whole axoplasmic transportation system is akin to the movement of goods by train along fixed tracks. It is important not to confuse axoplasmic transportation (protein movement along axons) with **neurotransmission** (the passage of an electrical impulse along axons). They are two very different concepts. Understanding neurotransmission is vital in grasping the main concepts of how the brain works and how drugs can modify its function.

Neurotransmission

Resting membrane potential

Neurotransmission is the passage of a nerve impulse (or **action potential**) along a neuronal axon. Before and after an action potential, the membrane is said to be at its **resting membrane potential** (Figure 3.3). Resting membrane potential involves a very distinct concentration of **ions** on both sides of the membrane. Ions are charged particles, either positively charged (+) particles called **cations**, or negatively charged (–) particles called **anions**. The particles themselves are atoms of elements such as sodium (forming a cation, Na$^+$), potassium (forming a cation, K$^+$), or chloride (forming a chloride anion, Cl$^-$). The ionic concentrations on both sides of the axonal membrane are shown in Figure 3.3. There is a sodium concentration outside the membrane (i.e. in the extracellular fluid), and a potassium concentration inside the membrane (i.e. in the cell cytoplasm). In addition to ions, there are compounds that also carry an electrical charge, notably proteins and phosphates (PO$_4$), both of which have three negative charges each. Compounds are larger than ions, and because of this larger size these compounds cannot pass through the membrane, and are therefore confined to the cytoplasm inside the membrane. If all the charges on each side of the membrane are added together (with each negative cancelling a positive), the net charge that remains after such cancellation is negative on the inside and positive on the outside. The *difference* between this overall

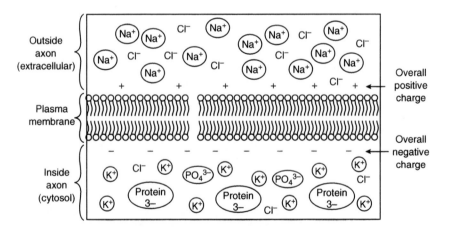

Figure 3.3 Resting potential in the neuronal membrane. Outside the membrane is a concentration of sodium, while inside is a concentration of potassium. The overall charge outside is caused mostly by the sodium, while the inside is negative because large negatively charged protein and phosphate (PO$_4^{3-}$) molecules cannot leave the axon.

negative charge *inside* the membrane and the overall positive charge *outside* the membrane is minus seventy thousandths of a volt (**–70 mV**, or minus seventy millivolts). This is the electrical value for the resting membrane potential.

Diffusion

The membrane of the neuronal axon is semipermeable, and as such it allows the occasional passage of ions one way or another. Sodium, for example, may tend to leak inward, moving down its concentration gradient from a high concentration outside to a low concentration inside. Potassium on the other hand, moving down its concentration gradient, may leak a little in the opposite direction. This is a natural movement for particles, which pass from a high to a low concentration in an attempt to equalise the concentration on both sides of the membrane (the process of **diffusion**). Diffusion of particles is the driving force for the movement of many substances both into and out of cells in many parts of the body.

Threshold potential

While leakage causes small fluctuations to occur at the resting potential of –70 mV, an action potential delivered from elsewhere will cause a rapid change. In fact, as soon as the resting potential reaches –50 mV, a rapid opening of sodium channels in the membrane allows a massive influx of sodium into the axon, creating a new action potential. This figure of **–50 mV** is called the **threshold potential** (Figure 3.4), and marks the opening of many sodium channels in the membrane. Channels that open at specific voltages in the membrane, such as the sodium channels described here, are known as **voltage-gated channels**. The sodium floods into the axon because, as a positive ion, it is attracted to the overall negative charge on the inside of the membrane (an electrical effect). Also, it will move rapidly down its concentration gradient (a chemical effect). The sodium influx is therefore an **electrochemical** event.

Depolarisation and repolarisation

As a result of the sodium influx, the membrane potential moves further away from threshold potential, to peak at **+30 mV**, and this is called **depolarisation** (Figure 3.4). As the membrane potential crosses **0 mV**, the membrane changes polarity – that is, the overall negative charge on the *inside* becomes positive, while the overall positive charge on the *outside* becomes negative (Figure 3.4). The inside of the membrane has gained many positive sodium ions and therefore becomes positive, while the outside has lost those same positive sodium ions and therefore becomes negative. At +30 mV (i.e. the peak of an action potential) potassium channels open and allow the rapid movement of potassium out of the axonal membrane. These potassium channels are also voltage-gated, but they open at a different voltage to the sodium channels. Potassium moves out for the same electrochemical reasons that sodium moved in. The positively charged potassium is attracted to the negative charge outside the membrane and is also flowing down its own concentration gradient, from high inside to low outside. This mass movement of potassium returns the membrane to resting potential, i.e. from +30 mV down to –70 mV again, a process called **repolarisation** (Figure 3.4). As 0 mV is crossed there is another reversal of membrane polarity, from the overall positive inside and negative outside of the action potential, to the overall negative

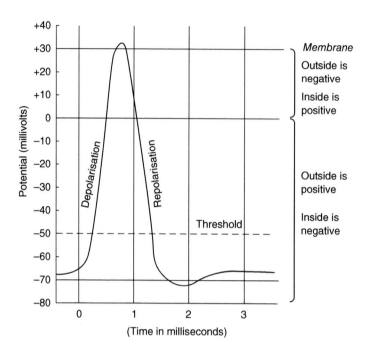

Figure 3.4 The action potential as seen on an oscilloscope screen. Resting potential is −70 mV. If sufficient depolarisation occurs for this value to reach −50 mV (threshold), an action potential will take place. Depolarisation is caused by sodium influx until +30 mV is reached. Repolarisation then occurs with a potassium efflux until resting potential is restored. As depolarisation and repolarisation cross 0 mV, the net charge on each side of the membrane reverses.

inside and positive outside of the resting potential. However, this restoration of resting potential occurs with the main ions, sodium and potassium, in the reverse positions from when the process started. Before another action potential is possible, the sodium must be returned to the *outside* of the membrane and the potassium returned to the *inside* of the membrane. The membrane has sodium-potassium pumps (Figure 3.5) that pump these ions across the membrane, against their concentration gradients, and thus return the two cations to their former concentrations, sodium outside and potassium inside the axon. The period of time needed for this to take place, and for the sodium and potassium channels to close, is known as the **refractory phase** (Figures 3.4 and 3.5). During this period the axon cannot produce another action potential (Marieb and Hoehn 2014).

Figure 3.4 shows the time scale, along the base axis, during which all these events take place. It is significant that the entire action potential occupies between two and three milliseconds (2–3 ms; i.e. two to three thousandths of a second), with a refractory phase lasting another millisecond. Thus, between one action potential and the next there is a time interval of about 4 ms, allowing a single neuron a capacity of up to 250 action potentials per second. The speed at which the nervous system works, in thousandths of a second, is faster than the blink of an eye, which to us appears to be instantaneous.

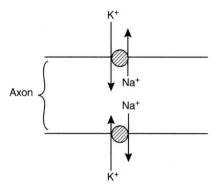

Figure 3.5 Sodium-potassium pumps are working during the refractory phase to restore the ions to the
    original positions; sodium is pumped out of the axon, potassium is pumped in.

Myelinated and unmyelinated axons

The action potential described also has to pass along the axon from cell to synapse. In an
unmyelinated axon, depolarisation at one part of the axonal membrane causes the membrane
just ahead to reach threshold and begin the process of depolarisation there. Repeating this
process continuously results in a wave of depolarisation that sweeps down the axon. This
will be followed by a wave of repolarisation, immediately behind depolarisation, during
which the resting potential is restored (Figure 3.6).

In a myelinated axon a different process causes the spread of an action potential down
the axon (Figure 3.7). Those segments of the membrane that are covered by myelin cannot
allow the passage of ions, and so will not be involved in the movement of an action potential.
However, the myelination has tiny gaps in it called the **nodes of Ranvier** where depolarisation and repolarisation take place. To describe what is happening, we will take a three-node
sequence from a myelinated axon (see Figure 3.7). In Figure 3.7 the active node has reached
threshold and will depolarise, i.e. reverse its polarity, while the other nodes are in resting
potential. The positive sodium entering at the active node is attracted to the negative on the

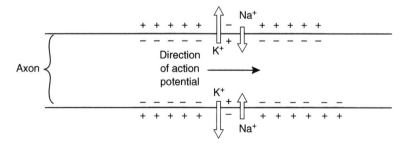

Figure 3.6 An unmyelinated axon. The impulse sweeps from left to right, caused by a sodium input,
    which reverses the membrane charge from resting to action potential, followed right behind
    by a potassium efflux, which restores the membrane resting potential charge.

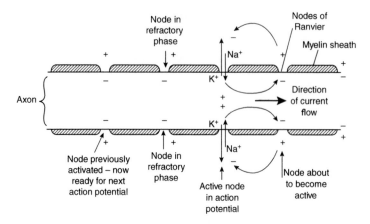

Figure 3.7 A section of myelinated axon showing saltatory action. The active node has a sodium influx followed immediately by a potassium efflux, i.e. an action potential. This positive input is attracted to the negative potential on the inside of the next node in the sequence, and this will rapidly reach threshold and action potential. The node behind the active node is in the refractory phase.

inside of the next node along, and will jump across the myelin internode to reach it. This movement of sodium causes the next node to reach threshold potential and depolarise. While sodium is entering this next node, the previous active node has reached repolarisation with the outflow of potassium. The process of sodium entering at a node and leaping over the internode to the next node is repeated along the length of the axon. This leaping over internodes is called **saltatory** ('jumping') action and speeds up the passage of an action potential down the axon. An action potential can pass along a fully myelinated axon at a speed of up to 120 metres per second compared to 2.3 metres per second along an unmyelinated axon. In either case the speed is fast, with action potentials passing through the full length of the body in a fraction of a second.

Synapses

Synapses (Figure 3.8) are the minute gaps (or **clefts**) occurring between the end of one neuronal axon and the membrane of the structure beyond. The **synaptic cleft**, which is between 20 nm and 50 nm across, separates the **presynaptic bulb** from the **postsynaptic membrane**. The presynaptic bulb is an expansion of the axon terminal. Within it there are many vesicles containing a chemical **neurotransmitter** destined to be released into the cleft. Neurotransmitters come in a variety of different forms (Chapter 4), but they all have in common the ability to bind to protein receptors attached to the postsynaptic membrane and thus cause a change within that membrane and the cell beyond. This happens when the neurotransmitter is released from the presynaptic bulb in response to the arrival of an action potential (Figure 3.9).

Action potentials sweeping down the axon involve the influx of sodium ions (Na^+), but on arrival at the presynaptic bulb the ionic influx changes to a different ion, i.e. the calcium ion (Ca^{2+}). This change to the double positive charge of calcium probably causes an even faster rise to +30 mV in the presynaptic bulb, triggering a sudden migration of the vesicles to

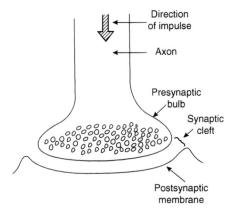

Figure 3.8 A synapse. The axon ends in a presynaptic bulb, which is filled with vesicles housing a neurotransmitter.

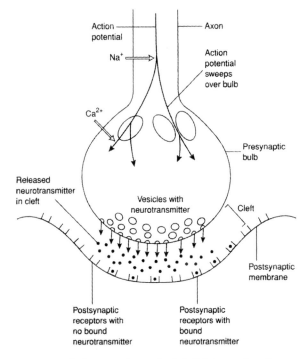

Figure 3.9 Events at a synapse during an action potential. Calcium enters the presynaptic bulb and the vesicles flood to the presynaptic membrane; the vesicles rupture and empty their contents into the synaptic cleft. Neurotransmitters can bind to receptors in the postsynaptic membrane and initiate a change in that membrane.

the presynaptic membrane. Here they rupture and empty their neurotransmitter contents into the cleft. These chemicals then flood the cleft and bind to receptor sites on the postsynaptic membrane. The binding of a neurotransmitter, even for only one or two milliseconds, causes important changes in the postsynaptic cell. After binding, the neurotransmitters are removed from the receptor. Some are broken down and disposed of by excretion via the cerebrospinal fluid (CSF) and the blood to the kidneys. Others are also degraded but reabsorbed back into the presynaptic bulb (called **reuptake**) and recycled. Some neurotransmitters are recycled in part via cells called **astrocytes** (see neuroglia, later in this chapter).

Excitation and inhibition

Some synapses are **excitatory** in function, while others are **inhibitory** (Figure 3.10). Excitatory synapses cause activity to occur beyond the postsynaptic membrane, often generating an action potential in the membrane of a second neuron. This is achieved by the binding of a neurotransmitter to receptors of the postsynaptic membrane that are linked to sodium channels in that membrane. The neurotransmitter causes the receptor to open the sodium channel; sodium then floods into the membrane from its high concentration outside the membrane, and starts a new action potential in the second neuron.

   Inhibitory synapses do the opposite. The postsynaptic receptors are linked to chloride (Cl⁻) channels, which open by the binding of neurotransmitter, allowing chloride to enter the membrane. Chloride moves down its concentration gradient from the higher concentrations found outside the membrane (Figure 3.3). The resting potential of that membrane, i.e. negative on the inside, becomes even more negative, ensuring that any action potentials in that neuron are impossible (i.e. they are inhibited). At first sight this may seem surprising. After all, the nervous system is designed to generate action potentials, so the blocking (or inhibition) of action potentials appears to go against the very purpose of the system.

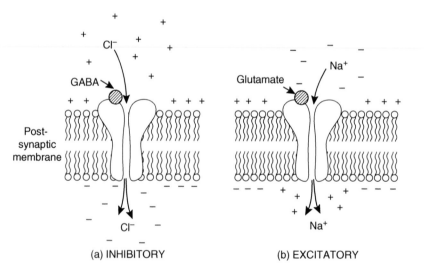

(a) INHIBITORY   (b) EXCITATORY

Figure 3.10 Two types of postsynaptic receptor. (a) An inhibitory receptor binding gamma-aminobutyric acid (GABA). This causes the opening of a chloride (Cl⁻) channel and chloride enters the postsynaptic membrane. The entry of this negative ion causes the resting potential to become even more negative, preventing any chance of an action potential in that membrane. (b) An excitatory receptor binding glutamate. This causes the opening of a sodium channel and sodium ions (Na⁺) to enter. The entry of a positive ion sets up an action potential in the postsynaptic membrane.

However, think for a moment about the motor car. It is designed to move (a car that does not move is a waste of time), yet one of the fundamental components is a braking system, designed to prevent any movement. Is that surprising? Of course not, since a car that cannot stop is deadly. And so it is with the brain. Uncontrolled, unchecked action potentials would be like a car going downhill with no brakes. Life for the person with no inhibitory synapses would be a living nightmare, and some mental health disorders are linked to low levels of inhibitory neurotransmitters (see Chapter 12 Epilepsy). With no inhibition, every action potential would cause some form of activity; and this would cause a state of brain overactivity. Compare the inhibitory synapses with the 'off' switch on a computer, where activation of this switch causes a shut-down of the system. Every system, including the nervous system, needs a form of deactivation mechanism at some point.

Neuromodulators

Neurotransmitters and their receptor binding sites are critical, not only to the function of the entire nervous system but also to the mechanism of action of many psychotropic drugs, and therefore a more detailed discussion of these chemicals and their receptors is given in Chapter 4. However, in addition to neurotransmitters, chemicals called neuromodulators are also produced at the synapse. The term '**neuromodulator**' can be applied to various substances that are often released along with a neurotransmitter. These neuromodulators have a generally wider effect on neuronal function than neurotransmitters for the following reasons:

1   Neurotransmitters are released in small quantities and act locally within the synapse in which they are released. Neuromodulators are released in larger quantities and spread out beyond the synapse from which they are released. They therefore influence many other synaptic connections over a larger area of the brain.
2   Neuromodulators appear to modify the response of receptors to the neurotransmitter.
3   Some neuromodulators may act by binding to **autoreceptors**, which are receptors situated on the presynaptic membrane of the bulb, thus modifying the release of neurotransmitters (Breedlove et al. 2010).

Neuromodulators are mostly **neuropeptides**, i.e. small proteins of the nervous system. However, several substances usually classified as neurotransmitters may have a neuromodulatory role by acting beyond the synapse from where they were released, e.g. **enkephalin** and **cholecystokinin** (see Chapter 4). Several groups of **hormones** are also peptides. Hormones have an even wider influence over the activity of the brain (as well as the body) by being released into the blood circulation. Hormonal influence over brain activity is discussed in Chapter 5.

Neuroglia

Astrocytes

Neuroglia, or glial cells, are the support cells of the central nervous system. They outnumber the neurons by nine to one (there are estimated 900 billion neuroglia compared with 100 billion neurons), but they do not create or transmit action potentials (impulses) as neurons do. Of this vast number of glial cells, the most common are the **astrocytes** (Figure 3.11), so called because of their star shape, created by many fine extensions pushing out in all directions.

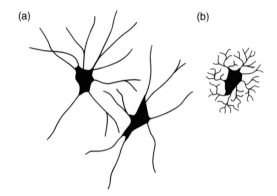

Figure 3.11 Astrocytes: (a) fibrous; (b) protoplasmic.

There are two forms of astrocyte; the **fibrous** form and the **protoplasmic** form. The fibrous form is largely found in the white matter of the brain. Fibrous astrocytes have fewer processes than their protoplasmic cousins, but their processes are long and straight, some with broad ends (like feet), which attach to blood capillaries or to the cells of the pia mater.

The fibrous astrocytes respond to brain tissue injury by growing in large numbers (a process called **gliosis**). Unlike most neurons, both kinds of astrocyte retain the ability to go through mitosis (cell division) for the duration of the person's lifetime. The protoplasmic forms appear mostly in the grey matter of the brain. Their processes are shorter but more numerous than in the fibrous type, each process being more extensively branched.

Astrocytes generally have a very close association with neurons, surrounding the cell bodies and synapses, as well as blood capillaries, with their processes. They appear to have a role to play during the moment when neurons are transmitting an action potential. Neuronal action potentials cause the adjacent astrocytes to increase their metabolism and at the same time to partly depolarise, although they do not themselves achieve an action potential. Potassium ions (K^+) flood out from the axonal membrane of the neuron as the action potential sweeps down towards the synapse, and the astrocyte takes up this extracellular potassium in order to stabilise the ionic environment around the neuron. Excess *extracellular* potassium is dangerous to the brain and, if it got into circulation, it would be dangerous to the heart. Potassium is normally kept concentrated *inside* the cells.

Astrocytes are also involved in the biochemistry of neurotransmitters. They are often found surrounding the synapse, where they prevent neurotransmitter leakage and assist in the removal, and in some cases the recycling, of neurotransmitters after these chemicals have fulfilled their task. One such form of neurotransmitter recycling that involves astrocytes is the production of glutamate from GABA within the cytoplasm of an astrocyte close to the GABA synapse. The glutamate thus created is passed back from the astrocyte to the neuron for the further synthesis of GABA (Figure 3.12). This is a good example of the supportive role of these cells.

Some astrocytes have been found to bind neurotransmitters to receptor sites attached to the astrocyte membrane, although the purpose of binding neurotransmitters to astrocytes is not fully known. In one example of this, glutamate, an important neurotransmitter in several

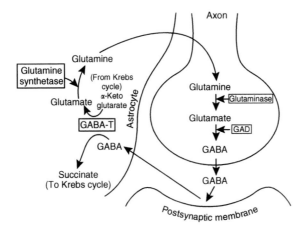

Figure 3.12 Astrocytes near a GABA synapse are partly involved in the GABA–glutamate synthesis cycle. The enzymes are in boxes: GABA-T = gamma-aminobutyric acid transaminase, GAD = glutamic acid decarboxylase.

brain areas such as the cerebrum, was able to bind to astrocyte receptors. Binding to these receptors caused the astrocyte to oscillate between high and low calcium levels within its cytoplasm. These calcium waves within the cell have been seen to pass on to other cells through membrane-to-membrane contacts between adjacent astrocytes. In one experiment, a calcium wave induced in one astrocyte by adding glutamate was witnessed to pass through 59 other attached astrocytes before it stopped. Such calcium surges must indicate a form of cell signalling about which much is still to be learnt. Other functions of astrocytes have been proposed from varying amounts of evidence. For example, the broad feet resting on blood capillaries suggest a possible nutritional role for these cells. It would not be possible for every one of 100 billion neurons to receive its own blood supply. Many neurons rely on nutrients being collected from the circulation by astrocytes and passed on to the neurons, with wastes possibly going in the opposite direction. Astrocytes also store glucose and pass this on to the neurons for energy purposes.

Astrocytes in the hippocampus are divided into **AMPA-type glutamate receptors** (**GluR** cells) and **glutamate transporters** (**GluT** cells). These have different structures and functions, and appear to be involved in epilepsy (see the section entitled The hippocampal involvement in seizures, in Chapter 12). GluT cells absorb glutamate, which is released from neurons, therefore terminating the stimulatory effect of glutamate (Chapter 4). They also have potassium (K^+) channels, thus reducing free potassium from around the neuron and reducing the neuron's excitation. GluT cells have junctions that connect them together in networks. These networks of GluT cells remove other ions from the around the neurons and move them to the blood for removal from the tissue. The other type of astrocyte, the GluR cells, have specialised receptors for binding multiple substances including glutamate. They do not have junctions between them and therefore they do not form networks. This means they are not able to remove ions from around the neurons. Their specific function remains unclear.

The importance of studying astrocytes is highlighted by this large number of diverse functions. Gliosis (excessive growth of glial cells) is somehow involved in brain repair, and this mechanism may have implications for mental health, such as in dementia. Also, the role of astrocytes in neurotransmitter recycling could be of importance in depression or anxiety, and the fact that they have neurotransmitter receptors now makes them possible targets for psychotropic drugs. Such future drugs may be used to modify mental activity by affecting astrocytes, with or without neuronal involvement, and it is possible that some current drugs may already be influencing mental activity through astrocyte involvement.

Other glial cells

The glial cells that form myelin sheaths around axons fall into two types, the **oligodendrocytes** within the central nervous system only, and the **Schwann cells** within the peripheral nervous system only. Myelination, as identified earlier, is essential for the saltatory passage of action potentials. Some neurons remain unmyelinated, but they are less numerous. Oligodendrocytes are small cells within the brain and cord, and during embryonic development each cell contributes myelination to several axons at once. Each Schwann cell, however, contributes myelination to only one segment of a single peripheral axon (Figure 3.1). Both types of cell leave gaps (the nodes of Ranvier) between the myelination patches where short sections of axon are exposed (Figure 3.1).

Glial cells include the following other types:

*   **Microglia**, small phagocytic cells of the central nervous system (i.e. the brain and spinal cord), which engulf and remove not only invading organisms but also remnants and debris of dead cells.
*   **Ependymal cells**, flat cells lining the brain's ventricular system and ducts, which provide a smooth surface for the CSF to flow over. They have cilia (minute hair-like processes) on the cell surface, which produce a sweeping action that aids the circulation of CSF.
*   **Satellite cells**, the smallest cells of the brain, associated with neuronal cell bodies and Schwann cells. They maintain the optimum chemical environment around neurons, and they appear to respond to inflammation and injury.

Ependymal cells fall into three main groups. The **ependymocytes** line the ventricles and central canal of the spinal cord. The **tanycytes** line the floor of the third ventricle and have processes touching blood capillaries; they may be involved in the movement of hormones from the blood to the adjacent hypothalamus. The **choroidal cells** cover the choroid plexus and promote the production of CSF.

During embryonic development of the nervous system, ependymal cells take on another role related to the migration of neurons within the neural tube (the embryonic stage of development of the central nervous system). They form a temporary framework along which the migrating neurons will move, away from the site of cellular mitosis. This framework is rather like a trellis along which a plant will grow. The process of neuronal migration is important for the correct location of neurons in the brain and the establishment of their subsequent synaptic connections (Chapter 2). If the wrong route is taken by neurons along the ependymal framework, inappropriate synaptic connections will be formed. This malformation is implicated in several mental health disorders, notably schizophrenia, and is discussed further in Chapter 10.

Key points

The neuron

- Neurons are the functional cellular unit of the nervous system. They have a cell body bearing dendrites and an axon.
- Axons are efferent pathways conveying action potentials to the synapse. They are mostly myelinated to speed up the passage of action potentials.

Neurotransmission

- The membrane begins at resting potential, with sodium concentrated outside the axon and potassium concentrated inside the axon.
- Action potentials are generated by a sodium influx into the axon, followed by a potassium output from the axon, which restores resting potential.

Synapses

- Synapses store neurotransmitters, which are released into the cleft on arrival of the action potential. Neurotransmitters then bind to the postsynaptic membrane and cause changes beyond that membrane.
- Synapses are either excitatory (causing changes such as action potentials in the postsynaptic membrane) or inhibitory (blocking such changes).

Neuroglia

- Neuroglia are the support cells of the nervous system. Astrocytes are the most numerous of the neuroglia, providing nutritional, ionic, and neurotransmitter support to neurons.
- Oligodendrocytes (within the brain and cord) and Schwann cells (within the peripheral nerves) provide myelination to axons.

References

Blows, W. T. (2000) The nervous system, part 1. *Nursing Times*, **96** (35): 41–44.

Blows, W. T. (2012) *The Biological Basis of Clinical Observations* (2nd edition). Routledge, Abingdon, Oxon.

Breedlove, S. M., Watson, N. V., and Rosenzweig, M. R. (2010) *Biological Psychology: An Introduction to Behavioural, Cognitive and Clinical Neuroscience* (6th edition). Sinauer Associates, Sunderland, MA.

Marieb, E. N. and Hoehn, K. N. (2014) *Human Anatomy and Physiology* (9th edition). Pearson Education Limited, Harlow, UK.

4 Neurotransmitters and receptors

- Introduction to neurotransmitters
- Receptors
- The amine neurotransmitters
- The amino acid neurotransmitters
- The peptide neurotransmitters
- Endogenous opioids
- Other neurotransmitters
- Key points

Introduction to neurotransmitters

Neurotransmitters are the chemical agents released from the presynaptic bulb into the synaptic cleft. They are sometimes referred to as the *primary messenger*, since they occur as free chemicals that move across a space (in this case, the cleft) and cause a change in another part (in this case, the postsynaptic membrane). Another term used for neurotransmitters is **ligand**, meaning a naturally produced agent that binds to a receptor and in so doing changes that receptor. The main change that occurs in receptors on binding of a ligand is an **allosteric** effect, i.e. a change of receptor *shape*. This change then has a further effect, the nature of which depends on which receptor is involved; it may be either within the membrane or beyond it in the cytoplasm of the cell.

Most neurotransmitters fall into three main groups: the **amines**, the **amino acids,** and the **peptides**. Amines are compounds containing the **amino group** (NH_2) and amines have the general structure RCH_2NH_2 where R is a variable portion (known as a **radical**) (Figure 4.1a). Variations in the radical give rise to different amines. Amino acids, the building blocks of proteins, are amines in which a **carboxyl group (COOH)** replaces one of the hydrogens on a carbon atom (Figure 4.1b). A peptide is a small protein, i.e. a small number of amino acids bonded together in a linear chain. Acetylcholine is a neurotransmitter of different origin and is discussed separately. **Catecholamines** are amines combined with a **catechol group** (Figure 4.1c), which consists of a carbon ring with two OH branches. A discussion related to each of the better-known neurotransmitters follows, as this information is relevant to an understanding of the neuropathology of the various mental health disorders and to neuropharmacology.

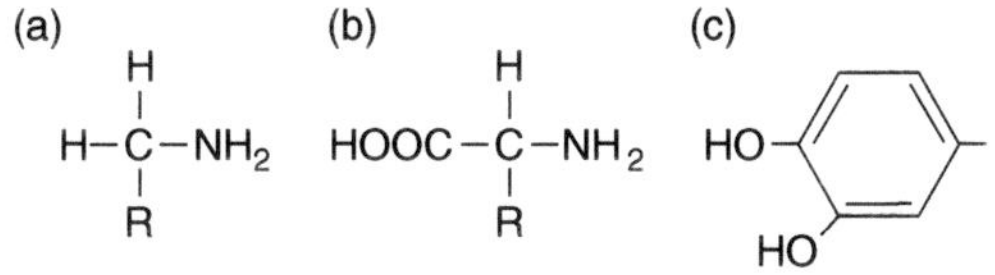

(a)

H–C–NH$_2$

(with H above C and R below C)

(b)

HOOC–C–NH$_2$

(with H above C and R below C)

(c)

(catechol ring structure with HO and HO groups)

Figure 4.1 The structure of three compounds: (a) an amine; (b) an amino acid; (c) the catechol group. NH$_2$ is the amino group; COOH is the carboxyl group; R is the radical (variable portion).

Receptors

Specific activity at the synapse is not due to the function of any particular neurotransmitter but to the function of the receptor to which it binds. By binding to different receptors, the *same* neurotransmitter is often seen to produce *different* effects. Receptors for any given neurotransmitter fall into several types (or groups) according to structure and function, and each receptor type usually has distinct subtypes. A good example is acetylcholine, which binds to two main types of receptor, either **nicotinic** or **muscarinic**, and these have subtypes (e.g. the muscarinic subtypes are M_1, M_2, M_3, M_4, M_5). Subtle variations in the way these subtypes respond to acetylcholine binding results in a wide range of activity for the neurotransmitter.

It is also important to recognise two other ways of classifying receptor sites:

1   According to their *location*. **Postsynaptic receptors** are part of the *postsynaptic* membrane of the cell that occurs beyond the cleft. Their purpose, when activated by neurotransmitter, is to effect some kind of change within that postsynaptic cell, such as the generation of a new action potential. Alternatively, **autoreceptors** are found on some *presynaptic* membranes or other parts of the neuron and therefore allow neurotransmitters to bind to the same neuron that releases it. Such autoreceptors are thought to provide feedback information to the neuron and the presynaptic bulb, in particular, to regulate (or control) any further neurotransmitter release.

2   According to their *function*. Some receptors are **ionotropic**. They control the opening or closing of a particular ion channel and can do this remarkably quickly, usually within milliseconds. When a neurotransmitter binds to a receptor, the receptor changes shape (the allosteric effect) and this opens a channel in the membrane, e.g. a sodium channel, allowing ions to pass through the membrane. The passage of sodium ions (or other positively charged cations) into the second neuron beyond the cleft will initiate a new action potential and therefore occurs at **excitatory** synapses (see Figure 3.10 in Chapter 3). The passage of chloride (a negatively charged anion) into a second neuron will prevent an action potential and therefore occurs at **inhibitory** synapses (Figure 3.10). Other receptors are **metabotropic** (Figure 4.2). They do not *directly* influence ionic channels but do cause changes in the metabolism of the postsynaptic cell.

The binding of a neurotransmitter to metabotropic receptors causes activation of a membrane-bound protein on the inside of the cell. This is the **G-protein**, abbreviated from *guanosine triphosphate (GTP) binding protein*, which may have an inhibitory (G_i) or a stimulatory (G_s) effect on cellular enzymes. In this way, metabotropic receptors, like ionotropic receptors,

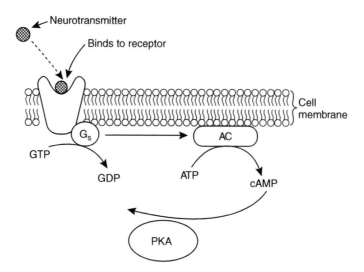

Figure 4.2 An excitatory metabotropic receptor. The neurotransmitter (first messenger) binds to the receptor outside the membrane. This activates a stimulatory G-protein (G_s), which binds guanosine triphosphate (GTP) and forms guanosine diphosphate (GDP). The activated G_s protein moves along the inner membrane, and collides with and activates adenylyl cyclase (AC). This in turn binds adenosine triphosphate (ATP) to form cyclic adenosine monophosphate (cAMP). cAMP is free to move into the cell (it is a second messenger) and activate protein kinase A (PKA), which can have a multitude of different effects on the cell. Compare with Figure 4.3.

can also be excitatory or inhibitory. However, because they operate through a different mechanism, they are slower than ionotropic receptors and their effects remain over a longer period of time. When the G_s protein is activated, it moves along the inside of the membrane until it contacts a membrane-bound enzyme called **adenylyl cyclase (AC)**. Allosteric activation of AC then occurs and this enzyme binds and splits intracellular ATP to form **cAMP (cyclic adenosine monophosphate)**. cAMP is known as a **secondary messenger** because it is free to move through the cell (unlike the G_s protein and AC, which are bound to the inside of the postsynaptic membrane). The primary messenger was the neurotransmitter, which was free to move around the synaptic cleft. The secondary messenger is free to move around the inside of the cell (within the **cytosol**). Secondary messengers like cAMP, and others such as **inositol trisphosphate (IP3)** and **diacylglycerol (DAG)** produced by some metabotropic receptors, then go on to influence other cellular functions. IP_3 opens calcium channels, whereas cAMP and DAG activate an enzyme known as **protein kinase (PK)**. When activated, PK regulates changes in the cell's metabolism. This may involve the opening of ion channels, causing changes in the ionic environment of the cell, the moderation of protein synthesis, or even the activation of specific genes leading to protein synthesis **(gene expression)** (Figure 4.2). Metabotropic receptors that activate G_i proteins are inhibitory because they block any activity of AC (Figure 4.3).

Receptors are actually proteins set into the cell membrane, and they have a specific role that is activated by the binding of neurotransmitter (Marieb and Hoehn 2014). Some receptors are attached to the outer surface of the membrane, while others are transmembranous

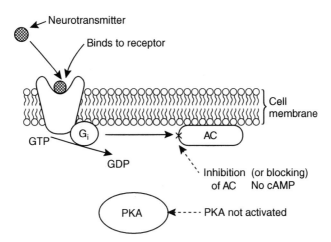

Figure 4.3 An inhibitory metabotropic receptor. The activated inhibitory G_i protein collides with adenylyl cyclase (AC), which is then deactivated and unable to form cyclic adenosine monophosphate (cAMP). As a result, protein kinase A (PKA) is not activated. Compare with Figure 4.2.

(i.e. they pass right through the membrane, appearing on both sides). Cells can of course produce proteins, so they can also produce receptors when necessary. This means that cells can **upregulate** their receptors by producing more of them, increasing the receptor density of their membrane and therefore binding more of the neurotransmitter. This is likely to be the consequence of reduced quantities of available neurotransmitter. Alternatively, cells can **downregulate** their membrane receptor density by slowing receptor production, especially if the neurotransmitter is in abundance. Measurements of receptor density on postsynaptic membranes give useful information about the levels of neurotransmitter present in the synaptic cleft. This is important because variations in the level of neurotransmitter can affect mental health, causing, for example, depression.

The amine neurotransmitters

Dopamine

Dopamine, noradrenaline, and adrenaline are three **catecholamine** neurotransmitters that share a common pathway of production (Figure 4.4). The starting point for the production of dopamine is the dietary amino acid **tyrosine**, which is converted by the neurons to **dihydroxyphenylalanine** (known as **dopa**) by the enzyme **tyrosine hydroxylase**. Further conversion to dopamine is by another enzyme called **dopa decarboxylase**. After use, dopamine is broken down in two sites, within the cleft and in the presynaptic bulb, by several enzymes including one called **monoamine oxidase (MAO)**, which is situated at the junction of the axon with the presynaptic bulb. The final metabolite, **homovanillic acid**, is excreted via the cerebrospinal fluid (CSF).

Dopamine activates several important pathways of the brain (Figure 4.5). From the brain stem nucleus known as the **ventral tegmental area (VTA)**, closely associated with the substantia nigra, two major dopaminergic (i.e. using and responding to dopamine) tracts pass

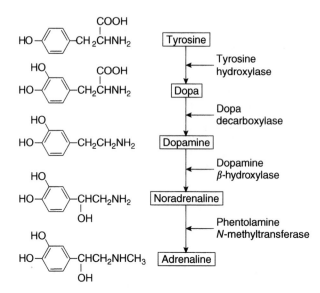

Figure 4.4 The formation of dopamine, noradrenaline, and adrenaline from the amino acid tyrosine. The names of the products are in boxes, and the enzymes (unboxed) label the arrows. The chemical structure of each product is shown on the left.

out to specific brain areas. Tracts passing to the **cerebral cortex** form the **mesocortical pathways**, and others to the **nucleus accumbens** of the **limbic system** form the **mesolimbic pathways** (Marieb and Hoehn 2014). Additional major dopaminergic pathways are the tracts from the **substantia nigra** in the midbrain to other main areas of the **basal ganglia**, forming the **nigrostriatal pathways**. Some authors join the nigrostriatal and mesolimbic pathways together under the term '**mesostriatal system**'.

In some sites of the brain, dopamine acts as an inhibitory neurotransmitter, although, as discussed, the function of neurotransmitters more often relates to the receptor that it binds to than to the ligand itself. In this capacity, dopamine is involved in inhibiting muscle tone, a function of the substantia nigra (see Parkinson's disease, page 288). It also inhibits breast milk production by blocking the release of the hormone **prolactin** from the anterior **pituitary gland** when the woman is not breastfeeding. Dopamine also plays a vital role in the function of the limbic system and is associated here with brain arousal. It is implicated in psychotic disturbances such as hallucinations in schizophrenia and manic-depressive psychosis, as well as being involved in the reward pathways associated with drug addiction (Blows 2000).

Dopamine receptors

Dopamine receptors are all metabotropic, i.e. working through a G-protein system. At least five subclasses of dopamine receptor are identified (**D_1, D_2, D_3, D_4**, and **D_5**). They are often grouped as the D_1-like subgroup (D_1 and D_5) because they are both excitatory, and the D_2-like subgroup (D_2, D_3, and D_4) because they are all inhibitory. D_1 and D_5 are both excitatory because they increase the level of cAMP in the cell. D_1 is the most abundant dopamine receptor in the

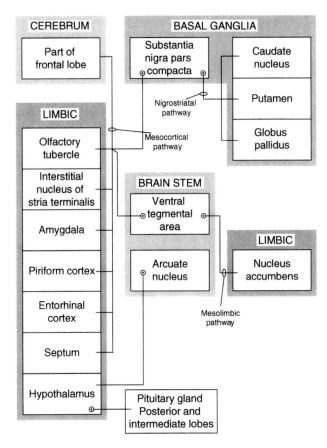

Figure 4.5 The main dopamine pathways of the central nervous system.

brain, especially the basal ganglia. D_2-like receptors are inhibitory because they reduce the level of cAMP in the neuron. D_2 is found in the basal ganglia, nucleus accumbens, and the VTA of the brain stem. The D_3 receptor is inhibitory and is found in the limbic system, and in particular the hypothalamus. D_4 is inhibitory and is mostly found in the cortex, hippocampus, amygdala, and nucleus accumbens. D_5 is excitatory and is found in the thalamus. D_6 and D_7 also exist, and they function in a similar way to D_1 and D_2. Their exact role in the brain is not yet established.

Noradrenaline

Noradrenaline (norepinephrine) is a catecholamine produced from dopamine by the action of the enzyme **dopamine β-hydroxylase (DBH)** (Figure 4.4). Noradrenaline is produced both as a hormone from the **adrenal medulla** and as a neurotransmitter in parts of the brain and at the **sympathetic** nerve terminals. The adrenergic brain pathways (i.e. those that use and respond to noradrenaline) centre primarily on the **locus coeruleus** in the brain stem (Marieb and Hoehn 2014). Tracts from this nucleus pass out to the cerebrum and limbic

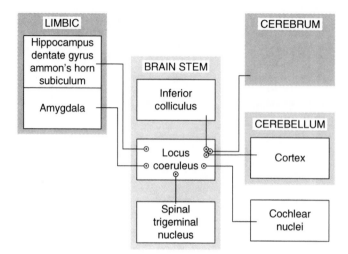

Figure 4.6 The main noradrenaline pathways of the central nervous system.

system (Figure 4.6) as part of the **diffuse modulatory systems** similar to serotonin pathways (see serotonin) (Blows 2000).

Adrenaline

Adrenaline (epinephrine) is the final stage in the production of catecholamine transmitters. Noradrenaline is acted on by the enzyme **phentolamine *N*-methyltransferase (PNMT)** to produce adrenaline (Figure 4.4). Adrenaline is well known as a *hormone* of the **adrenal medulla**, but as a *neurotransmitter* it is far less well understood. This is because it is found in low concentrations across many widespread sites in the brain. It does not usually occur in specific nuclei, and this pattern of diffuse distribution makes it difficult to study, resulting in a poor understanding of its neurotransmitter role in the brain.

Adrenergic receptors

Adrenergic receptors, i.e. those that bind and respond to noradrenaline and adrenaline, are either **alpha (α)** or **beta (β)**, with subtypes of each (α_1, α_2, β_1, β_2, β_3). They are all metabotropic, activating cellular changes through secondary messengers. The α_1 type is excitatory, and the activation of this receptor causes depolarisation by releasing calcium stored inside the cell. This receptor is found in the brain as a postsynaptic receptor and also in the vascular and intestinal smooth muscle and the heart. The α_2 type is inhibitory (i.e. it uses a G_i protein) and deactivates calcium channels, thus having the opposite effect to α_1 receptors. α_2 receptors are found in the brain as autoreceptors as well as postsynaptic receptors. They are also located in the same smooth muscles as α_1 and on the surface of platelets and nerve terminals.

Beta receptors, on activation by noradrenaline, increase the postsynaptic membrane response to other excitatory stimuli by indirectly affecting ion channels via a series of intermediate proteins that increase cAMP. Both β_1 and β_2 are found in the brain, whereas the β_3 type is located in adipose tissue.

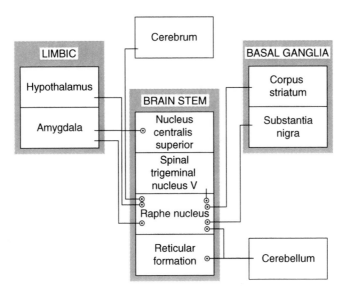

Figure 4.7 The main serotonin pathways of the central nervous system.

Serotonin

Serotonin, an important neurotransmitter, is part of the brain's **diffuse modulatory systems**. Nine nuclei (the **raphe nuclei**) in the brain stem send out serotonergic pathways (i.e. those using and responding to serotonin) to many parts of the cerebrum and limbic system (Figure 4.7). The serotonergic diffuse modulatory system has influence over a wide range of brain functions including regulation of mood, movement, appetite, sexual activity, sleeping, and some glandular secretions (Blows 2000). It therefore plays a vital role in the maintenance of mental health and will be discussed again when considering a number of conditions, such as depression and eating disorders.

Serotonin is also known as **5-hydroxytryptamine (5-HT)** and is originally derived from the dietary amino acid **tryptophan**. This crosses the **blood–brain barrier** into the brain, transported by a molecule called the **large neutral amino acid transporter (LNAA)**. The blood–brain barrier is a layer of cells between the circulating blood and the brain tissue that acts like a filter, allowing some molecules to pass into the brain but not others. As the LNAA transports several amino acids into the brain across this barrier, particularly tyrosine, valine, and leucine, the amount of tryptophan entering the brain is dependent on its concentration in the blood compared with the concentration of the other amino acids involved.

Neurons that use serotonin have the enzyme **tryptophan hydroxylase (TRPH)** in order to convert tryptophan to **5-hydroxytryptophan**, and this is further converted to serotonin by a second enzyme known as **aromatic amino acid decarboxylase (AAAD)**. **Vitamin B$_6$ (pyridoxine)** is vital in the function of AAAD, and thus is important overall in the production of serotonin (Figure 4.8). After its release into the synaptic cleft and after it has bound to postsynaptic receptors, serotonin is taken back into the presynaptic bulb (in a process called reuptake) and is metabolised. The enzymes that are responsible for this are **MAO** and **aldehyde oxidase**, resulting in a **metabolite** (waste product) called **5-hydroxyindoleacetic acid (5-HIAA)**. This is excreted first via the CSF, then to the blood, which carries it to the kidneys.

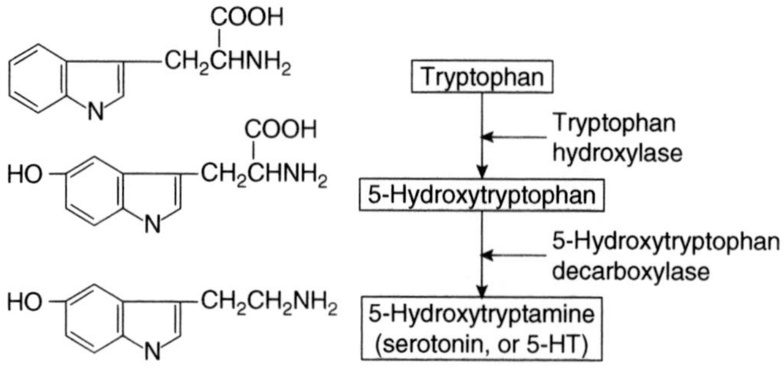

Figure 4.8 The formation of serotonin (5-hydroxytryptamine, or 5-HT) from the amino acid trypto-phan. The names of the products are in boxes, and the enzymes (unboxed) label the arrows. The chemical structure of each product is shown on the left.

Serotonin receptors

Serotonin receptors form many classes and subclasses, all of which are metabotropic. Table 4.1 shows the main classes and subclasses and their intracellular action on binding serotonin, where known. These intracellular actions may be involved in various mental activities and disorders as follows (Nolen-Heoksema 2007; Carlson 2012):

- Addiction involves 5-HT1A, 1B, 2A, 2C, and 3.
- Aggression involves 5-HT1A and 1B.
- Anxiety involves 5-HT1A, 1B, 1D, 2A, 2B, 2C, 3, 4, 6, and 7.
- Appetite involves 5-HT1A, 2A, 2B, 2C, and 4.
- Cognition involves 5-HT2A, and 6.
- Impulsivity involves 5-HT1A.
- Learning involves 5-HT1B, 2A, 3, 4, and 6.
- Memory involves 5-HT1A, 1B, 2A, 3, 4, 6, and 7.
- Mood involves 5-HT1A, 1B, 2A, 2C, 4, 6, and 7.
- Sexual behaviour involves 5-HT1A, 1B, 2A, and 2C.
- Sleep involves 5-HT1A, 2A, 2B, 2C, 5A, and 7.

Table 4.1 Classes of serotonin receptors and their intracellular actions. (Ex) = excitatory, (In) = inhibitory

Serotonin receptor class	Receptor subclasses	Intracellular role
5-HT1	5-HT1A, 1B, 1D, 1E, 1F	Decreases cAMP (In) with different effects. Some reduce AC activity
5-HT2	5-HT2A, 2B, 2C	Activates DAG and IP_3 (Ex)
5-HT3		Opens Ca^{2+} channels (Ex)
5-HT4		Increases cAMP (Ex)
5-HT5	5-HT5A	Decreases cAMP (In)
5-HT6		Increases cAMP (Ex)
5-HT7		Increases cAMP (Ex)

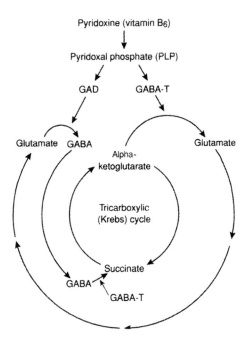

Figure 4.9 The synthesis of glutamate and gamma-aminobutyric acid (GABA). The two main enzymes involved are gamma-aminobutyric acid transaminase (GABA-T) and glutamic acid decarboxylase (GAD). Notice that vitamin B_6 is required to form pyridoxal phosphate (PLP), which is essential for both enzymes. Note also the involvement of the tricarboxylic (Krebs) cycle.

The amino acid neurotransmitters

Glutamate and GABA

Glutamate and **gamma-aminobutyric acid (GABA)** are important neurotransmitters found throughout the cerebral cortex, and they share a common synthesis pathway (Figure 4.9). Glutamate (also called glutamic acid) is a potent excitatory transmitter involved in consciousness. It is produced mostly during the daytime as a result of cerebral activity. The synthesis of glutamate is linked with the **tricarboxylic acid** (or **Krebs) cycle**, the energy cycle of the neuron. **α-Ketoglutarate**, a component of this cycle, is converted to glutamate by the enzyme **GABA transaminase (GABA-T)**. After use, glutamate is acted on by a second enzyme called **glutamic acid decarboxylase (GAD)** to produce GABA (Figure 4.9).

GABA is a major inhibitory neurotransmitter. After use it is converted to succinate by GABA-T (the same enzyme that acted on α-ketoglutarate). Succinate becomes another component of the tricarboxylic cycle. Both enzymes, GABA-T and GAD, rely on a cofactor called **pyridoxal phosphate (PLP)** in order to function. PLP itself relies on a supply of **pyroxidine** (vitamin B_6), and thus glutamate and GABA are both indirectly dependent on vitamin B_6 in the diet. GABA-T is most active in astrocytes located close to GABA synapses, whereas GAD is active in the presynaptic bulb of glutamate neurons (see Figure 3.12 in Chapter 3).

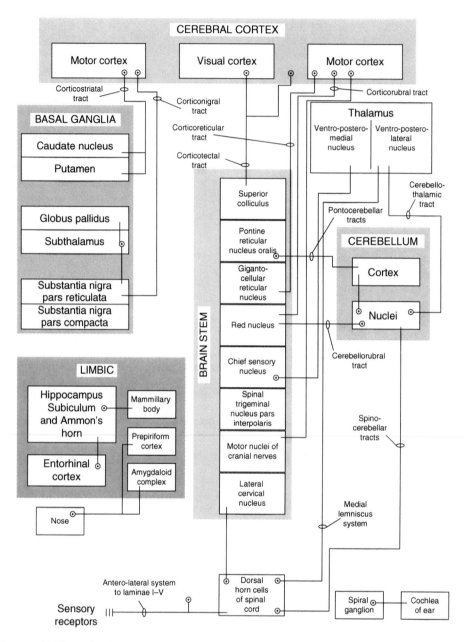

Figure 4.10 The main glutamate pathways of the central nervous system.

The major glutamate pathways of the brain are shown in Figure 4.10 and the major GABA pathways in Figure 4.11. A low GABA level in some areas of the brain is implicated as part of the cause of epilepsy, and some drug treatments of epilepsy (anticonvulsants) target the enzymes that regulate GABA production, and therefore increase GABA levels at the synapse.

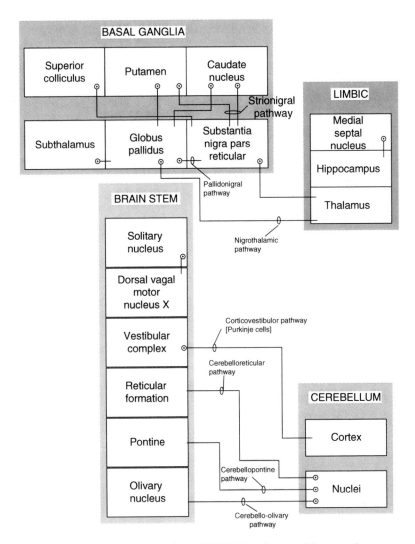

Figure 4.11 The main gamma-aminobutyric acid (GABA) pathways of the central nervous system.

Glutamate receptors

The term 'glutamate receptors' is used for those receptors that bind glutamate, but in reality other excitatory amino acids, such as aspartate, can also bind to and activate the same receptors. *Glutamate (excitatory amino acid) receptors* occur in seven known different classes (Carlson 2012), but only five classes are currently well understood. Each of these five is named after the artificial substance that is used as a ligand to bind to it in laboratory conditions. They are mostly ionotropic excitatory receptors linked to positive ion channels.

The **α-amino-3-hydroxy-5-methyl-4-isoxazoleproprionate (AMPA)** receptors are the most common type of receptor found in the brain. These ionotropic receptors are not specific to any particular positive ion, and they will allow the passage of calcium, potassium, and sodium.

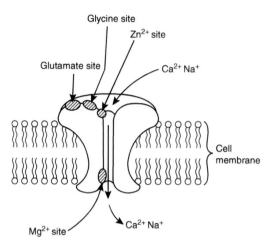

Figure 4.12 The NMDA glutamate receptor. Ca^{2+} is the calcium ion, Na^+ is the sodium ion, Mg^{2+} is the magnesium ion and Zn^{2+} is the zinc ion.

The **kainic acid**, or **kainate (K)** receptor is a nonspecific ion channel receptor allowing the passage of sodium and potassium, and causing depolarisation in the cell when activated. The distribution of K receptors is more limited in the brain than that of AMPA and NMDA receptors, and they have both a pre- and postsynaptic activity.

The ***N*-methyl-*d*-aspartate** (**NMDA**) receptor (Figure 4.12) is the most potent and best-understood of the excitatory amino acid receptors. It is mostly in the cerebral cortex, especially in areas concerned with learning and memory, such as the hippocampus. When inactivated, the ion channel that forms part of the receptor is both closed and blocked by a magnesium (Mg^{2+}) plug on its inner surface. Activation of the receptor requires the binding of both glutamate and glycine, which together cause allosteric changes that open the channel. Removal of the Mg^{2+} plug is achieved by voltage changes across the membrane, occurring when AMPA or K channels are opened farther along on the same membrane. In this way, NMDA receptors function in harmony with other excitatory amino acid receptors. Calcium movement through the open channel causes the biggest depolarisation, with sodium and potassium movements also occurring (Figure 4.12).

The metabotropic glutamate receptors are classified into eight subtypes (labelled $mGluR_{1-8}$) (Carlson 2012). These include the ACPD and the L-AP4 receptors, named after specific drugs that bind to and activate some of these receptors. They exist mostly within the central nervous system on neuronal dendrites, as well as on astrocytes and oligodendrocytes.

GABA receptors

GABA receptors are of two subtypes, **$GABA_A$** and **$GABA_B$**. The $GABA_A$ receptor (Figure 4.13) is ionotropic, where GABA opens a chloride channel in the postsynaptic membrane. When chloride (Cl^-) enters the cell, it hyperpolarises the membrane and therefore prevents action potentials (Figure 4.13). By blocking action potentials in this way, GABA is said to be inhibitory, and therefore reduces the overall activity of the brain. The $GABA_A$ receptor is the site of binding for several important drugs used in psychiatry, the benzodiazepines and the barbiturates, as well as binding alcohol.

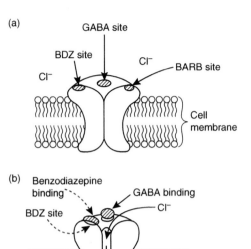

Figure 4.13 The gamma-aminobutyric acid (GABA) inhibitory receptor (GABA$_A$). (a) The closed receptor with no GABA binding. Notice the benzodiazepine (BDZ) and the barbiturate (BARB) binding sites. (b) The open receptor with GABA and benzodiazepine binding. The opening through the cell membrane is a chloride (Cl$^-$) channel.

The GABA$_B$ receptor is metabotropic, causing reduced AC activity and reduced levels of intracellular calcium.

Aspartate and glycine

Aspartate (Figure 4.14) and **glycine** are two nonessential amino acid neurotransmitters, and neurons can synthesise them as required (i.e. they are not directly obtained from the diet). Aspartate is, like glutamate, another excitatory neurotransmitter, acting through the NMDA receptor. Although aspartate is widely distributed throughout the brain, aspartate concentrations are generally weaker than those of glutamate, except in the ventral motor pathways of the spinal cord. Glycine is, like GABA, another mostly inhibitory neurotransmitter. The distribution of glycine in the central nervous system is similar to that of aspartate, being less widely distributed than GABA and somewhat less well concentrated in spinal motor neurons than aspartate.

The peptide neurotransmitters

Peptides are small proteins, and most peptide neurotransmitters are produced from **precursors** – that is, protein gene products from which the final neuropeptide is obtained by

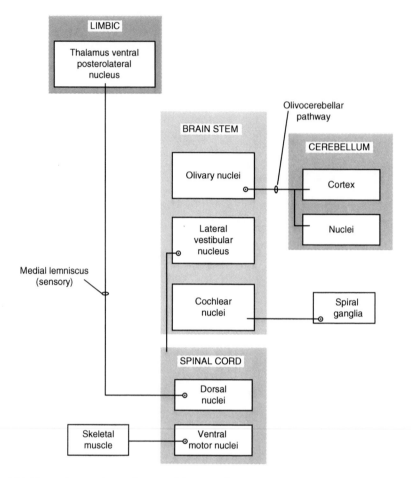

Figure 4.14 The main aspartate pathways of the central nervous system.

enzymatic action. These peptides are often found in both the digestive tract and the brain. In the brain they appear to be concentrated mostly in the hypothalamus. The hypothalamus is known for many functions, one of which is the control of appetite.

Cholecystokinin

Cholecystokinin (CCK) is a peptide found both in the digestive tract (where it regulates emptying of the gall bladder) and in the brain. It is derived from the precursor **procholecystokinin**, which is found in the cerebral cortex and the hypothalamus. A number of different CCKs are produced from this precursor, the best ones studied in the brain being **CCK4** and **CCK8**. Cholecystokinin in the hypothalamus is involved in regulating the inhibition of food intake once the stomach is full (a process called **satiation**), controlled by the **satiety centre** of the hypothalamus. The function of cholecystokinin in the cerebral cortex is less well understood, but is linked to memory, cognition, the mother–infant relationship, and pain threshold regulation. CCK8 is also concentrated in the hippocampus, amygdala, and the spinal cord. It is often found associated with dopaminergic neurons, notably in the nigrostrial pathway and the nucleus accumbens, where it must have a function related to the role of dopamine. Two receptor types are known, CCK_A (mostly found in the digestive tract, less in the brain) and CCK_B (mostly found in the brain, less in the digestive tract). CKK is generating greater interest now because there is evidence linking this neurotransmitter to several mental health disorders, notably anxiety, depression, and psychosis.

Neuropeptide Y

Neuropeptide Y (NPY) is a neurotransmitter known to occur in pathways connecting the **arcuate nucleus** (part of the basal **hypothalamus**) to the lateral hypothalamus. Release of NPY causes an increase in eating, the neurotransmitter itself being a powerful stimulator of food intake. There are two groups of neurons in the lateral hypothalamus activated by NPY: those that secrete **melanin-concentrating hormone (MCH)** and those that secrete **orexin**, both of which are peptides that stimulate appetite and lower body metabolism. As NPY has some control over normal food intake, disturbance of NPY may be related to some eating disorders (see page 190, Chapter 9). Of the five known receptors for NPY, only four (Y_1, Y_2, Y_4, and Y_5) are found in humans. They are metabotropic inhibitory receptors.

Vasoactive intestinal peptide

Vasoactive intestinal peptide (VIP) is a digestive system peptide that is also located in some neurons that use acetylcholine (e.g. the parasympathetic nervous system stimulation of salivary glands), where it potentiates the action of acetylcholine. It would appear that VIP in the brain is likely to have a neuromodulatory role, not causing direct effects itself but modifying the effects of other neurotransmitters. It appears to be active within the **suprachiasmatic nucleus**, a small area of the brain that controls the **circadian rhythms** (the natural daily rhythms of the body), in particular those linked to external light levels, e.g. the sleep–wake cycle (Chapter 16).

Substance P (now called neurokinin-1) and substance K (now called neurokinin A or neurokinin-2)

Neurokinin-1 (Substance P) and **neurokinin-2 (neurokinin A, substance K)** are two peptides derived from the same precursor molecule, the protein **protachykinin**.

Neurokinin-1 was the first neuropeptide discovered. It is the neurotransmitter of the grey matter at the back of the spinal cord (called the **dorsal horn**). Here it functions on the main pain pathways from the periphery to the spinal cord (i.e. the first sensory, or afferent, neuron). In the brain, neurokinin-1 is mostly concentrated in the substantia nigra, where it activates dopaminergic neurons, and in the hypothalamus; it is also found in association with serotonin neurons originating in the raphe nuclei (see Serotonin on page 61). Both neurokinin-1 and -2 bind to **neurokinin (NK) receptors**. Three such receptors are known – NK_1, NK_2, and NK_3 – all of which are metabotropic. Neurokinin-1 may have some influence on mood and thus on depression. Using drugs to block specific neurokinin-1 receptors, particularly NK_1, could therefore become a useful line of treatment in mood disorders (NK_1 is found in brain areas involved in stress and emotions). Neurokinin-2, although isolated and chemically analysed, and with at least one receptor found in the brain, is poorly understood in terms of brain activity.

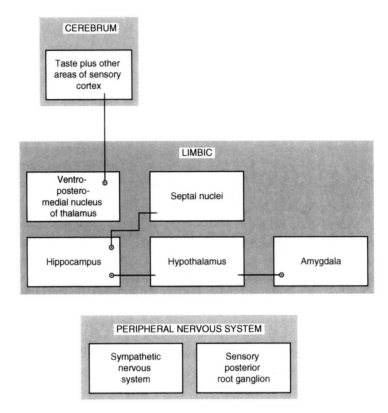

Figure 4.15 The main somatostatin pathways of the central nervous system.

Somatostatin

Somatostatin is a peptide found in various sites within the nervous system, such as the sympathetic nervous system (along with noradrenaline) and the thalamus (along with GABA). It is also present in the dorsal root ganglion of the first (peripheral) sensory neuron, the cerebral cortex, the limbic system, the hippocampus, the hypothalamus, and parts of the brain stem (Figure 4.15). It is also a peptide of the digestive system, where it inhibits the release of several digestion-related hormones. In the brain, somatostatin has a sedatory effect and increases the action of sedatory drugs such as the barbiturates. It appears to reduce the rate of firing of neurons, suppresses motor activity and inhibits the release of growth hormone from the pituitary gland. Several forms of the molecule are known to have activity in humans, notably somatostatin-14, somatostatin-25, and somatostatin-28, where the number represents the amino acid content of the molecule.

Endogenous opioids

The chemistry of the brain involves the production of opiate-like substances called **endogenous opioids**, proteins produced under pain or stress conditions that block pain at either **spinous** (spinal cord) or **supraspinous** (brain stem) levels. Several classes of endogenous opioids are now known. They are all metabotrophic.

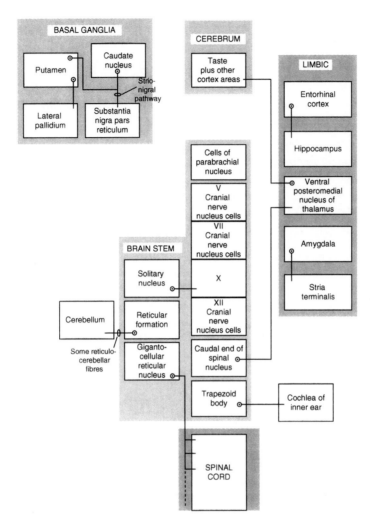

Figure 4.16 The main enkephalin pathways of the central nervous system.

The **enkephalins** (Figure 4.16) are very small peptides (five amino acids long) called **met-enkephalin** and **leu-enkephalin**, which are produced in response to minor pain, having an analgesic effect of about 2 minutes. They are largely found in the basal ganglia, limbic system, brain stem, and upper spinal cord. **Beta-endorphin (β-endorphin)** is a large peptide (31 amino acids long) produced in response to more severe pain with an analgesia effect of around 4 hours or so. It is found in the thalamus, hypothalamus, and brain stem.

The **dynorphins (dynorphin A, dynorphin B,**and others) are intermediate-sized peptides (18 amino acids long), found in the hypothalamus and brain stem, and the **endomorphines (endomorphine-1** and **endomorphine-2)** are both smaller peptides (9 or 10 amino acids long) found in the thalamus, hypothalamus, and basal ganglia. All of these naturally produced chemicals bind to opiate receptors in the upper cord and brain stem called **mu (μ)**, **delta (δ)**, and **kappa (κ)** receptors. Mu receptors may exist in two subtypes, μ_1 and μ_2, a

Table 4.2 The affinity of endogenous opiates for opiate receptors

Endogenous opiate	High affinity	Low affinity	Negligible affinity
Enkephalin	δ	μ	κ
β-Endorphins	μ, δ, κ_2	Other κ	
Dynorphins	κ	μ, δ	
Endomorphine	μ		

distinction based on possible variations that may occur between the mu receptors of the brain stem and the mu receptors of the respiratory centre. Delta and kappa receptors are similarly subdivided, with δ_1, δ_2, δ_{cx}, and δ_{ncx} proposed for delta, and κ_1, κ_2, κ_3 proposed for kappa. The delta receptor subtype d_{cx} is said to form a complex with mu receptors, whilst the δ_{ncx} does not form a complex with any other receptors.

Kappa receptor subtypes κ_1 and κ_2 have become a complex issue, with other further subdivisions of each subtype proposed. Research will continue in this area, mainly because of the devastating problems caused by heroin and other opiate addictions and the need to find a solution to this problem. The dynorphin receptors, for example, are somehow involved specifically in cocaine addiction. This work will eventually identify and classify many more subtypes of the opiate receptors with a view to finding antagonist drugs that will prevent the addictive opiate drugs from binding. The affinity of the endogenous opiates for the various opiate receptors, where this has been established, is shown in Table 4.2.

Nociceptin is a member of the endogenous opioid group that binds to its own specific receptor, called the **NOP receptor**, but does not bind well to the other opioid receptors. Therefore, the **nociception system** is often regarded as a separate system to the other opioids. NOP receptors are found widely throughout the brain and spinal cord. Nociceptin is an anti-analgesic, i.e. it increases pain perception by blocking the action of opioids. However, this may be useful in the future as a means of blocking the action of the opioid drugs taken during drug abuse (see Chapter 8). Drugs specifically designed to bind to the NOP receptor are currently under development. Nociceptin also dampens stress and anxiety (an anxiolytic effect) and helps to protect against the physical effects of stress (see Chapter 9). However, nociceptin also appears to have the less desirable effects of prolonging depression (see Chapter 11). And the role of nociception goes beyond that of the brain, as it appears to affect the regulation of the cardiovascular, renal, and immune systems.

Other neurotransmitters

Acetylcholine

Acetylcholine (ACh) is one of the earliest known synaptic ligands. Its production requires the enzyme **choline acetyltransferase (ChAT)**, which uses **choline** derived immediately from the extracellular fluid around the neuron and transfers to it an **acetyl group** to form ACh (Figure 4.17). Choline from dietary sources must be delivered to the brain by the blood, and therefore the supply of choline determines the amount of ACh that can be produced. Only **cholinergic** neurons (i.e. those that respond to ACh) contain ChAT and are therefore capable of producing ACh. These include **lower motor neurons (LMNs)** that use ACh at the **neuromuscular junction** (i.e. synapses between LMNs and muscle cells). ACh is produced in the neuronal cell body and moved to the synapse by axoplasmic transportation.

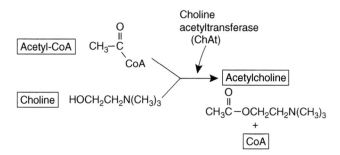

Figure 4.17 The synthesis of acetylcholine. The names of the products are in boxes with their chemical structure shown. The only enzyme (unboxed) labels the arrow.

After release into the synapse and binding to receptors, ACh is broken down while still within the cleft by another enzyme, **acetylcholinesterase (AChE)**. This releases the choline again from the molecule and much of this choline is returned to the presynaptic bulb and reused. The remaining **acetic acid** is excreted.

In the brain, acetylcholine is concentrated in the corpus striatum, with some found in the cerebrum, the nucleus accumbens, the limbic system including the hippocampus, and parts of the brain stem, especially some of the cranial nerve nuclei (Figure 4.18).

Cholinergic receptors

Cholinergic receptors, i.e. those that bind acetylcholine, occur in two forms, **nicotinic** and **muscarinic**. Muscarine and nicotine are plant alkaloids that bind to the respective receptor *under laboratory conditions*, and are therefore used to distinguish one receptor from the other. Obviously, *plant* alkaloids are not natural ligands of these receptors in the brain, they are just used to distinguish one receptor type from another. The nicotinic (N) receptor is ionotropic, causing the *direct* opening of membrane channels used by a range of cations, mostly sodium (Na^+) and calcium (Ca^{2+}). Nicotinic receptors are found mostly within the spinal cord, in the autonomic nervous system (ANS) and at the neuromuscular junction, but are less commonly found in the brain. Subtypes of nicotinic receptors are the N-m (muscle type), found at the neuromuscular junction, and the N-n (neuronal type), found at the ganglion synapse of the ANS.

The muscarinic (M) receptors are metabotropic; they regulate potassium ion channels *indirectly* by first affecting the secondary messenger **cAMP**, and this in turn affects the ion channels. The subtypes of muscarinic receptors are M_1, M_2, M_3, M_4, and M_5. The functions of these subtypes vary, but they generally cause excitation in the postsynaptic membrane. They are more common than nicotinic receptors in the brain, occurring both as postsynaptic and autoreceptors.

Histamine

Histamine is known as a chemical agent outside the brain that induces inflammation when released from storage in mast cells or platelets. It is synthesised from the dietary amino acid **histidine** using the enzyme **histidine decarboxylase**, which requires **vitamin B$_6$ (pyroxidine)** to function. Histamine is also known as a neurotransmitter in the brain, but because it cannot cross the blood–brain barrier from the body to the brain, histamine must be synthesised

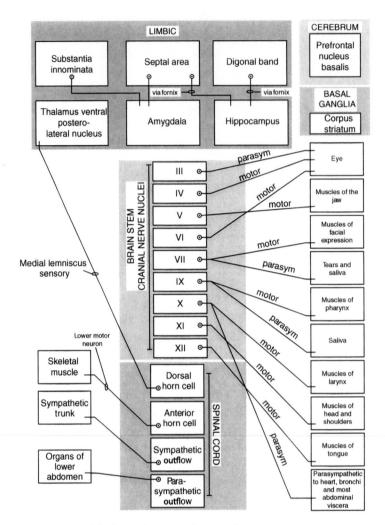

Figure 4.18 The main acetylcholine pathways of the central nervous system.

within the brain. The hypothalamus has the greatest concentration of histidine decarboxylase found in the brain. Since the amino acid histidine can cross the blood–brain barrier, histamine can be produced in areas of the brain that have this enzyme, particularly the hypothalamus. Histamine is also found in a pathway extending from the brain stem to the cerebral cortex via the *median forebrain bundle* and in the hippocampus (Figure 4.19). Histamine is involved in the brain's control of alertness, part of the sleep–wake cycle, and in the mechanisms that regulate nausea and vomiting in the brain stem.

Histamine receptors

Histamine receptors are of four known classes, H_1, H_2, H_3, and H_4. They are all metabotropic and some are found in brain tissue. The H_1 receptor is found in both the brain stem and

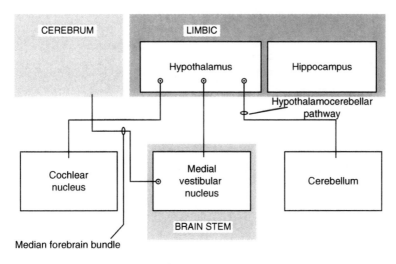

Figure 4.19 The main histamine pathways of the central nervous system.

cerebral cortex, the two areas linked by the histaminergic *median forebrain bundle* mentioned above. Because of histamine's role in the control of alertness of the cerebrum, antihistamines (or H_1 antagonists), which are able to cross the blood–brain barrier, can cause drowsiness as a side effect. The H_1 receptor is also involved in regulation of circadian rhythms. H_2 receptors are found largely outside the brain on hydrochloric acid (HCl)-producing cells of the stomach wall, where the binding of histamine increases HCl production. In the brain, H_2 receptors are found in the same sites as H_1. H_3 receptors are found in the brain as a presynaptic autoreceptor on histaminergic neurons, allowing feedback to the presynaptic bulb to inhibit histamine release. H_4 is not involved in brain activity but controls histamine release from mast cells.

Key points

Neurotransmitters and receptors

- Neurotransmitters are the chemical agents released from the presynaptic bulb into the synaptic cleft.
- Most neurotransmitters fall into three main groups: amines, amino acids, and peptides.
- The same neurotransmitter is often seen to produce different effects by binding to different receptors.
- Some receptors are postsynaptic, part of the *postsynaptic* membrane; others are autoreceptors on the *presynaptic* membranes or other parts of the neuron.
- Autoreceptors are thought to provide feedback information to the presynaptic bulb to regulate further neurotransmitter release.
- Some receptors are ionotropic; they control the opening or closing of a particular ion channel.
- Other receptors, described as metabotropic, cause changes in the metabolism of the postsynaptic cell.

Amine neurotransmitters

- Dopaminergic neurons and receptors are found in the basal ganglia (the nigrostriatal pathway) and the limbic system (mesolimbic pathway), and are involved in mental health symptoms and drug treatments.
- Serotonergic and adrenergic neurons and receptors are found in the diffuse modulatory pathways of the brain stem, and are involved in the cause and drug treatment of mood disorders.

Amino acid neurotransmitters

- Gamma-amino butyric acid (GABA) is an important inhibitory neurotransmitter, which is partly implicated in epilepsy.
- Enzymes that control GABA levels are targets for some anticonvulsant drugs.
- The GABA$_A$ receptor is a major site for the action of some drugs used in psychiatry.

References

Blows, W. T. (2000) Neurotransmitters of the brain: serotonin, noradrenaline (norepinephrine) and dopamine. *Journal of Neuroscience Nursing*, **32** (4): 234–238.

Carlson, N. R. (2012) *Physiology of Behaviour* (11th edition). Pearson Education, Harlow, UK.

Marieb, E. N. and Hoehn, K. N. (2014) *Human Anatomy and Physiology* (9th edition). Pearson Education, Harlow, UK.

Nolen-Heoksema, S. (2007) *Abnormal Psychology*. McGraw-Hill, Boston, MA.

5 Hormones and behaviour

- Introduction: hormones, form and function
- The pituitary hormones
- The thyroid hormones
- Hormones from the adrenal cortex
- Hormones from the adrenal medulla
- Sex hormones and the differences between male and female brains
- Behaviour
- Key points

Introduction: hormones, form and function

Hormones are chemical messengers: they move from one part of the body to another in the blood and have an effect, often stimulatory, on a *target* organ or tissue. The brain is the target organ for a range of hormones that have influence over neuronal growth and development as well as function.

Hormones are the products of **endocrine glands**, which are glands that secrete their products directly into the blood. Hormones are of two basic types, the protein hormones (the **peptides**) and the lipid (or fat-based) hormones (the **steroids**). In order to work, a hormone must first bind to a receptor site that is associated with the target cell. Cells without receptors for a specific hormone are not targets for that hormone. Peptide hormones are too large to penetrate the cell membrane and must therefore bind to receptors on the cell surface. Steroid hormones can pass through the membrane and bind with receptors within the cell cytoplasm or the nucleus (Figure 5.1). Receptors for hormones, like those for neurotransmitters, are usually proteins, coded by and synthesised from gene sequences within the target cell **deoxyribonucleic acid (DNA)**. DNA is the molecule housed inside the nucleus of most cells and forms the genes, the blueprints on which all cellular proteins and other characteristics are based. Cells therefore have the ability to increase (upregulate) or decrease (downregulate) their receptor numbers by activating or deactivating the appropriate genes. This affects the sensitivity of that cell to the effects of the hormone, as upregulation binds more hormone and downregulation binds less hormone.

On binding to the receptor, the hormone–receptor complex effects changes within the cell, usually by binding to a **gene promoter** sequence on the DNA and initiating transcription of the gene (Figure 5.2). **Gene transcription** involves the assembly of an **RNA (ribonucleic acid)**

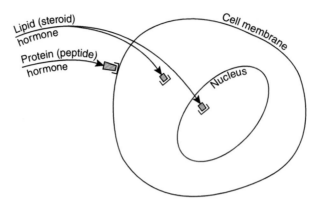

Figure 5.1 Hormones and receptors. Protein (peptide) hormones are too large to enter the cell, so they bind to surface receptors. Lipid (steroid) hormones are smaller and so they can enter the cell and bind to receptors inside the cytoplasm or nucleus.

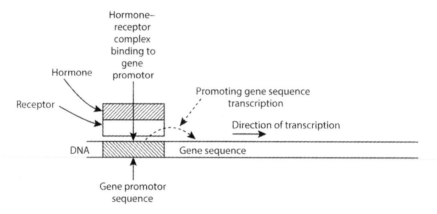

Figure 5.2 The complex of hormone and receptor affects gene transcription by interacting with the gene promotor sequence of the deoxyribonucleic acid (DNA).

molecule, the first step in protein synthesis. In this way hormones arriving at the cell trigger a wave of protein synthesis, which will alter in some way the activity of that cell. In neurons this change in activity is likely to influence the response of the cell to action potentials or to neuro-transmitters, or alter the cell's metabolism in some way.

As the functional component of the endocrine system, hormones are regulated by **feed-back mechanisms** that influence their production and release from the gland. This feedback is mostly of the **negative** kind, i.e. a rise in the hormone levels in the blood causes the produc-tion and release of the hormone to fall. The opposite is also true: low blood hormone levels allow greater production and release of the hormone. In this way, a stable blood level should be achieved. Such feedback mechanisms are a part of general **homeostasis** by which the body maintains a stable internal environment that promotes optimum function of its organs. Homeostasis is critical in many areas such as temperature control, and electrolyte, fluid, and acid–base balance. Many observations are carried out on patients in order to monitor the function and effectiveness of specific homeostatic mechanisms: observations such as recording the pulse rate, blood pressure, and temperature (Blows 2012). Homeostasis operates through the two major communication systems of the body, the endocrine and nervous systems. Close collaboration between these two systems is responsible for regulating most of the functions of the cells and tissues through a wide variety of situations, a collaboration known as the **neuroendocrine response**. Disturbance of homeostasis causes biochemical and other imbalances, which seriously upset the normal functioning of various organs, not least the brain. Some disorders of homeostasis involving hormones can cause mental symptoms for which the hormonal levels of the blood require investigation.

The pituitary hormones

The pituitary hormones were listed in Chapter 1 because they are subject to hypothalamic control.

Some disorders of the pituitary gland can disrupt the function of other endocrine glands, and the resulting change in hormonal levels can cause mental symptoms. Important examples of this are changes in **thyroid-stimulating hormone (TSH)**, which controls levels of thyroid hormone in the blood, and in **adrenocorticotropic hormone (ACTH)**, which influences adrenal cortex function by stimulating cortisol production (Figure 5.3).

The thyroid hormones

The thyroid hormones are produced by the thyroid gland, which is situated in the neck, on top of the trachea and below the larynx. Hormones from this gland occur in two forms,

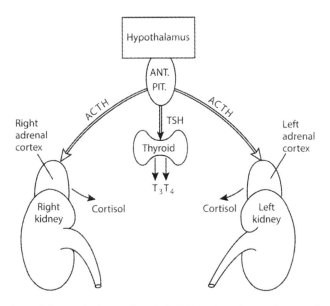

Figure 5.3 The hypothalamo–pituitary–adrenal (HPA) axis, where adrenocorticotropic hormone (ACTH) from the anterior pituitary stimulates cortisol production. The hypothalamo–pituitary–thyroid (HPT) axis, where thyroid-stimulating hormone (TSH) stimulates the release of the thyroid hormones T_3 and T_4.

triiodothyronine (T$_3$) and **tetraiodothyronine (T$_4$)** (Figure 5.3). **Iodine** is a major component of these thyroid hormones and the two forms have three and four atoms of iodine per molecule, respectively. Production of T$_3$ and T$_4$ is dependent on the levels of **thyroid-stimulating hormone (TSH)** produced by the pituitary gland. T$_3$ and T$_4$ are essential for the growth, development, and metabolic function of many tissues, especially the brain.

In normal tissues, these hormones maintain a normal metabolic rate, but changes in mental function appear if the levels of thyroid hormone are too low or too high. Disorders of thyroid level may be *primary* (i.e. affecting the gland itself), or *secondary* (i.e. caused by abnormal changes in TSH level from the anterior pituitary gland). Blood tests for T$_3$\T$_4$ plus TSH levels will indicate which is the problem.

Hypothyroidism, in which the blood level of thyroid hormone is too low, is sometimes called **myxedema**. It is most common in females over the age of 40 years. Failure to produce enough of this hormone can result in a number of symptoms that could be misinterpreted as a true mental disorder. Patients with myxedema suffer lethargy, depression, personality changes, and psychotic episodes known as **myxedema psychosis** or *myxedema madness*. This is manifested as paranoia, hallucinations, and delirium.

Hypothyroid disorders are occasionally associated with depressive mood disorders and about 10% of depressed patients with lethargy are also hypothyroid. Thyroid hormone treatment is sometimes used in addition to antidepressant drugs to improve the patient's response to the antidepressant therapy. Such a combination is sometimes used in those patients who quickly rotate between the depressed and manic phases of bipolar depression. The mood stabilising drug lithium can predispose to hypothyroid states, especially if used for long-term therapy, and therefore monitoring of thyroid function during lithium treatment is important to avoid complications. Neonatal hypothyroidism puts the newly born infant at risk of developmental brain function failure, known as **cretinism**, a serious problem that can be corrected if recognised from birth and treated with thyroid hormone.

Hyperthyroidism is the production of excess thyroid hormone by the thyroid gland. **Thyrotoxicosis** is an umbrella term incorporating a number of disorders involving high thyroid levels. It refers to the release of excess hormone into the blood at very high toxic levels. In these disorders the patient may show a degree of anxiety, agitation, and delirium, with nervous excitability, irritability, insomnia, and other psychotic manifestations, largely due to the thyroid hormone causing excessive overactivity of the sympathetic nervous system. If the hormone excess is severe, memory loss and disorientation can occur, with manic excitability, delusions, and hallucinations. Stress seems to be a causative factor, theoretically due to excessive use of the endocrine system during childhood trauma (e.g. loss of parents, economic hardship, rivalry with siblings) (Sadock et al. 2009). It becomes important, therefore, for all patients suffering from 'anxiety' to have their blood thyroid hormone and TSH levels measured to exclude a thyroid problem, especially if they show physical symptoms such as a goitre (swelling of the thyroid gland in the throat) or exophthalmus (protruding eyes) as seen in the thyrotoxic disorder called **Grave's disease**.

Hormones from the adrenal cortex

The adrenal glands, situated on top of the kidneys, have an *outer* **cortex** and an *inner* **medulla**. The cortex produces several steroidal hormones based on cholesterol derived from the blood (Figure 5.4). There are several hormonal groups produced by the cortex, including the **mineralocorticoids** (those hormones active on minerals), the **glucocorticoids** (those hormones

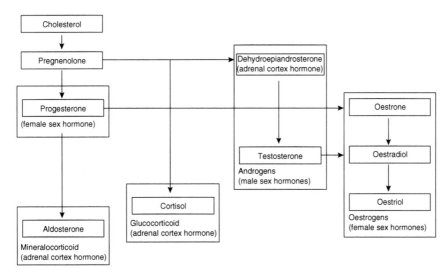

Figure 5.4 Flow diagram of the production of various steroidal (lipid-based) hormones from cholesterol in the adrenal cortex, including cortisol, aldosterone, the female oestrogens, and the
male androgens.

influencing blood glucose levels), and the sex hormones for males (**androgens**) and females
(**oestrogens**) (Figure 5.4).

Cortisol is a glucocorticoid, the production of which is stimulated by ACTH from the
anterior pituitary gland. Cortisol has several functions, notably raising the blood glucose
level by its anti-insulin effects, and it helps to protect cells against the adverse effects of
stress. Excess cortisol occurs in the disorder Cushing's syndrome or as a result of prolonged
corticosteroid drug treatment. Treatment by drugs is of course a medical activity, and when
the action of doctors or nurses causes disease it is described as iatrogenic, i.e. disease caused
by medical intervention. Iatrogenic disorders should be avoided as much as possible, but
some iatrogenic problems are unavoidable. In the case of disorders caused by drugs, this can
be avoided or reduced by adjusting the dose level.

Cushing's syndrome occurs more often in women than in men and causes a similar state
to that of bipolar depression (Breedlove et al. 2010), with insomnia, loss of emotions and
energy, and attempted suicide in about 10% of untreated patients. Alternatively, the patient's
mood may swing into euphoria, agitation, mania, and delirium, with psychotic symptoms
such as hallucinations. Depression may also follow withdrawal from long-term steroid
therapy, this being one of several reasons for a keeping the period of steroid treatment as
short as possible and reducing the dose gradually rather than a sudden reduction of dosage.
Some women with Cushing's syndrome may show a degree of **masculinisation**, growing
unwanted hair and losing their menstrual periods (**amenorrhoea**), and this can add to their
depression. Men with this condition can become impotent and lose their hair.

Addison's disease is an insufficiency in cortisol production from the adrenal cortex. Lack of cortisol results in the patient becoming tired, lethargic, and depressed and
sometimes showing psychotic symptoms. This person may also develop delirium and confusion. Generally the mental symptoms are milder that those seen in Cushing's syndrome.

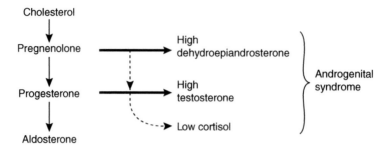

Figure 5.5 Adrenogenital syndrome, caused by excessive androgens (testosterone and dehydroepian-drosterone) in conjunction with low cortisol.

The problem may not reside in the adrenal gland itself but could be a failure of adreno-corticotropic hormone (ACTH) from the pituitary gland. Treatment with corticosteroid supplements is essential for life.

Production of cortisol is also severely reduced in a condition called **adrenogenital syndrome** (Figure 5.5). The poor secretion of cortisol can be caused by low activity of either of the enzymes **21-hydroxylase** or **11β-hydroxylase**, both of which are essential for the metabolic pathway that leads to cortisol (Figure 5.4). The loss of these enzymes is a **con-genital** defect – that is, the person is born with the enzyme error, the consequences of which are a corresponding increase in the synthesis of androgens. In the female fetus this causes Addison's disease, the excess androgens having a masculinising effect at the same time. The 'girl', while being genetically female, develops male-like external genitalia, making gender difficult to determine **(pseudohermaphroditism)**. The excess testosterone produced may also have a masculinising effect on the girl's brain, causing a mental conflict of identity or 'self'. In a male fetus with this condition, the Addison's disease is accompanied by advanced sexual development, i.e. puberty, at an early age.

A similar condition, **adrenogenitalism** (Figure 5.6), occurs in the fetus when the pituitary gland produces too much ACTH. The excessive stimulation of the adrenal cortex results in

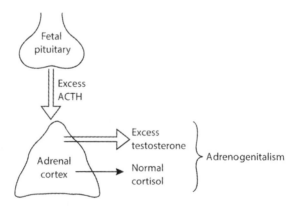

Figure 5.6 Adrenogenitalism, caused by excessive ACTH driving testosterone production to excess, while cortisol remains normal.

higher than normal production of testosterone, the main male androgen. Cortisol production in this situation remains normal, because all the enzymes involved in the steroid hormone pathways are functioning. The stimulation of the cortex causes **hyperplasia** (excessive cellular growth) within the cortex of the gland. This is an **autosomal recessive** disorder, again causing masculinisation of the female fetus (pseudohermaphroditism) with male-like external genitalia. The male fetus with this condition has excessive sexual development, except for smaller-than-average testes, which remain underdeveloped owing to the negative feedback from the high adrenal testosterone. Testosterone stimulates growth, so androgenital children of both sexes are generally taller than their peers, but as bone growth is stopped prematurely they are therefore shorter than average as adults. The mental effect is again one of conflict concerning sexual identity and this may need to be addressed by both physical and psychological treatment.

Hormones from the adrenal medulla

The hormones produced by the adrenal medulla are the **catecholamines**, adrenaline and noradrenaline (epinephrine and norepinephrine). Adrenaline has sympathomimetic activity – that is, it increases the functions of the sympathetic nervous system (Figure 5.7). The physical symptoms of excessive stimulation of the sympathetic nervous system include an increase in the heart rate, sweating, tremor, and insomnia. The mental symptoms include apprehension, or even fear, leading to panic, all of which give a clinical picture of anxiety attacks. Differentiation between excessive catecholamine production and true anxiety may be achieved by measuring the blood adrenaline levels, although anxiety itself may cause increased release of this hormone. A rare cause of high levels of adrenaline in the blood is an adrenaline-producing tumour of the medulla called a **pheochromocytoma**.

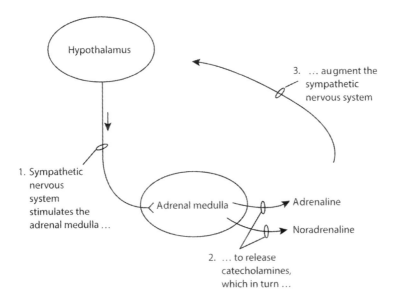

Figure 5.7 The sympathetic nervous system, controlled by the hypothalamus, can increase the production of catecholamines (adrenaline and noradrenaline) from the adrenal medulla. These, in turn, augment the sympathetic nervous system.

Sex hormones and the differences between male and female brains

The **oestrogens** and **androgens** are the sex hormone groups for females and males respectively. There are three oestrogen hormones and several androgen hormones. The female oestrogens are **oestradiol, oestrone**, and **oestriol**. The male androgens are mainly **testosterone** and **dehydroepiandrosterone (DHEA)**. However, besides testosterone, other androgens include **androstenedione, androstenediol**, and **androsterone** (Figure 5.4). Oestradiol is the most potent of the oestrogens, whereas testosterone is the most potent of the androgens. They are all synthesised from **cholesterol** via a pathway that includes the production of the other steroidal hormones, **cortisol, progesterone**, and **aldosterone** (Figure 5.4). Following puberty, the female ovary produces most of the oestrogen, and the male testes produce most of the testosterone. However, in addition, trace quantities of both the oestrogens and the androgens are produced and released from the **adrenal cortex** in both sexes. Females produce small quantities of androgens and males produce small quantities of oestrogens. This is a vestige of the past life of the growing fetus, when the adrenal cortex was the only producer of these substances. Both these hormonal groups have a multitude of target tissues and organs around the body, including the brain, where they have a profound influence on functional and sexual organisation. A lack of testosterone, supported by oestrogen, influences a 'feminine' brain, while testosterone forms a 'masculine' brain. It is important to note that these hormonal organisational effects happen at very precise and critical moments in fetal brain development. After this critical point the hormonal influence over the brain is of a different nature; that of influencing behavioural patterns, in particular sexual behaviour, and mood. High levels of testosterone are known to influence aggression in males, whereas oestrogen reduces aggression.

Low levels of testosterone appear to result from stress and are linked to nervousness, bad temper, and depressed moods in men (the **irritable male syndrome**) (Nowak 2002). Postmenopausal loss of oestrogen in women can lead to anxiety, loss of confidence, forgetfulness, and even depression.

Male and female brain

Hormones, mostly the androgens and oestrogens but others too, influence from before birth the sexual differences that are noted between male and female brains. The environment also has a massive impact on the way that gender variations in the brain are moulded throughout childhood (see also Chapter 2) (Eliot 2010). The physical differences in the brain are generally small. Males have larger brains than their female peers throughout all the stages of life, and female brains reach full development earlier than male brains. However, this has no bearing on intelligence or cognitive abilities.

The hypothalamus is involved in sexual behaviour and perinatal exposure to androgens in the male was thought to cause a larger **preoptic region** of the hypothalamus than in females, i.e. the anterior hypothalamus having significant **sexual dimorphism** (dimorphism = *two shapes*, two different shapes between the sexes). However, a new study (Tan et al. 2015) has created significant doubt about this, and there now appears to be no hypothalamic difference between the sexes. The preoptic region was called the **sexually dimorphic nucleus**, but this may now change. Structural variations are achieved through exposure to sex hormones before, during, and after birth.

While male brains are physically larger than female brains, women have a greater concentration of grey matter cells (neurons) in the areas concerned with communication. Out of the

Table 5.1 Sex differences in the brain in terms of task performance. The differences found are usually very small

Male-orientated brain (skills at which males are better than females)	Female-orientated brain (skills at which females are better than males)
• Spatial tasks, especially rotational skills • Mathematical reasoning • Navigational skills (e.g. map reading) • Target-directed skills, such as guiding or intercepting projectiles (e.g. dart throwing)	• Perceptual speed, i.e. rapid identification of matching items • Arithmetical calculations • Precision manual skills (e.g. embroidery) • Verbal fluency • Recall of landmarks along a route

six layers of cells, two of the layers show more neurons per unit volume in females than in males. These areas are the **dorsolateral prefrontal cortex** (involved in memory and initiative: 23% more cells) and the **superior temporal gyrus** (involved in listening: 13% more cells). The female brain has more volume in the **frontal lobes** and the **limbic association cortex** (linked to emotional areas), while male brains show greater volume in the **parietal lobe** (special perception). Male brains show a larger **amygdala** and a greater degree of **lateralisation** than those of females. Lateralisation is designating one hemisphere for a task rather than both. On a day-to-day basis this makes no difference, but it could be a handicap in circumstances in which the designated hemisphere becomes damaged. In this situation in males the task is often lost altogether, whereas females can switch to the other hemisphere. A typical example is damage to the speech centre in the left hemisphere, where **aphasia** (loss of speech) occurs four times more often in males (who cannot switch to the right side) than in females (who can often make the switch). Lateralisation does not necessarily make the performance of a skill any better or worse. In female brains there is increased overlap between the hemisphere functions for the verbal skills and women do better in these skills than men. There are also other physical differences in the brain between the sexes, the significance of which, if any, is not entirely understood:

• The female posterior **corpus callosum** (connecting the left hemisphere with the right hemisphere) is bulbous and wide compared with that in the male, which is cylindrical and uniform in width throughout its length. In fact, the male brain is said to be more connected front to back within the hemispheres, and the female brain more connected side to side between the two hemispheres. There is little significance attached to this, other than small increases in perception and action in males, and small increases in analytical process in females. The differences are small because both sexes have some degree of both lateral and front to back connections, and these connections can change throughout life.

• The female brain is more tightly packed with grey matter, especially in the speech areas of the temporal lobe.

• The amygdala responds differently to emotional situations between the sexes, with males using largely the right side of the amygdala, and women the left side. This results in men remembering the overall emotional event, while women can recall more details. Results such as this could have implications for the treatment of post-traumatic stress disorder (PTSD; see Chapter 9).

- Male brains have, on average, 52% higher production of serotonin (Chapter 4), and this may be one reason why women are more prone to depression than men (Chapter 11).
- Female brains may also be affected by oestrogen in a surprising way: the hormone may be boosting dopamine levels in the brain areas involved in drug abuse (Chapter 8). This may be the reason why women progress to full drug dependence more often than males do.

This topic is subject to significant research, and the picture of brain differences is likely to change, or even become irrelevant. Already one study has indicated that only about 10% of human brains show typical male features, and another 10% show typical female features. The remaining 80% have a mix of both features in varying degrees, so the picture is not clear-cut, and the concept of male and female brains may already be redundant (Joel et al. 2016).

Behaviour

Many aspects of life have some control or influence over behaviour, and the role of biology is now recognised as a major factor in the way we behave. Behaviourists are scientists that identify a particular behaviour that is of interest, or of social significance (e.g. drug abuse) and try to find causes. Physiologists and geneticists investigate the biology of specific behaviours.

The brain is the governing organ that determines our behaviour, and this is influenced strongly by developmental aspects (especially environmental stimuli), hormones (some aspects of hormonal influence on behaviour have already been looked at in this chapter) and genes.

Genes do not directly determine behaviour. Their role is to code for many varied proteins, which are components of much of the body's structure and metabolism. Genes in the brain code for a large number of different protein receptors that bind hormones and neurotransmitters, and changing these receptors has significant influence on brain function, especially behaviour. A good example is a variation of a gene that codes for a dopamine D_2 receptor called the **A1 allele**, associated with one specific behavioural pattern, alcoholism. The behaviour patterns of alcoholism and drug abuse are examined in more detail in Chapter 8.

Developmental aspects have been discussed in Chapter 2, where we saw that the influence of **environmental factors** moulds the mind. For example, consider a child and its mother, who are playing on the floor when a spider runs from under the chair. The child's mother is scared of spiders and climbs on a chair screaming. The older child may infer from this that the correct response to a spider is to climb on a chair and scream. This is called **learnt behaviour**, where children learn how to behave in various situations by copying from example. Children and adults both learn aspects of behaviour from good or bad experiences. A child knocked over in a park by a large dog may, as a result, fear dogs for life, and adjust their behaviour to avoid them. The opposite is also true, as in drug addiction, where initial exposure to drugs may lead to further drug-seeking behaviour. As seen in Chapter 2, both good and bad experiences, especially in early life, has profound good or bad influences on both brain development and future behaviour. When considering both ends of the behavioural spectrum, i.e. good and bad, both charitable and criminal activities can be seen to be influenced by learnt behaviours.

Aggression

As seen earlier in this chapter, exposure of the fetus to androgens such as testosterone causes masculinisation of the brain (prenatal androgenisation). However, the highest testosterone levels in males occur between the ages of 16 and 30 years, peaking around 25 years of age. Testosterone has been described as the fuel that drives a number of behaviour patterns, especially aggression. **Innate drives** are those motivating forces that are built in from birth, i.e. those from within, and testosterone fulfils that criterion in relation to aggression. Evidence has linked violent crime with high testosterone levels. At puberty, exposure to high levels of testosterone causes males to increase their aggressive tendencies, including sexual aggression. Apart from this innate drive, other theories of aggression include: (1) the frustration model, where a frustrated need leads to aggression to satisfy that need; and (2) aggression as a learnt behaviour. There is probably some degree of all these theories in any act of aggression.

The three types of aggression are:

1   **offence**, where aggression is used against another person, often without provocation;
2   **defence**, where aggression is used as protection against offence;
3   **predation**, where aggression is used to gain something. In the animal world this is used to gain food (e.g. the lion attacks a gazelle), but in the human world predation is used mostly to gain money or goods (e.g. theft and mugging) or other needs (e.g. rape).

Aggression is also strongly linked to the levels of serotonin in the brain. Evidence indicates that serotonin has a calming (inhibitory) effect on an individual, reducing impulsive behaviour in particular, and therefore aggression is linked to low levels of serotonin. Reduced levels of serotonin correlate particularly well with aggression to oneself (i.e. suicide) and with impulsive aggression towards others. Corresponding changes in serotonin receptors, consistent with serotonin receptor structural abnormalities, have been found in the frontal lobes of those committing violent suicide. Such receptor changes reduce the effectiveness of the serotonin present. The poor function of the serotonin system may be due to an error in the gene that codes for **tryptophan hydroxylase**, a key enzyme in the synthesis of serotonin.

Another neurotransmitter involved is dopamine. Both serotonin and dopamine are destroyed after use by an enzyme called **monamine oxidase A (MAO-A)**, and mutated versions of this gene (a mutation sometimes called the '**warrior gene**') appear to be predisposing individuals to violent crime and gang membership, especially when combined with a history of maltreatment as a child (see Chapter 2). The warrior gene mutation causes underactivity of the gene, resulting in a lack of the enzyme required to break down the dopamine, which then rises in quantity (a '**dopamine hyperactivity**'). *MAO-A* is a gene on the X chromosome, and this means that males have only one X chromosome, i.e. one version of this gene, whereas females have two X chromosomes (two versions of the gene) (see Chapter 6). It would be very unlucky for a female to have this mutation in both copies of the gene, so they most likely have one normal gene. Male carriers of the 'warrior gene' mutation of MAOA have no normal version available, and this means that, driven by high dopamine levels, they are more likely to join gangs and perhaps carry a weapon. It should be pointed out that this applies mostly in provocative situations, indicating that aggression is a combination of factors, not just biological, and that the environmental situation is a major factor.

Another gene mutation that could be involved in aggression is the *CDH13* (**cadherin 13**) gene, the normal version being involved in the control of impulsive behaviour. Mutations of the gene may be responsible for a loss of this control.

The areas of the brain involved in aggression are also becoming apparent (Figure 5.8). The effect of androgens on aggression between males appears to be mediated through part of the hypothalamus called the preoptic area. Androgens early in life (prenatal testosterone in males) appear to organise and sensitise this and other areas of the brain involved in aggression later in life. Testosterone later in life (pubertal testosterone, again in males) appears to activate these same areas. Offensive aggression appears to be mediated through the **ventral tegmental area (VTA)** in the brain stem, while different parts of the **periaqueductal grey (PAG)** are associated with defensive and predatory aggression. These areas are themselves moderated by inputs from the hypothalamus, the septum and the amygdala (Figure 5.8). Examples of this are defensive and predatory aggression. Defensive aggression can be activated by stimulation of the medial hypothalamus, whereas predatory aggression can be activated by stimulation of the lateral hypothalamus. The frontal lobe inhibits impulsive behaviour, including aggression to some extent, but this is reduced during puberty (see Chapter 2).

While testosterone is significantly lower in females than in males, some women receive exposure to higher levels than others, and the women thus exposed, either as a fetus or later in life, show increased aggressive tendencies towards others. Excessive alcohol often induces higher levels of testosterone in women, which the female brain is not used to, and they therefore misbehave in public, often aggressively, as a result.

Pregnant women with higher testosterone levels than average are more likely to have daughters described as 'tomboys', i.e. interested in male-orientated, rather than female-orientated lifestyle. The opposite also appears to be true, with higher-oestrogen mothers having daughters with very feminine ways. Clearly the child is being influenced by the tera-togenic effect of the mother's hormone, and in the case of testosterone this organises and sensitises pathways involved in aggression.

Oestradiol, the main female oestrogen, causes a reduction in aggression and a general calming effect on the brain. It is possible that hormonal shifts that result in a lowering of oestradiol just prior to menstruation may have some bearing on the premenstrual syndrome, a state of irritability and increased aggression that occurs a few days before a menstrual period.

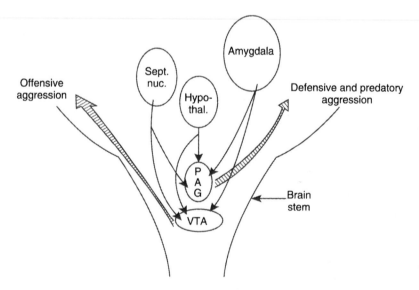

Figure 5.8 Aggression. Inputs from the septal nucleus (Sept. nuc.) and amygdala to the periaqueductal grey (PAG) cause defensive and predatory aggression; inputs to the ventral tegmental area (VTA) cause offensive aggression.

A neurotransmitter called **arginine-vasopressin (AVP)**, which is active in the amygdala, helps to regulate maternal aggression, a behavioural pattern aimed at making sure the child survives. Stress is also directly related to aggression, as violence is a very stressful social experience for both the aggressor and the victim. Brain neurotransmitters and immune cytokines change alarmingly during stress, and this increases vulnerability to depression and immune-related disorders. Couples in a relationship may react to stress in a manner in which the woman may display relational aggression towards their partner. This involves less belligerent aggressive attacks, such as social manipulation, spreading rumors and gossip, refusing to speak to their partners, damaging their property, and other such activities (Lilienfeld and Arkowitz 2010).

Antisocial and criminal behaviour

Murder, especially *serial murder*, is a form of offensive aggression that has also sparked a great deal of interest. Neuroscientists want to be able to answer the question: *What goes on inside a serial killer's mind?* Now some answers are coming to light. Murderers appear to lack the level of **prefrontal lobe** activity seen in law-abiding subjects. In the absence of adequate prefrontal lobe activity, the emotions are unmodified in any way by conscious reasoning. Some work carried out on male murderers has shown an actual loss of prefrontal neurons, particularly those neurons responsible for learnt remorse, conscience, and social sensitivity. These men have been categorised as suffering from **aggressive impulse personality disorder**, or **antisocial personality disorder (ASPD)** (Nolen-Hoeksema 2007; Carlson 2012).

ASPD is characterised by: impaired relationships with other people; deceitfulness; lying; lack of emotion; lack of fear of danger; lifelong antisocial behaviour and irresponsibility; violent crime; little, if any, remorse for others and an indifference to their suffering; low tolerance for frustration; boredom and an inability to endure boredom.

About 3% of people in the population are thought to suffer from ASPD, most of them being men. Two types of ASPD are recognised: that with (ASPD+P) and that without (ASPD-P) psychopathic tendencies. There is a strong genetic influence, with **monozygotic** (identical) twin studies indicating 50% concordance, and **dizygotic** (non-identical) twin studies showing 20% concordance. Deficits in the frontal and temporal lobes in ASPD (causing poor concentration and an inability to form concepts and goals and to perform sound reasoning) coupled with low serotonin (where low levels are linked to impulsiveness and aggression) appear to be the main pathological problems. The specific brain problems occur with the dorsal and ventral prefrontal cortex, the amygdala, and the angular gyrus, all brain areas required for making moral decisions. There are also reductions in volume of two parts of the front lobe; the **middle frontal gyrus** (18% less volume) and the **orbital frontal gyrus** (9% less volume). Because of this, these people tend also to be of a lower educational status.

Psychopath (ASPD+P) is the term often used to describe those persons who are generally more disturbed than those with ASPD-P. They show no emotions, being cold and callous towards other people. They can gain pleasure from inflicting suffering on others; they are often violent, cruel, and malicious. On the surface they may appear charming, confident, and charismatic with a grandiose sense of self-worth. They are also dogmatic in their opinions, and engage freely in unacceptable and criminal activity. People with ASPD-P have been described as 'hot-headed' whereas those with ASPD+P have been described as 'cold-hearted'. About 0.5% of the UK population are thought to be psychopathic (but between 15 and 20% of the UK prison population). Psychopaths have been found to have a deformed and malfunctioning amygdala, with an 18% reduction in the volume of this part of the brain due to a thinning of its cortex. The amygdala is the emotional centre, so they are not processing emotions correctly. There are also anomalies in the frontal and temporal lobes, especially the prefrontal cortex, which normally restrains impulsive and aggressive behaviour. It appears that this restraint is lost in psychopaths. The prefrontal cortex and temporal lobes show reduced grey matter volume in people with ASPD+P, but not in those with ASPD-P, and connections between the prefrontal cortex and the amygdala are fewer than expected. The result of this is a malfunctioning circuit involving the amygdala and the frontal areas of the brain. Normally this circuit allows the amygdala and frontal lobes to work together to control emotions and behaviour, but this fails to happen in psychopaths, leaving them devoid of empathy, guilt, and embarrassment. Dopamine levels are also significantly raised in psychopaths. The brain appears to be structured towards obtaining constant reward at any cost, through the dopaminergic pathways, and this is often achieved by antisocial behaviour, which involves taking risks.

Murderers also show altered levels of other chemicals in the brain. Testosterone appears to be the fuel that drives predetermined behaviour in men as well as aggression. That predetermined behaviour pattern is probably controlled by other factors such as genetics. If the behaviour pattern involves aggression, high levels of testosterone can drive the aggression to the point of murder. Alarmingly high levels of testosterone in some men have been associated with violence involving the rape and murder of women, sometimes multiple women – a problem called **sexual sadism**.

Apart from testosterone, two other chemicals, the neurotransmitter serotonin and the hormone oxytocin, also appear to be involved in severe forms of violence. The neurotransmitter serotonin normally has an inhibitory effect on violent behaviour. Killers often have low levels of serotonin, and the combination of high testosterone with low serotonin becomes an explosive mixture that can result in particularly nasty impulsive violent murders that may be repeated multiple times. Low serotonin in an adult appears to be associated with disruption of the family during that person's childhood. Separation of the child from the mother is the key disrupting factor, and this is where oxytocin becomes important. As indicated in Chapter 2, environmental factors, in particular bonding of the child with its mother, appears to *mould the mind*, providing stimulus for synaptic connections within the serotonergic pathways of the brain. Bonding is a big factor during breastfeeding, a time when oxytocin is produced by the mother. Oxytocin has been called the 'moral molecule', as it promotes cooperation and bonding within a group. It is said to be the 'key to empathy' by stimulating selflessness. Contrary to this, testosterone promotes selfishness. Without this maternal love and support; and the bonding between family and friends throughout childhood, the resulting effects of low oxytocin could cause the brain to become devoid of vital serotonin.

Some murderers also have high levels of a substance called **cryptopyrol**, a chemical normally found in the liver and obtained from the breakdown of **erythrocytes** (red blood cells). Increased levels of cryptopyrol have a similar activity in the brain to that seen in use of the drug **lysergic acid diethylamide (LSD)**. LSD has the effect of a hallucinogen, i.e. distorting the sensory systems, causing the subject to see the world as a jumble of abnormal sensory inputs.

The fact that there are brain changes related to aggression raises issues such as: *Can murderers be held responsible for their crimes if they have errors in their brain?* and *If there is no cure for their brain disorder, should murderers ever be released from custody?*

This is an ethical debate beyond the scope of this book, but these issues will be of greater importance as more pathological discoveries are made.

Cannibalistic behaviour, which is rare, may be simply a response to the need for food in a situation where there is a risk of starvation. Cannibalistic tendencies have been associated with some modern murders, and evidence of cannibalistic practices has recently been found in some ancient archeological sites (McKie 1998). Cannibalism may be caused by physical damage to the frontal lobes, possible from a head injury. It does not seem likely at present that any of this neuroscientific 'evidence' creates the grounds for excusing the perpetrators of their crime by claiming they are 'sick' (Ahuja 2002).

Healthcare professionals need to be able to manage aggression effectively for their own safety and the safety of others, particularly children, who are unable to protect themselves. Aggression in the public arena and in the workplace is now an escalating problem, and medical personnel are in the front line for physical and verbal abuse (Liu 2004). The **CASE de-escalation model** for coping with a potentially violent situation is an initiative of the University of Sheffield in the UK, and involves an education programme for healthcare workers. Walker et al. (2002) describes the calming, assessing, self, enabling (CASE) de-escalation model and gives instructions on the prevention and safe management of aggressive situations. Much aggression and violence is associated with excessive consumption of alcohol and drugs, and this complicates the situation. The emphasis must be placed on personal safety and getting help at the earliest opportunity.

Key points

Hormones

- Hormones are chemical messengers; they have an effect on a *target* organ or tissue.
- The brain is the target organ for many hormones, influencing neuronal growth, development, and function.
- Hormones come from endocrine glands, and are of two basic types: proteins (called peptides) and lipids (called steroids).
- A hormone must bind to a receptor site on the target cell.
- The hormone–receptor complex changes the cell by binding to DNA, and causing transcription of a gene.

Thyroid hormones

- Thyroid hormone occurs in two forms, triiodothyronine (T_3) and tetraiodothyronine (T_4). Iodine is a major component of this hormone.
- Hypothyroidism (or myxedema) is too-low level of thyroid hormone in the blood, which causes depression, lethargy, personality changes, and psychotic episodes (myxedema psychosis or myxedema madness).
- Lithium can cause hypothyroidism, and patients should be monitored for thyroid function.
- Neonatal hypothyroidism, leading to brain developmental failure, is known at cretinism. It is corrected by treatment with thyroid hormone.
- Hyperthyroidism (thyrotoxicosis) is excess thyroid hormone in the blood causing memory loss, disorientation, manic excitability, delusions, and hallucinations.

Adrenal cortex hormones

- Cortisol is a glucocorticoid from the adrenal cortex. Production is stimulated by adreno-corticotropic hormone (ACTH) from the anterior pituitary gland.
- Excess cortisol causes Cushing's syndrome, with depression-like symptoms, insomnia, energy loss, and emotional flattening. Sufferers may have mood swings with euphoria, and delirium with hallucinations.
- Addison's disease is a lack of cortisol, causing tiredness, lethargy, and depression, and sometimes delirium and confusion.
- Oestradiol is the most potent of the female oestrogens, and testosterone is the most potent of the male androgens.
- An absence of testosterone, coupled with oestrogen, creates a 'feminine' brain, whereas the presence of testosterone forms a 'masculine' brain.

Adrenal medulla hormones

- The hormones produced by the adrenal medulla are the catecholamines, adrenaline and noradrenaline (epinephrine and norepinephrine).
- Adrenaline has sympathomimetic activity – that is, it increases the functions of the sympathetic nervous system.

Differences between male and female brains

- Differences between male and female brains are created by both hormonal and environmental exposure.
- The sexually dimorphic nucleus is part of the hypothalamus that shows differences between the sexes.

Behaviour

- Behaviour is determined by multiple factors, notably developmental aspects, environmental stimuli, hormones, neurotransmitters, and genes.
- The three forms of aggression are offence, defence, and predation.
- Aggression is influenced by hormones such as testosterone and oestrogen, and neurotransmitters, especially serotonin.
- Healthcare professionals need to be able to manage aggression effectively for their own safety and the safety of others, particularly children.
- Frontal and temporal lobe problems plus low serotonin appear to be the main pathological problems in antisocial personality disorder.
- A malfunctioning circuit involving the amygdala and the frontal areas of the brain is the main problem in psychopaths.
- Testosterone appears to be the fuel that drives aggression.

References

Ahuja, A. (2002) Bad brain or bad person? *The Times* (T2 Science) 22 April: 10.
Blows, W. T. (2012) *The Biological Basis of Clinical Observations* (2nd edition). Routledge, Abingdon, Oxon.

Breedlove, S. M., Watson, N. V., and Rosenzweig, M. R. (2010) *Biological Psychology: An Introduction to Behavioural, Cognitive and Clinical Neuroscience* (6th edition). Sinauer Associates, Sunderland, MA.

Carlson, N. R. (2012) *Physiology of Behaviour* (11th edition). Pearson Education, Harlow, UK.

Eliot, L. (2010) The truth about boys and girls. *Scientific American Mind*, **21** (2): 22–29.

Joel, D., Berman, Z., Tavor, I., Wexler, N., Gaber, O., Stein, Y., Shefi, N., Pool, J., Urchs, S., Margulies, D. D., Liem, F., Hangg, J., Jancke, L., and Assaf, Y. (2015) Sex beyond the genitalia: the human brain mosaic. *PNAS*. DOI 10.1073/pnas.1509654112.

Lilienfeld, S. O. and Arkowitz, H. (2010) Are men the more belligerent sex? *Scientific American Mind*, **21** (2): 64–65.

Liu, J. (2004) Concept analysis: aggression. *Issues in Mental Health Nursing*, **25** (7): 693–714.

McKie, R. (1998) The people eaters. *New Scientist*, **157** (2125): 43–46.

Nolen-Hoeksema, S. (2007) *Abnormal Psychology* (4th edition). McGraw Hill International Edition, New York, NY.

Nowak, R. (2002) Men behaving sadly. *New Scientist*, **173** (2332) (2 March 2002): 4.

Sadock, B. J., Sadock, V. A., and Ruiz, P. (2009) *Kaplin and Sadock's Comprehensive Textbook of Psychiatry* (9th edition). Lippincott, Williams and Wilkins, Baltimore, MD.

Tan, A., Ma, W., Vira, A., Marwha, D., and Eliot, L. (2015) The human hippocampus is not sexually-dimorphic: meta-analysis of structural MRI volumes. *NeuroImage*, **124**: 350. DOI: 10.1016/j.neuro image.2015.08.050.

Walker, J., Wren, J., and Skalycz, A. (2002) Safety first. *Nursing Times*, **98** (9; 28th Feb): 20–21.

6   Genetic disorders affecting mental health

- Introduction
- Chromosomes and genes
- Disorders of inheritance
- Autosomal disorders
- Sex chromosomal abnormalities
- Genetic disorders
- Key points

Introduction

An understanding of the genetic component of many diseases is crucial to unraveling the pathology of the disease and improving its management. This is particularly true in the case of mental health disorders. Key people in the management of these disorders will need a fundamental knowledge of the subject if they are to engage in counseling, drug therapy, and research intended to improve treatment and care. This chapter provides an introduction to human genetics and an overview of the genetic aspects of various disorders.

Chromosomes and genes

The human **karyotype**, or chromosome 'set', is made up of the 46 **chromosomes** normally found irregularly arranged in the cell's nucleus, but artificially arranged by researchers as shown in Figure 6.1. Forty-four of these chromosomes (1–22) pair up to make 22 pairs of **autosomes**, which regulate many different body activities. The chromosomes making up the final pair are the sex chromosomes – X and Y in males, X and X in females. All the chromosomes carry our genes, some of the largest (e.g. chromosome 1) carrying around 2000 genes! The total number of genes that code for proteins present in the karyotype is estimated between 20,000 and 25,000.

Of each pair of chromosomes, one is inherited from the mother, the other from the father, i.e. 23 chromosomes from each parent. Each pair of autosomes therefore consists of two chromosomes that are structurally the same, carrying an identical arrangement of corresponding genes. For this reason they are known as **homologous autosomes** (*homologous* = similar, corresponding to). The genes that occur on one chromosome of a pair also occur in the same positions on the other chromosome of the same pair; thus chromosome 1 from

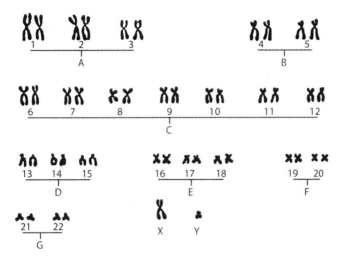

Figure 6.1 The normal human karyotype (this is a male, as denoted by the Y chromosome). A normal karyotype has 46 chromosomes, 22 pairs of autosomes (1 to 22), and one pair of sex chromosomes.

the mother holds the same genes as chromosome 1 from the father, and so on. Within any homologous pair of chromosomes, the gene pairs are alternate versions of the same gene on each chromosome. The word **allele** is used to represent alternative versions of the same gene, one on each chromosome pair. They are the same gene, but because they come from different parents they are likely to carry different **traits**. The difference between *genes* and *traits* is highlighted by the following example: the genes for eye colour carry different traits according to which parent it comes from. From the mother, the genes could carry the trait for blue eyes, whereas from the father the genes may carry the trait for green eyes. So, eye colour is the function of genes, and blue or green are the traits. If two different eye colour traits are present in the same karyotype, which one will become the true colour of the eye in that individual? In other words, which gene will be expressed into the **phenotype** (the features of the physical body)? The answer to the question depends on which gene is dominant and which is recessive. **Dominant** genes are always expressed into the phenotype when present at either one or both alleles (i.e. from one or both parents) (Figure 6.2). The gene traits of dominant genes therefore become a physical feature of the person. When the same genes (and the same traits) are present at both alleles they are described as **homozygous**. When different genes (and therefore different traits) are present at the alleles they are described as **heterozygous**. **Recessive** genes are only expressed into the phenotype when they are present at both alleles, i.e. when no dominant gene is present (Figure 6.3). A recessive gene at only one allele will not be expressed and the alternative dominant gene will determine the physical trait. However, the recessive gene will be passed on to the next generation. Two different dominant traits, one at each allele, may both be expressed into the phenotype as **codominant** genes, resulting in some kind of mixture of both traits in the phenotype of the individual.

Genes demonstrate varying degrees of **penetrance** – that is, the amount to which each individual gene contributes to the completed body (the phenotype). Genes showing complete penetrance achieve maximum influence over the phenotype. Incomplete penetrance occurs

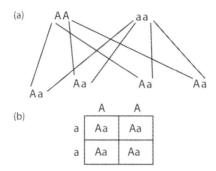

Figure 6.2 Dominant gene inheritance. A capital letter represents a dominant gene; a small letter represents a recessive gene. Homozygous parents (*AA*, i.e. both dominant genes; or *aa*, both recessive genes) will have offspring that are all mixed (*Aa*, i.e. mixed dominant and recessive). Shown as a cross-over and as a Punnett square.

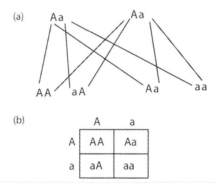

Figure 6.3 Recessive gene inheritance. A capital letter represents a dominant gene; a small letter represents a recessive gene. Heterozygous parents (*Aa*, i.e. mixed dominant and recessive genes) have 25% chance of having an *AA* offspring (i.e. pure dominant genes), 50% chance of having an *Aa* offspring (i.e. mixed genes), and 25% chance of having an *aa* offspring (purely recessive). This last child shows recessive traits (or a recessive genetic disorder) that has missed one or more generations. Shown as a cross-over and as a Punnett square.

where the gene's activity is reduced, resulting in a weaker influence on the phenotype. Dominant genes will often show a high degree of penetrance whenever they are present, but recessive genes will have little or no penetrance unless they exist at both alleles (i.e. no dominant gene is present). The amount of penetrance that a *mutated* (or abnormal) gene demonstrates is an indication of its influence on the severity and course of several important mental health disorders. However, those genes of low-level penetrance may still be passed on to future generations of the same family, where the gene's penetrance may be altered and increased. Genes are stretches of **deoxyribonucleic acid (DNA)** found within the chromatin that makes up the chromosomes, and this DNA provides a code for producing specific proteins. Through the DNA, genes determine three important things about proteins: the type of protein that will be produced; the amino acids that will be present in the final protein; and the sequence of those amino acids in the protein.

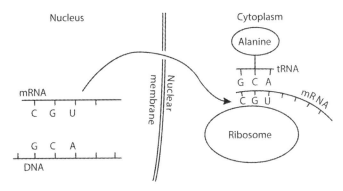

Figure 6.4 The genetic code for alanine. GCA (guanine–cytosine–adenine) on the DNA codes for the amino acid alanine by first forming the opposite code on messenger RNA (mRNA). The opposite of G is C, but the opposite of A is U (uracil) in RNA. U replaces the T (thymine) used in DNA. The mRNA leaves the nucleus and binds with a ribosome. Transfer RNAs (tRNAs) bear the same codes of bases as the original DNA codons (triplets of bases) in the DNA in the nucleus; of the case shown here it is GCA, coding for alanine. Repeating this along the DNA molecule, with different codes for different amino acids, forms a string of amino acids at the ribosome called a protein.

DNA comprises four chemical bases: **adenine (A)**, **thymine (T)**, **guanine (G)**, and **cytosine (C)**, usually represented by their first letter, as shown in brackets here. These bases form groups of three along the DNA called **codons**, and each codon codes for one specific amino acid in the final protein; for example, the codon GCA (guanine, cytosine, and adenine) codes for the amino acid alanine (Figure 6.4). The types, numbers, and sequence of the codons determines the type, numbers, and sequence of the amino acids in the completed protein. Strands of DNA, together with its structural proteins, make up **chromatin**; and two chromatin strands, joined at a point called the **centromere**, form a chromosome.

Genes have a particular site where they are found on the chromosome, called the gene **locus** (or gene slot). This locus is specified by giving the chromosome number first, followed by the arm of the chromosome (p = short arm; q = long arm), and then the banding number, which is the site along that arm where the gene is located (see Figure 6.5). The arms of chromosomes show light and dark bands, and it is the number of the band, counting away from the centromere, where the gene is located. The centromere is the point at which the two chromatin strands join. This gives us the final number of the locus. As an example, take the gene locus 15q21.3, which means it is on the 15th chromosome (see the karyotype in Figure 6.1), in the long arm (q) at the site found at band numbered 21.3, counted away from the chromosome's centromere. The higher the number, the farther from the centromere the gene is sited (see Figure 6.5).

The proteins derived from the genetic code are of various types. They could be, for example:

- **structural** proteins involved in building the cells of the body;
- **enzymes** involved in the metabolism of cells;
- **hormones** involved in the regulation of body functions;
- **antibodies** involved in the defence systems of the body.

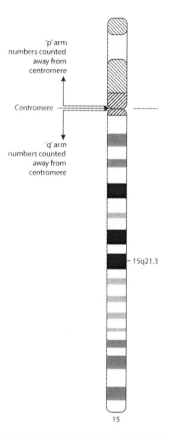

'p' arm
numbers counted
away from
centromere

Centromere

'q' arm
numbers counted
away from
centromere

15q21.3

15

Figure 6.5 The gene locus. Genes are localised by a code using first the chromosome number (here it is chromosome 15), then the arm, represented by 'p' for the short arm, 'q' for the long arm, and then the number counted away from the centromere. So 15q21.3 identifies the long arm of the 15th chromosome at point 21.3 from the centromere.

This list is incomplete, but it shows the vital importance of genes in the construction, function, and defence of the body and why gene errors can be so devastating to the individual. Most gene errors are mutations – changes occurring in the bases of the DNA, resulting in a false code and therefore an error in the protein produced from that code. This faulty protein will no longer function properly. Mutations occur as a result of damage to DNA, caused either by chemicals or by radiation, i.e. beyond the capabilities of the DNA repair enzymes. These excellent enzyme systems (which we share in common with the elephant!) can repair most of the mutations that occur, but sometimes the damage involves DNA that is missing or is beyond repair. Mutations that are inherited from generation to generation are rarely repaired and may often go on to cause diseases.

Mutations include the following DNA errors (see Figure 6.6):

1   **Point mutations**, where a single base is swapped for another, incorrect, base. This has the effect of coding for the wrong amino acid in the protein, which therefore suffers a loss of function to varying degrees (Figure 6.6a).

2   **Translocations**, where some DNA of one chromosome has switched position with another stretch of DNA from a second chromosome. As an example, a 9:21 transloca-tion means that chromosomes 9 and 21 have switched parts of their DNA with each other. The DNA is now in the wrong place and activation of these codes is likely to cause either a faulty protein or no protein product at all (Figure 6.6b).

3   **Deletions**, where some DNA is lost and chromosomes are therefore incomplete. The loss of some, perhaps many, genes will be detrimental to the function of the body, since some vital proteins cannot be produced (Figure 6.6c).

4   **Inversions**, where DNA is turned upside down in the chromosome and may be coded backwards, causing disruption of both the code and the protein that results (Figure 6.6d).

5   **Frame shifts**, where the codon is read incorrectly one base to the left or right of the correct reading frame. As an example, if the DNA sequence was . . . AACGCATT . . . , the normal codon reading, from left to right, might be AAC, then GCA, and so on. However, a frame shift might read (again, left to right) ACG, CAT . . . , i.e. it would be read incorrectly, one base along to the right. It could also be read one base along to the left, i.e. CGC, ATT, and so on. The result of either shift is the incorrect reading of the codes, leading to the wrong amino acids being selected and the protein being wrongly constructed (Figure 6.6e).

6   **Base sequence repeats** (the so-called *stuttering gene*), where one codon is repeated many times – often hundreds of times – resulting in a long chain of one type of amino acid on the end of the protein. This is seen in several mental health and neurological con-ditions, notably Huntington's disease and fragile X syndrome. The mechanism of how this error causes neurological and mental health problems is not fully determined. Not only do base sequence repeats occur as familial disorders (passed on through multiple generations of the same family), they also show the phenomenon of anticipation, i.e. an addition of further repeats to the DNA with each successive generation. This causes the disorder to start earlier with each new generation of that family, who also show increas-ingly severe symptoms as the repeat sequence gets longer (see Huntington's disease, page 295) (Figure 6.6f).

7   **Duplication**, where a sequence of DNA is copied (as part of a chromosome) and added onto the previously existing arm of a chromosome (Figure 6.6g).

8   **Unstable sequence**, where a very large repeated base sequence, similar to but much longer than that found in 'duplication' above, causes a complete loss of gene function. Fragile X syndrome is such a condition, resulting in some degree of intellectual disability.

Disorders of inheritance

Autosomal gene mutations are responsible for a number of genetically inherited disorders (i.e. those genes present at birth) and genetically acquired disorders (i.e. those where an individual develops a gene error during their life due to the damage and mutation of a pre-viously normal gene). However, environmental factors are also likely to play an important role in some mental health disorders, and these disorders are therefore usually classified as **polygenic**, in which several genes are seen as interacting with one or several environmental factors to cause the disorder. In this sense, genes play a role that *increases the susceptibility* of an individual to develop a particular disorder, rather than causing the disorder directly. Whether the person develops the disorder or not may depend on the environmental factors they encounter.

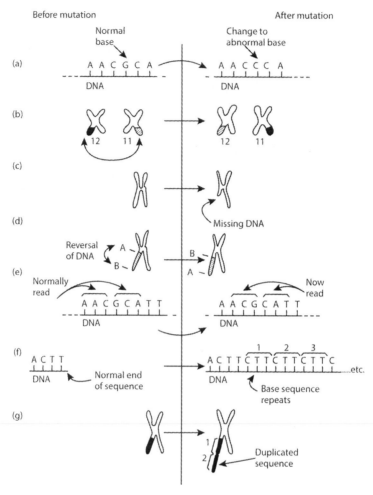

Figure 6.6 Genetic mutations. The left column shows before the mutation, the right column is after the mutation. (a) In a point mutation one base on the DNA is changed to a different one, creating a different code, which introduces a different amino acid into the protein. (b) Translocation, in which a DNA sequence is swapped over between two chromosomes (shown here as an 11:12 translocation). (c) Deletion, in which a DNA sequence is lost entirely. (d) Inversion, in which a DNA sequence is reversed on the same chromosome (and thus will be read backwards). (e) Frame shift, where the normal DNA reading is moved one or more bases along (shown here as a single base shift normally read AAC, but now read ACG). This changes the amino acids in the protein. (f) Repeated base sequence, where the same base code is repeated many times (here it is CTT), resulting in a long tail of one kind of amino acid on the protein. (g) Duplication, where a DNA sequence is copied and attached to the end of a chromosome.

Inherited genetic disorders are said to be familial; that is, they are found in successive generations of the same family. In the case of *inherited* disorders, the gene error is passed on from parents to offspring through the sperm or ovum. In studies involving families affected by an inherited gene disorder the researcher will look at percentage risks between first-degree

Table 6.1 Proportions of genes in common between relatives of different degrees

Relationship to affected person	Approximate percentage of shared genes
Monozygotic (MZ or identical) twin	98
Dizygotic (DZ or non-identical) twin	50
First-degree relative (sibling, parent, son, daughter)	50
Second-degree relative (grandparent, aunt, uncle)	25
Third-degree relative (e.g. cousin)	12.5

relatives (parents, brothers, sisters, sons, or daughters) of an affected person. Studies of second-degree relatives (grandparents, aunts, or uncles), or even third-degree relatives (e.g. cousins) of an affected person may also be of value in understanding the nature of the gene and its inheritance pattern. Studies of twins are particularly important when studying genetic inheritance, especially of monozygotic (identical) twins who have about 98% of their genes in common. Table 6.1 shows the approximate proportions of genes shared between an affected person and their various relatives. From this it can be seen that dizygotic (non-identical) twins share the same amount of genes as ordinary brothers or sisters.

For a discussion on the genes related to a specific mental disorder, see the chapter on that disorder; for example, the genes involved in depression are discussed in Chapter 11, those for schizophrenia in Chapter 10, and those for dementia in Chapter 14. Genes involved in Huntington's and Parkinson's diseases are discussed in Chapter 13.

The most important difference between a genetic disorder and a chromosomal disorder is the number of genes involved (i.e. it becomes a problem of magnitude). In genetic disorders there may be one or just a few genes at the root cause of a particular disease, whereas chromosomal disorders involve abnormalities of a whole or part of a chromosome, adding up to perhaps several thousand genes.

Autosomal disorders

Two major chromosomal errors can result in mental health disorders: those that involve whole chromosomes and thus affect the number of chromosomes in the karyotype (e.g. trisomies and monosomies), and those that affect part of individual chromosomes without influencing the karyotype number (e.g. deletions).

Several chromosomal abnormalities can occur that result in an abnormal karyotype chromosome count (the normal value being 46 chromosomes). A **trisomy** is the occurrence of one extra chromosome attached to a pair, giving a karyotype of 47 chromosomes (Figure 6.7). A **monosomy** is the occurrence of only one chromosome instead of a pair; one chromosome is missing, giving a karyotype of 45 chromosomes (Figure 6.7). People with some trisomies or with most monosomies do not survive; those bearing these chromosomal abnormalities are subject to spontaneous natural abortion during pregnancy, i.e. a miscarriage caused by nature. This is because either too much genetic material is present (trisomies) or not enough is present (monosomies) to be compatible with life. It is possible that individual cells within one person can differ in the presence or absence of a trisomy. Those sufferers with all their cells containing a trisomy are called 'full trisomies', and those with a mix of trisomy and non-trisomy (normal) cells are called 'mosaic trisomies'.

The trisomies that can *survive* to birth are those of autosomes 8[1], 9, 13, 16[2], 18, 20[2], 21, and 22[1], (1 = survival is rare; 2 = survives as a mosaic only). Autosomal monosomies are

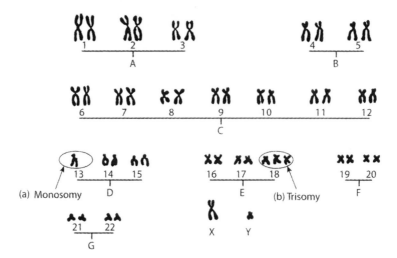

Figure 6.7 The human karyotype showing monosomy (here seen at chromosome 13) and trisomy (here seen at chromosome 18).

almost entirely fatal as a fetus. The only exception may be monosomy 21. Only a few full monosomy 21 have been reported, and only one lived beyond their first birthday. Mosaic monosomy 21 have survived more often.

Trisomy 8, or **Warkany syndrome 2** (three number 8 chromosomes), results in an individual who is abnormally shorter or taller than average (due to variations in growth patterns), no facial expressions, multiple physical abnormalities, especially of the musculoskeletal system (e.g. a large skull), low set ears, bulbous-tipped nose, heart and palate defects, eye abnormalities, deep hand and foot creases, and some degree of intellectual disability. Most sufferers are mosaic for trisomy 8 (abbreviated to T8mS), with full trisomy 8 causing early death. The severity of the syndrome in survivors depends on how many cells are affected and how many are normal within the mosaic mix.

Trisomy 9 (three number 9 chromosomes) can be in full or mosaic form. The symptoms vary widely but include abnormal skull shape, disorder of the nervous system, and a degree of intellectual disability. The heart, kidneys, and musculoskeletal system may be involved.

Trisomy 13 (three number 13 chromosomes) is called **Patau syndrome**. This occurs about once in every 5000 live births and (like Edwards and Down syndromes) the risk of Patau syndrome is increased with advancing maternal age at the time of pregnancy. It causes a wide range of severe physical abnormalities (e.g. heart, kidney, and eye defects, microcephaly, low-set ears, cleft palate, extra fingers, abnormal feet) with profound intellectual disability. Half of those born with this syndrome die within one month of their birth.

Trisomy 16 (three number 16 chromosomes) occurs in full or mosaic form. Full trisomy 16 is incompatible with life and causes most of the miscarriages from chromosomal errors occurring during pregnancy. Trisomy 16 live births are mosaics only. The features of mosaic trisomy 16 are premature birth, defects in growth, lung and heart abnormalities, a short neck, high forehead, and scoliosis (a specific curvature of the spine).

Trisomy 18 (three number 18 chromosomes) is called **Edwards syndrome**. This is more common than Patau syndrome, and second only to Down syndrome in prevalence, being

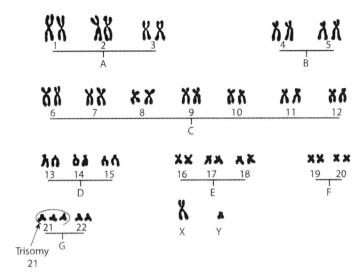

Figure 6.8 Down syndrome karyotype, showing trisomy at chromosome 21.

present in around one in 3000 conceptions, but one in 6000 live births, due to death of the fetus before birth. The incidence rises with increased maternal age at the time of pregnancy. It causes various physical abnormalities (heart, kidney, and other organs), failure of growth (developmental delay) and intellectual disability. **Microcephaly** (a small head) with other cranial abnormalities are characteristic. Survival rate is poor, about 50% dying before birth (mostly due to the cardiac malformations) with about 30% of those surviving up to birth dying before their first birthday.

Trisomy 20 (three number 20 chromosomes) occurs in full or mosaic form, with full (non-mosaic) trisomy 20 (NMT20) causing early fetal death and miscarriage during the first trimester of pregnancy from gross physical abnormalities. Mosaic trisomy 20 is often detected prenatally, but the resulting child often appears normal, or has minor abnormalities, at birth. A consistent set of abnormalities has now been established. These are spinal defects, sloping shoulders, poor muscle tone, recurrent constipation, and significant learning disabilities.

Trisomy 21 (three number 21 chromosomes) is known as **Down syndrome** (Figure 6.8). This is more common than other trisomies, occurring on average in about one in 600 live births. The incidence of a Down syndrome rises with increasing maternal age: the older the mother is at the time of pregnancy the greater is the risk of Down syndrome. A typical risk pattern is seen in Table 6.2.

Table 6.2 Changes in the incidence of Down syndrome with maternal age

Maternal age at conception of child (years)	*Approximate incidence of Down syndrome*
15 to 29	1 in 1250 to 1 in 1100 live births
30 to 34	1 in 900 to 1 in 500 live births
35 to 39	1 in 385 to 1 in 140 live births
40 to 44	1 in 100 to 1 in 40 live births
45 and over	1 in 25 live births

As with some of the other trisomies, the extra chromosome is caused mostly by a **nondysjunc-tion**, where ovarian cell division results in abnormal separation of the chromosomes and one ovum retains both of the chromosomes 21. The older the woman becomes, the greater becomes the risk of nondysjunction. The single ovum then has two chromosome 21, and the addition of a third chromosome 21 from the sperm on fertilisation completes the trisomy. Incidentally, should the normal sperm fertilise the other half of that ovum division – the half with no chromosome 21 – it would generate a monosomy 21 (having only the paternal chromosome 21).

Down syndrome results in a wide range of physical abnormalities and varying degrees of intellectual disability, from mild through to severe. The physical abnormalities include a round skull on a short, broad neck, a flattened face and a prominent epicanthus of the eye (the upper lid fold close to the nose is anchored lower down, giving an oriental or 'Mongolian' appearance, a feature responsible for the term *mongolism,* which is sometimes inappropri-ately used). Other features are a large, furrowed tongue in a small mouth, a single crease in the palm of the hand (known as a simian crease), and a long plantar crease down the sole of the foot extending from an enlarged gap between the first two toes. There may also be increased extensibility of the limbs due to poor muscle tone. Varying degrees of congenital heart defects can occur, and cataracts (opacity of the lens of the eye, causing blindness), squints, and nystagmus (rapid uncontrollable lateral eye movements) are more common in trisomy 21 than in the average person.

The intellectual disability can be anything from very mild to quite severe (Sadock et al. 2009). At the mild end of the spectrum, Down syndrome children communicate and learn quite well and become relatively independent adults. They can perform quite intricate tasks and cope with jobs that are not too demanding. They are often happy and enjoy participating in activities such as learning a musical instrument, singing, and dancing. Before the advent of modern social conditions and life-saving treatments such as antibiotics, Down syndrome children often died from neglect, undernutrition, and infections. Now, many are living into adulthood, when they begin to face another problem. The middle-aged Down syndrome adult (i.e. 30 to 40 years of age) often shows evidence of dementia of the type related to Alzheimer's disease. Chapter 14 explores Alzheimer's disease in some detail, and the con-nection with chromosome 21, relating this to Down syndrome.

The ability to remove the third chromosome from a Down syndrome cell culture in the laboratory was demonstrated for the first time in 2012. The team used a virus to deliver a spe-cial gene to the third chromosome 21, which was then rejected from the cell. Although this is not expected to be a cure, it may have clinical applications for the future in reducing some of the effects of the disorder (Li et al. 2012). In other research, new drugs are being developed that appear to correct the development of the cerebellum (which is said to be 40% smaller in Down syndrome mice) with a corresponding improvement is learning and memory. If these drugs can be used in humans, the benefits may allow trisomy 21 people to lead a better life (Das et al. 2013; Laidman 2014).

Trisomy 22 (three number 22 chromosomes) occurs in full or mosaic forms. Full trisomy 22 is the second most common cause of spontaneous miscarriage during pregnancy after full trisomy 16. Mosaic trisomy 22 causes a long list of physical abnormalities, including micro-cephaly, intrauterine growth retardation, craniofacial malformation (abnormal development of the head and face), limb deformities, heart and vascular disorders, and arrested mental development.

Mosaic monosomy 21 (only one number 21 in some cells) rarely survives as a live birth, with only a few cases reported. They have a collection of medical problems including microcephaly, skull, brain and facial deformities, abnormalities of the digits, poor muscle tone, and both intellectual and physical disability.

A constant physical abnormality in many of these disorders is **craniofacial malformation**, such as cleft lip and palate (incomplete closure of the upper lip and roof of the mouth), or more rarely cyclopia (a single eye in the forehead often associated with an absent forebrain). Cleft lip and palate is a birth defect that is encountered regularly, and the majority of these occur in otherwise normal babies (i.e. they are not suffering from a chromosomal syndrome, and therefore they are 'non-syndromic'). In chromosomal 'syndromic' cleft lip and palate, the upper jaw defect forms part of the multiple features that make up the syndrome.

The formation of the head and face is a complex biological phenomenon that is controlled by multiple genes, most of which are only now being discovered. Because the brain, head, and face develop together as a unit, any defect in the development of one will impact on the development of the others. Although the brain forms from the head end of the neural tube, the bones, cartilages, and connective tissue of the skull, and the peripheral nervous system of the head are all derived from cranial neural crest cells. The face grows forward from both sides and fuses down the midline. It is the failure of this midline fusing process that causes cleft lip and palate.

New work is revealing the genes and their protein products that link the development of the brain with embryonic skull and facial construction (Cohen 2000). It is beyond the scope of this chapter to discuss them all, but one important gene involved in this process has several vital roles. This is the **sonic hedgehog homolog (*SHH*)** gene, which is one of three so-called Hedgehog proteins. *SHH* acts as a **morphogen**, i.e. a cell signalling molecule that governs the nature of tissues, e.g. controlling cell differentiation, during embryonic development. *SHH* is involved in the development of many embryonic systems, in particular the midface (e.g. controlling the width of the face) and frontal areas of the brain. Mutations of *SHH* cause a collection of disorders called **holoprosencephaly**, i.e. failure of development of the face and frontal brain lobes, which includes cleft lip and palate.

Sex chromosome abnormalities

The genetic determination of an individual's sex relies on the inheritance of a combination of the sex chromosomes, X and Y. The XX combination produces a female and the XY combination produces a male. 'Maleness' therefore requires the presence of the Y chromosome, while 'femaleness' requires the absence of the Y chromosome.

Several genes are involved in creating the male condition, one of which is very close to the centromere on the Y chromosome (Figure 6.9). This is the **sex-determining region Y (*SRY*)** gene, a gene that codes for a transcription factor. Transcription factors are proteins that bind to DNA and begin to trigger the process of RNA assembly, i.e. the process called transcription, leading to protein synthesis. The *SRY*-encoded transcription factor switches on testicular development in the primitive gonad at about week 6 or 7 of gestation. Up to that point the gonads were undifferentiated, being neither testes nor ovary.

The **Eve principle** is the term often given to the condition in which the absence of the Y chromosome always causes the undifferentiated gonads to become ovaries (i.e. female). This could be regarded as the default state. The Y chromosome (and the corresponding androgens) must be present to produce the male condition (i.e. the gonads become testes), and therefore the need to add the Y chromosome to the basic female condition to produce a male sex is often called the **Adam principle**.

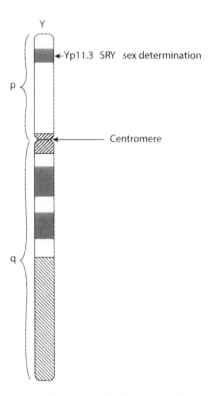

Figure 6.9 The male Y chromosome, showing the *SRY* (sex determination) gene locus at Yp11.3.

XXY males are described as having **Klinefelter's syndrome** (Figure 6.10). The additional X chromosome changes the normal karyotype of 46 chromosomes into the abnormal number of 47. Klinefelter's syndrome is the result of fertilisation involving either diploid sperm or diploid ova. 'Diploid' in this context means that the sperm or ovum carries *both* the sex chromosomes instead of just one; thus one ovum would carry XX, or one sperm would carry XY. On fertilisation with a normal Y sperm, the XX ovum would become XXY. Fertilisation between an XY sperm and a normal X ovum would also result in XXY (see Figure 6.10). Klinefelter's syndrome occurs in 1 in 600 live births and, because the Y is present, the child is always male. Males with this condition are usually tall, often thin, with poor sexual development and have a mild degree of intellectual disability. It would appear that if more extra X chromosomes are present, e.g. XXXY or XXXXY, the greater the degree of intellectual disability (McCance et al. 2010).

    Figure 6.10 also shows an XXX combination, which is the inappropriately named **superwoman syndrome**. This is another 47-chromosome karyotype, caused by a trisomy X. As for the male in Klinefelter's syndrome, the XXX female sometimes has poor sexual development and a mild intellectual disability, but people with this syndrome are able to live relatively normal lives in society. Superwoman syndrome is rarer than Klinefelter's syndrome, occurring in 1 in 1600 live births. Again, as with Klinefelter's syndrome, any additional X present causes greater degree of intellectual disability. Very rare cases of XXXX and XXXXX syndromes have been reported, where more X chromosomes cause much greater degrees of intellectual disability (Visootsak et al. 2007).

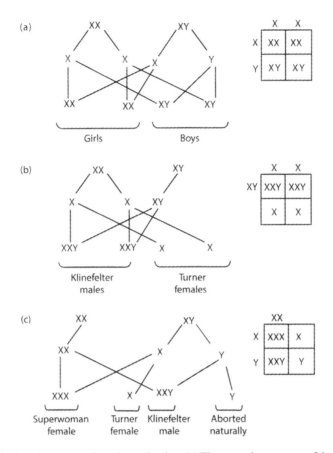

Figure 6.10 Inheritance patterns of sex determination. (a) The normal cross-over of the female XX and male XY to produce a 50% chance of either sex. (b) Abnormal male clustering together of the XY chromosomes, giving sons with Klinefelter's syndrome, or daughters with Turner's syndrome. (c) Abnormal female clustering together of the XX chromosomes, giving sons that either have Klinefelter's syndrome or are incompatible with life and will spontaneously abort, or giving daughters who may be superwoman syndrome or Turner's syndrome. All three are shown as cross-overs or Punnett squares.

As shown in Figure 6.10, the single X (monosomy X) female also occurs, giving a 45-chromosome karyotype. Monosomy X is **Turner's syndrome**, characterised by a short female with poor sexual development and some minor physical abnormalities, including a depressed sternum and a webbed neck. However, with one X present these females have normal intellectual development. Turner's syndrome happens in about 1 in 3000 live births.

XYY males do occur as well, because nearly 1% of all sperm carry the YY chromosome combination, which may fertilise a normal single X ovum to cause XYY. It perhaps happens in 1 in 1000 live births. These males have attracted a great deal of research because this particular genetic combination has been associated with aggression and criminal behaviour. The XYY combination was first reported in 1961 and its association with violent criminal behaviour was made in 1965. Today, much of this original work on XYY is seen to be inappropriate and flawed because of sample bias, as most of the work focused on male prison

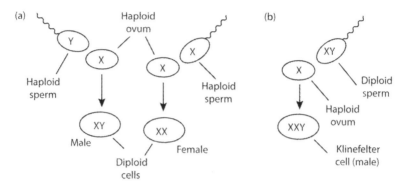

Figure 6.11 Sperm meets ovum. (a) Normally the sperm carries one sex chromosome (either X or Y) and this meets the ovum that carries one X chromosome to produce a fertilised ovum with XX or XY. (b) Sometimes an abnormal sperm carries both XY and meets a normal ovum to give a fertilised ovum with XXY. Normal sperm fertilising abnormal XX ovum to give either XXX or XXY also occurs occasionally (not shown).

populations. We now know that less than 1% of all XYY men become prisoners and that less than 2% of male prisoners are XYY. Leaving prison populations aside, XYY may cause some small increase in antisocial behaviour when compared with the normal XY or even XXY combinations. Other characteristics of the XYY male include above-average height, XYY are around 1.82 metres compared to the XY average of 1.67 metres. Even as a child of 6 years, the XYY male is taller than 90% of his peers of the same age. Sexual development is normal, but there may be a degree of poor coordination, delayed language skills, and some learning difficulties. These males generally perform less well in intelligence quotient (IQ) tests than their XY counterparts, approximately on a par with XXY males.

Very rarely, XYYY and even XYYYY males have been reported, but unlike the additional X chromosomes, the additional Ys have little or no effect on intellectual development.

The X chromosome

The X chromosome is much larger than the Y chromosome, and this means that it carries many more genes. Even when the number of X chromosomes is normal, it can be the source of a significantly large number of rare but important intellectual disability syndromes caused by gene mutations (Figure 6.12). Table 6.3 lists the better-known X-linked syndromes that result in some degree of intellectual disability and also illustrates the large number of intellectual disability syndromes associated with the X chromosome. Notice in Figure 6.12 that there are a number of intellectual disability syndromes positioned in clusters on the chromosome, the loci of the major ones being Xp22.3–p22.2; Xp11.3–p11.21 (close to the centromere); Xq21.3–q24 and Xq28.

An important point concerning the X chromosome is the fact that females have two X chromosomes whereas males have only one. This means that any particular gene error on one X chromosome is likely to be matched by a normal gene on the other X chromosome in females (the mutation occurring at only one allele), whereas in males the X chromosome gene error has no such normal counterpart. This results in X-linked gene disorders being generally much

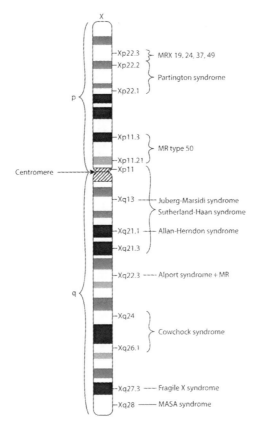

Figure 6.12 The X chromosome. Several important intellectual disability syndromes are located on both the p (short) and q (long) arms.

more severe in males than in females. Males suffer the full disease, which may prove fatal in some cases. On the other hand, females may have only mild symptoms or even remain asymptomatic (having no symptoms at all). However, females will still be able to pass on the faulty gene to their offspring, and if this is a son he is likely to suffer the severe form of the illness. It is very rare (and very unlucky) for a female to have the faulty gene on both X chromosomes (i.e. at both alleles). This only happens if both parents have the disorder, i.e. they both carry the same faulty gene. In this case, the disorder in this female would be severe.

Earlier in this chapter the term *phenotype* was described as the body, i.e. the physical features caused by the genotype (*genotype* = genes present in the cell). Another way of stating this is to say that the genotype consists of the genes locked up in the cell nucleus, while the phenotype is the bodily features (tall, short, brown hair, etc.) created by expression of the genes. Other terms included in Table 6.3 are **adducted thumbs** (where the thumbs lie bent inwards across the palm of the hand); **aphasia** (the inability to speak); **brachycephaly** (a congenital skull malformation in which the head is short but wide); **dysarthria** (a difficulty with speech due to poor speech muscle control); **dystonia** (an abnormal posture of a limb or the trunk with slow and twisting movements); **elliptocytosis** (an increase in the number of **elliptocytes**,

Table 6.3 X-linked syndromes involving intellectual disability

Gene locus	Syndrome name or code (if any)	Phenotype
Xp22.3–22.2	MRX19, 24, 37	
Xp22.3–22.2	MRX49	Mild to moderate ID
Xp22.3–21.3		ID in males only
Xp22.2–p22.1	Partington syndrome	Male only, mild to moderate ID, dystonic hand movements, dysarthria
Xp21–q13		Varying degree of ID
Xp11–q21.3	Sutherland–Haan X-linked ID syndrome	Short stature, small testes, microcephaly, brachycephaly, ID
Xp11.3–p11.21	MR type 50	Moderate ID
Xq13	Juberg–Marsidi syndrome	Probably males only. Growth delay, facial anomalies, deafness, ID, and microgenitalism
Xq21.1	Allan–Herndon syndrome	Severe ID, muscle and movement anomalies, head abnormalities
Xq22		Female epilepsy, ID
Xq22.3		Alport syndrome (multiple physical deformities and disorders, worse in males) with ID, elliptocytosis, midface hypoplasia
Xq24–26.1	Cowchock syndrome	Neuropathy, deafness, and ID. Worse in males
Xq26–27		Male moderate ID, facial abnormalities and large testes
Xq27.3	Fragile X syndrome	See text
Xq28	MASA syndrome	ID, aphasia, shuffling gait, adducted thumbs
X	Chudley MR syndrome	Moderate to severe ID, short stature, mild obesity, hypogonadism, facial abnormalities

ID = intellectual disability. X = X chromosome (MRX with a number refers to a specific intellectual disability syndrome). p = short arm. q = long arm. See text for other definitions of terms.

i.e. oval instead of round **erythrocytes**, or red blood cells, in the blood); **gait** (the method of walking); **hypogonadism** (underdevelopment of either testes or ovum); **hypoplasia** (abnormal reduction in the numbers of cells causing underdevelopment of an organ); **microcephaly** (a small head with a small brain); and **neuropathy** (a disorder of the nerves).

Fragile X syndrome (Figure 6.13) is an intellectual disability syndrome caused by a trinucleotide repeat gene mutation within the **fragile X mental retardation 1 (*FMR1*)** gene at Xq27.3, where the same three genetic bases are repeated many times. The repeated bases in this case are CGG (i.e. cytosine–guanine–guanine), where CGG codes for the amino acid arginine. Up to 53 such repeats occur normally, but any number of repeats from 55 to more than 200 are found in this syndrome. When expressed, the normal gene would code for a protein, known as **fragile X mental retardation protein (FMRP)**, which binds with RNA (ribonucleic acid) and moves it around the neuron. RNA locks onto a ribosome, where translation of the RNA code into a protein (protein synthesis) takes place. FMRP is required for the successful binding of RNA to a ribosome. In fragile X syndrome, however, the excessive CGG repeats block gene expression, with the consequent loss of the normal FMRP protein and a subsequent loss of RNA binding ability. This leads to failure of the cell's protein synthesis functions, and in neurons this causes varying degrees of intellectual disability (Figure 6.13). Males appear to be more affected than females, with 1 in 4000 males and 1 in 8000 females

NORMAL GENE ON X CHROMOSOME

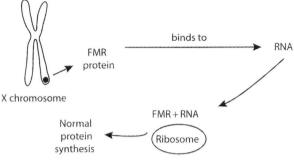

ABNORMAL EXCESS OF CGG REPEATS

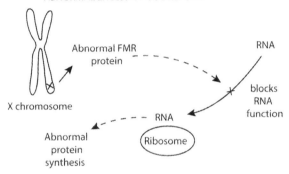

Figure 6.13 Fragile X syndrome. A gene on chromosome X codes for the FMR protein, which appears to be important for RNA binding at the ribosome (top). In fragile X syndrome faulty DNA at the *FMR* gene causes failure of normal FMR protein, which in turns reduces RNA's ability to bind at the ribosome (below). Failure of RNA binding reduces the cell's protein production ability, and the neuron will suffer from the loss.

having the disorder, but only 30–40% of affected females have some degree of intellectual impairment. Less commonly, other symptoms occur, notably enlarged testes at puberty, large ears, a prominent jaw, some enlargement of the head in a few affected males, finger joints that extend farther than expected owing to loose connective tissues, and aortic and heart valve disorders. Speech may be delayed and high pitched. There is also a link with **autistic spectrum disorder (ASD)** as people with fragile X syndrome also show autistic-like symptoms (see Chapter 15).

Fragile X syndrome appears also to disrupt the function of a natural **cannabinoid protein** (an **endocannabinoid**) called **2-arachidonoylglycerol (2-AG)**, which binds to the CB1 cannabinoid receptor, and is important in improving the efficiency of synapses within the cerebral cortex and corpus striatum.

Trinucleotide repeats, which are also sometimes called stuttering genes (look back at Figure 6.6f on page 100), are of growing importance in mental health, and are implicated in other disorders such as Huntington's disease and schizophrenia.

Genetic disorders

Apart from whole chromosomes or parts of chromosomes, a single gene or a few genes on autosomes or the X chromosome may be responsible for specific disorders involving mental health disturbance. The types of abnormal genes (mutations) are shown in Figure 6.6 (see page 100).

Deletions (Figure 6.6c) involve the loss of a genetic sequence, i.e. a number of DNA bases, often due to breakages during cell division. Cri-du-chat ('cry of cat') syndrome involves the deletion of part of the short arm of chromosome 5 (5p15.2) (Faraone et al. 1999). This gene codes for catenin delta-2, a protein that is specific to neurons and is involved significantly in neural motility during the very early stages of nervous system development. Children born with this condition show intellectual disability and severe physical abnormalities, such as microcephaly (small head and brain), low-set ears, and oblique palpebral fissures (openings of the eye). The disorder gets its name from the cat-like crying sound children with this syndrome make, but this gradually disappears as they get older.

Williams syndrome is caused by the loss of a small fragment of genetic material from one of the seventh chromosomes, a loss of about 15 or so genes at 7q11.23. The other seventh chromosome is present and complete. The incidence of this condition is about one in every 20,000 births worldwide. It causes a minor degree of intellectual disability, resulting in lower than average intelligence test scores. The surprise, however, is the remarkable musical talent that many people with this disorder display. Williams syndrome people can often perform, remember, and even compose music to a very high degree of competency (Lenhoff et al. 1997). Several genes that are missing from the deleted segment are involved in brain development, but their mechanism of action is not fully known. The musical ability can be partly explained by studies of the brains from Williams syndrome people that show an extensive expansion of part of the temporal cortex called the **planum temporale**. This expansion is also found in gifted musicians without this syndrome (see the section on music in Chapter 9). However, other areas of the brain in Williams syndrome are reduced to below normal size.

Epigenome and genomic imprinting disorders

Epigenetics (which means 'beyond genetics') is a relatively new science that studies the molecular effects that control gene activation and thus cell differentiation without changing the genes themselves. The genes that code for proteins are referred to as the **genome**, but the epigenetic mechanisms that include various chemical markers and the DNA that does not code for proteins, is the **epigenome**. Similar to the genome, the epigenome is vulnerable to environmental assaults from radiation, chemicals, pathogens, and parasites, and ageing, causing epigenetic errors (mutations) that can lead to disordered control of the genome and thus disease.

Imprinting is the epigenomic process by which gene activation is controlled in the fetus by influences from both the mother and the father separately. Both influences are vital for normal brain development, the mother influencing brain areas concerned with language and thinking, and the father influencing brain areas concerned with growth, control of food intake, and reproduction. Imprinting determines if a gene will be activated or switched off without changing the genetic code of that gene. It is useful to think of it as genetic switching, turning genes on or off. Between them, the parents create a balanced pattern of gene activation that usually results in a normal brain; but sometimes it can go wrong. Genetic **imprinting patterns** (i.e. the pattern of inactivated genes within the genome) housed within the ovum or the sperm cells is called **genomic imprinting**.

Genomic imprinting works through the addition of a molecule (a **methyl group**, or **CH₃**) to the gene, which effectively switches the gene off, i.e. it reduces the **penetrance** of that gene to zero (Figure 6.14). Both parents' genomic imprinting patterns influence the fetal development of the offspring, but if that offspring were a girl she would ultimately pass only her mother's imprinting pattern onto her own offspring. Similarly, a boy would pass the imprinting pattern of his father onto his offspring. This is because the ovum carries the imprinted gene pattern from the mother only (the father's imprinting pattern is removed), whereas the

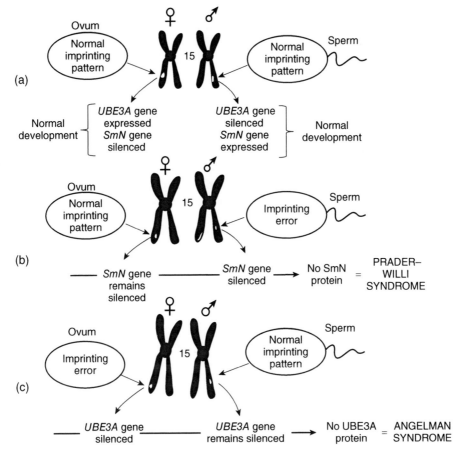

Figure 6.14 Normal imprinting and imprinting errors in Angelman and Prader–Willi syndromes. (a) The male and female copies of the genes located on chromosome 15 at 15q11–q12 are controlled by normal imprinting patterns inherited from both parents. While the male gene for SmN protein is active, the female gene is silenced by the imprinting pattern; while the female *UBE3A* gene is active, the male gene is silenced by imprinting. (b) Mutation errors in the imprinting pattern inherited from the male parent reduces SmN protein production from the male gene; the female gene remains silenced so cannot make up the difference in the amount of SmN protein available, causing Prader–Willi Syndrome. (c) Mutation errors in the imprinting pattern inherited from the female parent reduces production of the UBE3A enzyme from the female gene at the same location. The male *UBE3A* gene remains normally silenced by the male imprinting pattern, so cannot make up the difference, causing Angelman syndrome.

sperm carries the imprinted gene pattern from the father only (the mother's imprinting pattern is removed). Because the male and female imprinting patterns are different, any disorder involving an imprinting pattern will affect the offspring differently depending on which parent had the error.

Prader–Willi syndrome and **Angelman syndrome** are good examples of this. The genes involved in both of these syndromes are of part of chromosome 15, i.e. the gene locus 15q11. The problem in Prader–Willi syndrome appears to be limited to 15q11, while in Angelman syndrome the problem is wider, to include 15q11 and 15q12, and sometimes even part of 15q13. It appears that the difference between these syndromes depends on which parent the imprinting error was obtained from. If the imprinting error is inherited from the mother (the maternal line of inheritance), the resulting syndrome in the offspring is Angelman syndrome; but if the imprinting error is from the father (the paternal line of inheritance) it is Prader–Willi syndrome (Figure 16.14).

Prader–Willi syndrome involves a gene called **small nuclear ribonucleoprotein N** (***SNRPN***). It codes for a protein called **SmN** (a **small nuclear ribonucleoprotein subunit**). This is involved in the processing of messenger ribonucleic acid (mRNA), the molecule required to carry the DNA code to the ribosome for protein synthesis. SmN is particularly expressed in the brain. Disturbance in the activation of this gene could be a cause of inappropriate protein synthesis in specific neurons, leading to abnormal development of the brain or malfunction of those neurons. Normally, the paternal copy of the gene is active, the maternal copy being silenced by imprinting. However, if the paternal gene is abnormally imprinted (switched off) or deleted, there is no active gene, the female copy remains switched off, and this causes the symptoms. The deletions are probably due to the fact that this particular DNA sequence has two points that are susceptible to breakage.

Angelman syndrome is a deletion (70% of cases) or imprinting error (30% of cases), which involves a gene called ***UBE3A***. This gene codes for an enzyme that attaches a protein called **ubiquitin** to cell structures for normal degradation. Normally in the brain the maternal gene is active, while the paternal gene is silenced by imprinting. When the female gene is abnormally silenced by an imprinting error, or is deleted, Angelman syndrome occurs because the paternal gene remains imprinted and thus inactive (Figure 6.14).

Angelman syndrome is characterised by severe motor impairment, e.g. **ataxia** (poor coordination of movement and loss of balance), **hypotonia** (loose, floppy muscles), and intellectual disability, including failure of speech and epilepsy. Other abnormal characteristics include a large mandible, which may protrude forward (**prognathism**), a large open mouth (**macrostomia**) with protruding tongue, excessive laughter (appears happy), puppet-like movements, and hyperactivity.

Prader–Willi syndrome also shows symptoms of hypotonia and intellectual disability. In this syndrome the sufferer develops what appears to be a **hyperphagia**, i.e. an excessive appetite, which could lead to overeating and obesity. In fact, they appear to eat anything, even to the point of eating clothing, curtains, paper, and other non-edible substances. However, the current opinion is that these patients are not actually eating these inedible substances, they are using the mouth as another sense organ, i.e. taste is as important to recognition of objects as is sight and touch. People with this condition have small hands, small feet, and a short stature, coupled with reduced levels of gonad function (**hypogonadism**) due to under-secretion of gonadotrophic hormones from the pituitary gland. Children with this condition may show defiant behaviour. Both syndromes are rare; Prader–Willi syndrome, for example, affects fewer than one person in 10,000 (Sadock et al. 2009), and Angelman syndrome affects one person in 15,000 to 20,000.

A good example of changes within epigenetic imprinting by an environmental factor is the parasitic organism that causes **toxoplasmosis**. The organism is *Toxoplasma gondii*, a single-celled protozoan that can invade human cells, including brain cells, and secrete foreign proteins that alter the cell's chemistry, including gene expression. Among other things, these proteins can remove the gene methylation (i.e. remove the imprinted methyl group from a gene), thus removing the block that held the gene silent. It then becomes active, with effects that could include raising the levels of neurotransmitter, especially in those parts of the brain regulating social and sexual activity. Cells not directly invaded by the parasite can also harbour the foreign proteins that have been injected into the cell from passing *T. gondii*. This kind of epigenetic change in brain cells may have serious effects on brain functions and therefore on behaviour patterns. The parasite can be acquired from cat faeces and soil contaminated by faeces, because the organism has part of its life cycle inside the cat's gut (Hill and Dubey 2002).

Lissencephalic disorders

The Lissencephalic disorders (*lissos* = 'smooth', *encephalon* = 'brain'; i.e. the 'smooth brain' disorders) includes a number of microdeletions (very small genetic deletions), which result in a degree of intellectual disability and other symptoms. In these disorders, abnormal neuronal migration occurs during fetal development, resulting in a smooth cortex, i.e. a significant loss of the normal folding into sulci and gyri, together with varying changes of cortical cell layers. Neuronal migration is described in Chapter 2. A gene that is vital in the control of cortical cell structure, called the lissencephaly gene (**LIS1**), is on chromosome 17 (17p13.3). This gene is probably involved in cell signalling during fetal neuronal migration of the cerebrum. The microdeletion of this gene is a major cause of these 'smooth brain' disorders. Other genes have also been found: **LIS2** at 7q22; **LIS3** at 12q12-q14; **LISX1** at Xq22.3-q23, and **LISX2** at Xp22.13. Lissencephalic disorders are usually divided into type I ('classical'), and type II (variant, or **Walker's lissencephaly**).

- **Type I lissencephaly** shows a smoothing of the brain surface with disruption of the cell structure (cytoarchitecture) causing a thick, four-layered cerebral cortex (normally, the cerebral cortex has six distinct cell layers). The cerebellum is basically normal. The clinical features are intellectual disability, diplegia (bilateral paralysis, and fits. Type I lissencephaly is more likely to be sporadic in origin, rather than inherited. Sporadic genetic changes involve the affected individual only and are not passed on to subsequent generations through the sperm or ova. **Miller–Dieker syndrome (MDS)**, which is caused by a microdeletion at gene locus 17p13.3 (the lissencephaly gene), results in severe intellectual disability with other neurological deficits (e.g. difficulty in swallowing), and growth deficiency with craniofacial defects (sometimes called the 'Miller–Dieker face') involving a prominent forehead, a short, upturned nose, protruding upper lip and small jaw. Death usually occurs within the first year of life.
- **Type II lissencephaly** shows a smoothing of the brain surface with disruption of the cytoarchitecture in a manner that results in no distinct cell layers. The main features of type II are severe neurological dysfunction from an early age, eye abnormalities, and hydrocephalus. Type II lissencephaly is thought more likely to be genetically inherited than type I. The disorders that fall into the type II category are those that cause various forms of muscular dystrophy (muscle wasting with weakness) due to the neurological dysfunction. **Walker–Warburg syndrome (WWS)** is a cause of severe intellectual and psychomotor disability, but it is also part of this group of muscle disorders known as

the congenital muscular dystrophies (CMD), in which muscle weakness, loss of muscle tone, and muscle contractures are predominant symptoms. Walker–Warburg syndrome shows an autosomal recessive inheritance pattern and is linked to five genes at loci 14q24.3, 9q34.1, 9q31, 22q12.3-q13.1, and 19q13.3. It should not be surprising that a brain lissencephaly causes muscle problems, as the main motor cortex that controls skeletal muscle movement is part of the cerebrum (Brodmann 4).

A deletion close to that seen in Miller–Dieker syndrome occurs at 17p11.2, resulting in the **Smith–Magenis syndrome**. This causes brachycephaly (short, broad skull caused by early closure of the coronal skull suture and excessive lateral skull growth), a prominent forehead, a broad face and nasal bridge, heart defects, hyperactivity, and fits. Maladaptive behaviour causes problems such as self-harm and sleep pattern disturbance (Dykens and Smith 1998).

Viruses in our brain DNA?

Among the billions of base pairs in our human DNA there resides about 5% DNA from retroviruses that have become incorporated in our genome over millions of years of evolution. They are particularly important in the brain and they have been passed down through successive generations in the same way as our own genes have. These viral genes do not code for any proteins, but they do form part of our epigenetics; i.e. providing an essential role in regulating gene expression. It is possible, therefore, that the viral genes could malfunction through mutation just as human genes do, and that could cause mental health problems. It is too early to tell yet, but they could prove to be targets for future treatments.

Key points

Chromosomes and genes

- The human karyotype is made up of 46 chromosomes.
- Autosomes are chromosomes 1 to 22 in the human karyotype, i.e. 22 pairs of autosomes.
- The chromosomes making up the final pair are the sex chromosomes – X and Y in males, X and X in females.
- Each pair consists of two chromosomes that are the same, called homologous chromosomes.
- Two alternative versions of the same gene are called alleles, one allele on each chromosome.
- Being from different parents, these alleles are of different traits.
- Whether a gene is expressed into the phenotype or not depends on whether it is dominant, recessive, or codominant.
- Genes demonstrate varying degrees of penetrance, or how much each individual gene contributes to the completed body (the phenotype).
- The DNA determines what proteins will be produced, the amino acids they will contain, and their sequence in the protein.
- Genes are found on the chromosome at sites called the gene locus (or gene slot), written by giving the chromosome number first, then the arm of the chromosome: 'p' for short arm and 'q' for long arm.
- Mutations are DNA errors, e.g. point mutations, translocations, deletions, frame shifts, inversions, base-sequence repeats, and fragile sites.

Disorders of inheritance

- Inherited genetic disorders are often familial, i.e. found in successive generations of the same family.
- First-degree relatives of an affected person are their parents, brothers, sisters, sons, or daughters; second-degree relatives are their grandparents, aunts, or uncles; and third-degree relatives are those such as cousins.
- Monozygotic (MZ) twins are identical twins, i.e. most of their genes are the same; dizygotic (DZ) twins are non-identical twins, i.e. about half of their genes are the same.

Autosomal disorders

- A genetic disorder may involve one gene or a few genes, but a chromosomal disorder involves abnormalities of whole or part of a chromosome, adding up to perhaps several thousand genes.
- A trisomy is one extra chromosome attached to a pair; a monosomy is only one chromosome instead of a pair.
- When all the cells contain a trisomy it is known as a full trisomy, but if there is a mix of trisomy and non-trisomy cells this is called a mosaic trisomy.

Sex chromosome abnormalities

- The sex chromosomes are X and Y, where XX corresponds to female and XY to male.
- 'Maleness' requires the Y chromosome, whereas 'femaleness' occurs in the absence of the Y chromosome.
- X-linked gene disorders are more severe in males than in females.
- XXY male is Klinefelter's syndrome and XXX is superwoman syndrome.
- These conditions are trisomies, i.e. three chromosomes in place of two (47 chromosomes in the karyotype).
- XYY males also occur.
- Monosomy means one chromosome in place of two (giving 45 chromosomes).
- Monosomy X is Turner's syndrome.
- The X chromosome is the source of a large variety of gene mutations that cause intellectual disability syndromes, albeit that they are generally rare.
- Fragile X syndrome is an intellectual disability syndrome caused by a trinucleotide repeat.

Genetic disorders

- Cri-du-chat syndrome (cry of cat syndrome) is caused by a deletion of part of the short arm of chromosome 5.
- Williams syndrome is caused by the loss of about 15 genes from 7q11.23.
- Prader–Willi and Angelman syndromes are both caused by imprinting errors or deletion of part of chromosome 15 at the gene locus 15q11.
- Lissencephalies, the 'smooth brain' disorders, include a number microdeletions resulting in intellectual disability and other symptoms.
- These disorders include Miller–Dieker and Walker–Warburg syndromes.

References

Cohen, P. (2000) Shaping up. *New Scientist*, **165** (2227): 16.

Das, I., Park, J.-M., Shin, J. H., Jeon, S. K., Lorenzi, H., Linden, D. J., Worley, P. F., and Reeves, R. H. (2013) Hedgehog agonist therapy corrects structural and cognitive deficits in a Down syndrome mouse model. *Scientific Translational Medicine*. DOI: 10.1126/scitranslmed.3005983.

Dykens, E. M. and Smith, A. C. M. (1998) Distinctiveness and correlates of maladaptive behaviour in children and adolescents with Smith–Magenis syndrome. *Journal of Intellectual Disability Research*, **42** (6): 481–489.

Faraone, S. V., Tsuang, M. T., and Tsuang, D. W. (1999) *Genetics of Mental Disorder, a Guide for Students, Clinicians and Researchers*. The Guilford Press, London.

Hill, D. and Dubey, J. P. (2002) *Toxoplasma gondii*: transmission, diagnosis and prevention. *Clinical Microbiology and Infection*, **8** (10): 634–640.

Laidman, J. (2014) Drugs for Down syndrome. *Scientific American Mind*, **25** (18). DOI: 10.1038/scientificamericanmind0314-18a.

Lenhoff, H. M., Wang, P. P., Greenberg, F., and Bellugi, U. (1997) Williams syndrome and the brain. *Scientific American*, **277** (6): 42–47.

Li, L. B., Chang, K.-H., Wang, P.-R., Hirata, R. K., Papayannopoulou, T., and Russell, D. W. (2012) Trisomy correction in Down's syndrome induced pluripotent stem cells. *Cell Stem Cell*, **11** (5): 615. DOI: 10.1016/j.stem.2012.08.004.

McCance, K. L., Huether, S. E., Brashers, V. L., and Rote, N. S. (2010) *Pathophysiology, The Biological Basis of Disease in Adults and Children* (6th edition). Elsevier–Mosby, London and Oxford, UK.

Sadock, B. J., Sadock, V. A., and Ruiz, P. (2009) *Kaplin and Sadock's Comprehensive Textbook of Psychiatry* (9th edition). Lippincott, Williams and Wilkins, Baltimore, MD.

Visootsak, J., Rosner, B., Dykens, E., Tartaglia, N., and Graham, J. M. (2007). Behavioural phenotype of sex chromosome aneuploidies: 48,XXYY, 48,XXXY, and 49,XXXXY. *American Journal of Medical Genetics Part A*, **143A** (11): 1198–203.

7 Pharmacology

- Introduction
- Pharmacokinetics
- Pharmacodynamics
- Pharmacotherapeutics
- Pharmacogenetics
- Key points

Introduction

The study of drugs is called **pharmacology** (*pharm* = 'drug'; *ology* = 'study of'), and involves the chemistry of the agents themselves, their passage through the body (**pharmacokinetics**), how they work in the body (**pharmacodynamics**), how they are used and administered in clinical practice (**pharmacotherapeutics**), and even how they can interact with genes and gene products (**pharmacogenetics**).

Pharmacokinetics means 'drug movement' and documents the passage of drugs through the body, from point of entry to point of exit. Pharmacodynamics studies the way drugs act in the body. A useful, if simplified distinction between pharmacokinetics and pharmacodynamics is that the former looks at *how the body handles the drug*, while the latter looks at *how the drug handles the body*.

Drugs are a major component in mental health treatment. Healthcare professionals are often responsible for the prescription and delivery of drug therapy, so it is vital that they have a good understanding of why a particular drug is prescribed, how drugs work, and how they are administered safely.

The major classes of drugs used in mental health are as follows (each class of drugs is covered in more detail in the chapters indicated):

- **Sedatives (hypnotics)**, have a calming effect at standard doses, and only cause sleep at higher doses (Chapter 16).
- **Anxiolytics** are anti-anxiety drugs. The word *anxiolytic* means 'anxiety breaking' (Chapter 9).
- **Antipsychotics**, alter behaviour without affecting consciousness (Chapter 10).
- **Antidepressants** are drugs used for the relief of depression (Chapter 11).
- **Antimanics** are mood-stabilising drugs (Chapter 11).
- **Stimulants** increase brain activity (Chapter 8).
- **Anticonvulsants** are drugs used to prevent fits (Chapter 12).

Pharmacokinetics

As noted earlier, pharmacokinetics means 'drug movement', i.e. the passage of drugs through the body, from the point of entry to the point of exit. For example, oral medication is affected by the processes of digestion, absorption, transportation by the blood, liver function, tissue storage, and excretion (Sadock and Sadock 2008). These are normally considered in the four stages of pharmacokinetics: absorption, distribution, metabolism, and elimination.

Absorption

This is the means by which drugs enter the body, and it varies according to the route of administration. The fastest absorption rate by far is by **intravenous (IV)** injection, in which absorption into the venous blood is instantaneous. **Intramuscular (IM**, direct injection into a muscle) and **subcutaneous (SC**, an injection just under the skin), and the oral method of administration have much slower rates of absorption. Because it would be impractical to administer all drugs by injection, the oral route becomes the method of choice wherever possible. Table 7.1 considers the various routes of drug administration.

Absorption of drugs from the digestive tract (mostly from the small bowel, or **ileum**) is affected by various factors. Bowel **motility**, the movement of the bowel that pushes the contents along, may vary according to health. Increased motility (as in **diarrhoea**) may prevent most of the absorption because the contents are propelled too quickly through the bowel. The opposite is also true: poor bowel motility (as in **constipation**) may prevent absorption as drug **transit**, i.e. movement through the bowel, is slowed down. Vomiting prevents drug absorption because oral drugs will be expelled too quickly if vomiting occurs soon after the drug is taken. Under normal bowel conditions, different drugs are absorbed differently. Lipid (fat-based) drugs absorb better than water-based drugs. The reason for this is that lipid drugs can pass through the cell membrane (which is also lipid) easier than water-based drugs. Nonlipid drugs have to find a water channel in the membrane in order to pass through, and this delays absorption. Charged particle drugs (i.e. those with positive and negative charges, called **polar** molecules) are not as well absorbed as nonpolar molecules. Drugs are best absorbed at their own **pH**; thus acidic drugs are mostly absorbed from the stomach, and alkaline drugs are best absorbed from alkaline areas of the bowel. Above all, oral medication must survive the digestive process. The fact that so many drugs remain unaffected by digestive enzymes is surprising, and lucky for us, otherwise all drugs would have to be given by injection. Imagine what life would be like if we had to give painkillers by injection just to stop a headache! Sadly, insulin is one drug that does not survive digestion, and this must be given by injection.

On absorption, oral drugs pass into the **hepatic portal vein** and are transported to the **liver**. The liver is the main site for drug metabolism, and so a percentage of the absorbed drug will be chemically changed by metabolism as it passes through the liver. The volume of drug changed by the liver occurs *before* any of this drug has reached the general circulation, and therefore *before* the drug has had the chance to do its job. This process of early metabolism by the liver is called **first pass metabolism**, and the percentage of the drug affected varies with different drugs. First pass metabolism only applies to oral medication, as administration by injection does not involve the hepatic portal vein. Finally the drug gets into the general circulation from the liver via the **hepatic vein**.[1] The amount of active drug arriving in the general circulation, either directly (by injection) or via the liver (from oral intake), is called the **bioavailability**. Because of variable amounts of first pass metabolism,

Table 7.1 Routes of drug administration

Route of administration	Comments
Oral	The most frequently used method of drug administration, because it is easy, can be used anywhere (e.g. at home), and is not embarrassing or painful. Absorption is generally very good and within an acceptable time frame. Medication given by this route, however, is the only route subject to **first pass metabolism** (see text).
Intravenous (IV)	Involves injection directly into a vein. Absorption into the blood is therefore instantaneous, but it is often inconvenient and may be painful.
Intramuscular (IM)	Involves injection directly into a muscle. Absorption into the blood is slower than by IV, as it requires the blood to collect the drug from the muscle, which acts as a temporary reservoir. **Depot** drugs are exceptionally slow in absorption because the drug is combined with an oil base that inhibits absorption, so the injections only need to be given weekly or even monthly.
Subcutaneous (SC)	Injection of drug given just under the skin into the dermis. Used for administration of slowly absorbed drugs that cannot be given by other means, e.g. insulin, which would be destroyed if given by mouth, and would act far too fast if given by IV or IM injections.
Intrathecal	Injection directly into the spinal canal during a procedure called a lumbar puncture. Not often used except to treat **meningitis** (inflammation of the meninges, the membranes covering the brain).
Rectal	Drugs incorporated into a suppository. Rectal administration is limited in use because of hygienic concerns and because it can be embarrassing. It is best used for treating local conditions of the rectum, e.g. constipation. Rarely it is used to give medication for symptoms of system disease where other routes are unavailable.
Inhalation	Inhaled medication directly into the lungs. Useful for treating lung conditions such as asthma. Small quantities of the drug are absorbed into the blood, but this is less than the oral route and therefore causes fewer side effects.
Topical	Medication rubbed into the skin in ointment or as a cream, or as patches stuck to the skin for long periods. With patches, small amounts are absorbed into circulation gradually, so it needs long periods of skin exposure, e.g. over 24 hours, for it to have a systemic effect. As creams and ointments, topical medication has a great value in treating local skin conditions, e.g. eczema.
Sublingual	Medication given under the tongue, not swallowed. The medication is absorbed directly into the mouth mucosa. The drug usually causes a quick beneficial response via this route.

the bioavailability varies from one oral drug to the next. The greater the extent of first pass metabolism occurring, the lower the bioavailability. Entry into general circulation is the starting point for distribution.

Distribution

Distribution describes the manner by which drugs are transported around the body. Most drugs by far are transported in the general blood circulation, but a small number of drugs are transported in the lymph. When drugs arrive in the blood plasma most are rapidly bound to blood proteins. The most common protein in the blood is **albumin**, so most drugs bind to

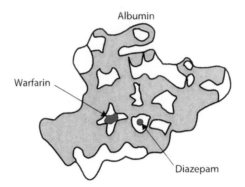

Albumin

Warfarin

Diazepam

Figure 7.1 Drugs binding to albumin. This simplified and stylised albumin molecule is binding diazepam and warfarin at different sites. See also Figure 7.6.

this. A few drugs bind to specific proteins, such as **glycoproteins**, **lipoproteins**, and **gammaglobulins** found in smaller quantities in the blood. A small amount of the drug remains unbound, i.e. dissolved in the plasma. Protein-bound drugs are not available for use, i.e. they are inactive, and therefore temporarily lose their bioavailability, until they are gradually released from the protein. These blood proteins are acting as a kind of drug 'bus', transporting drugs to their site of use, and also creating a drug reservoir. As drugs become detached from the protein they regain their activity, i.e. they become bioavailable (Figure 7.1).

Target tissues are those cells on which the drugs have an effect. **Nontarget tissues** are those cells unaffected by the drug. So **psychoactive** drugs will have an effect on the brain (their target tissue), but have no effect on other organs, such as bones or the bowel (nontarget organs). Tissues are regarded as target or nontarget depending on the presence or absence of **receptors** on the cell surface that can bind the drug. If the tissue has receptors on the cell surface that bind a specific drug, that tissue becomes a target for that drug.

Drugs entering the tissues from circulation may be further bound to tissue protein (e.g. muscle) or tissue fat (e.g. adipose). This binding creates another tissue reservoir and again temporarily removes the drug's bioavailability until the drug is gradually released from that reservoir. This drug reservoir storage is dependent on the amount of muscle and adipose present in the tissues, and these change slowly with age. It will also be affected by being excessively obese or muscular, or by being too thin. The elderly and children store drugs differently from the average adult.

Metabolism

Metabolism is the chemical alteration, or **biotransformation**, of drugs prior to removal from the body. This is necessary in the vast majority of cases because the drug, as administered, is not suitable for excretion as it stands. Drugs often need to be made more **hydrophilic**, i.e. more water soluble (*hydrophilic* means 'water-liking'). The best-absorbed drugs are lipid (fat-based) drugs, but we excrete water (as urine), not fat, so a change to the drug is necessary. There is also a need to make the active drug less active, so again, some chemical change is necessary. The final result of these chemical changes is known as a **metabolite** (*metabolite* = 'end product of metabolic change'). The metabolite is the usual product for excretion.

So the usual scenario for most drugs is:

Active drug → metabolism → inactive metabolite

However, a few variations do occur, such as:

Active drug → metabolism → active metabolite

Here, because the metabolite is also active, it carries on the function of the original drug until excreted. Another variation is:

Inactive drug (called a *prodrug*) → metabolism → active metabolite (often considered to be the drug).

The vast majority of drug metabolism occurs in the liver. Much smaller amounts of metabolism may occur in the circulation or in the kidney. Liver metabolism uses **enzyme systems** (several enzymes working together), which, like a conveyer-belt system, carry out chemical changes on the original drug. Two main phases of liver metabolism are:

- **Phase I**, the biotransformation of a drug to a more **polar** metabolite ('polar' meaning to give it an electrostatic charge, which allows it to blend better with water, as water molecules themselves are polar), and this then becomes easier to excrete through the kidneys. This phase uses enzyme systems, particularly a system known as **cytochrome P-450** (**CYP**, or **P450**), which is involved in the metabolism of many drugs. In humans, these enzymes are proteins found on the inner membranes of **mitochondria** or in the **endoplasmic reticulum** (**ER**) of cells. Mitochondria and the endoplasmic reticulum are cellular components involved in metabolism. The CYP enzyme system is involved in about 75% of drug metabolism.
- **Phase II**, the **conjugation** of the drug, or end product of phase I, with an endogenous substance. Conjugation means joining one substance (the drug or phase I product) with a second substance (mostly a natural product of the liver). This reduces the activity of most drugs.

Elimination

Elimination of drugs is mostly through the **renal system**, i.e. the **kidneys**, where the drug metabolites become a component of urine. Far less often, some drugs may be eliminated through the bowel in faeces, or very rarely through the skin in perspiration and in breast milk. Anaesthetic gases are mostly eliminated though the lungs during exhalation.

Renal excretion requires the drug metabolites to have some specific properties. First, the metabolites must be water soluble in order to mix with the urine. Fat-soluble substances cannot become a component of urine. Second, the metabolite molecular size must be small enough to pass through the holes in the **glomerular membrane** of the **nephron**. These holes are about 3 nanometres (nm) in diameter, so any molecules larger than this may have problems being filtered.

The rate of metabolism and the rate of excretion are the main factors that determine a drug's half-life. **Half-life** is the standard time it takes for the body to repeatedly clear 50% of

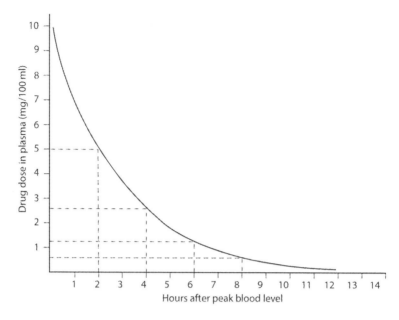

Figure 7.2 Illustration of a drug half-life. In this example, the drug half-life is 2 hours. By 2 hours after peak blood level, metabolism has removed 50% of the drug from the plasma (in this case, from 10 mg/100 ml to 5 mg/100 ml). By a further 2 hours, 50% of the remaining drug (5 mg/100 ml) is removed (down to 2.5 mg/100 ml). By another 2 hours again, 50% of the remaining drug (2.5 mg/100 ml) is removed (down to 1.25 mg/100 ml), and so on.

the blood plasma concentration of a drug. The half-life is best explained using a diagram, so consider the following example, as illustrated in Figure 7.2.

Drug X has reached maximum plasma concentration (regarded as 100%) a short time after consumption. Drug X has a half-life of 2 hours, which means that over the first 2 hours from this peak concentration the drug plasma concentration is reduced to half (50%). Over the second period of 2 hours (up to 4 hours from peak concentration), this 50% plasma concentration will be reduced by half (half of 50% is 25%). Over the third period of 2 hours (now up to 6 hours from the peak plasma concentration), the plasma concentration will again be reduced by half (half of 25% is 12.5%), and so on. The liver is removing the drug from the blood for metabolism, and the kidneys are removing the metabolites from the blood for excretion. The half-life of drugs varies widely, with some drugs having *very short* half-lives (less than 1 hour), or *short* half-lives (1 to 6 hours), or *intermediate* half-lives (6 to 12 hours) or *long* half-lives (12 to 24 hours), or *very long* half-lives (more than 24 hours). This has pharmacotherapeutic implications, because generally shorter half-life drugs may need to be given more often (possibly several times a day) whereas longer half-life drugs are given less frequently (possibly once daily).

If a drug metabolite cannot be excreted through the renal system into the urine, the alternative is for excretion from the bowel in the faeces. The metabolite leaves the liver in the bile, i.e. via the bile duct into the duodenum. From here it goes through the digestive tract and gets incorporated in the faeces. However, the bowel is the organ of absorption, so some of the metabolite will be reabsorbed back into the hepatic portal vein and return to the liver. The metabolite is again put into the bile, and passes into the bowel. So a 'bowel→liver→bowel'

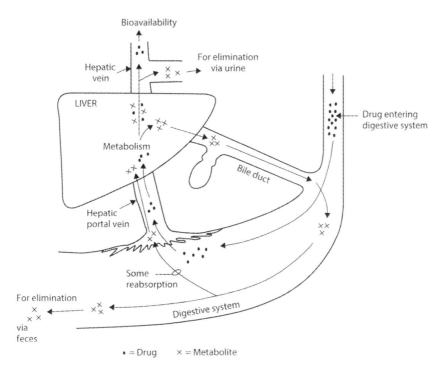

Figure 7.3 The enterohepatic cycle. Drug entering the digestive system from oral ingestion is absorbed and removed to the liver via the hepatic portal vein. First pass metabolism partly reduces this dose, producing some metabolite for excretion. Normally the metabolite would pass into general circulation and be excreted from the kidneys. Nonmetabolised drug enters the general circulation, and is known as the bioavailability. Occasionally the kidneys cannot excrete the metabolite so the liver must excrete it through the bile. This is emptied into the digestive system and thus excreted in the faeces. Some reabsorption of the metabolite will take place from the bowel back to the liver, which then recycles it via the bile once again. Each bowel–liver cycle reduces the amount reabsorbed by a small quantity.

cycle (the **enterohepatic cycle**) is set up, but with each cycle a small percentage of the metabolite is excreted (Figure 7.3). In this way the amount of drug metabolite in the body is gradually reduced with each cycle until zero or only a trace remains.

Pharmacodynamics

Pharmacodynamics is the study of the way drugs act in the body. Psychotropic drugs (i.e. those that act on the brain) work by altering the brain chemistry – mostly by acting on receptors or on ion channels.

Drugs acting on receptors

Receptors are present on brain cell surfaces, where they bind with the naturally produced chemicals called **neurotransmitters** and **neuromodulators** (see Chapter 4). These chemicals

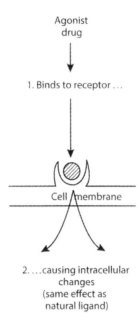

Agonist
drug

1. Binds to receptor . . .

Cell membrane

2. . . .causing intracellular
changes
(same effect as
natural ligand)

Figure 7.4 Agonist drugs are those that bind to a receptor and activate the receptor in the same way as the natural ligand would.

act by binding to the receptor and then triggering a sequence of changes within the cell. These changes can be made rapidly through **ionotropic** receptors, or over a longer period of time through **metabotropic** receptors (Chapter 4). The changes may also be to increase cellular activity (**excitatory**) or decrease cellular activity (**inhibitory**).

Two main types of drug act on brain receptors: the **agonists** and the **antagonists**.

Agonist drugs (such as the dopamine agonist **bromocriptine**) bind to specific receptors (bromocriptine binds to dopamine receptors) and stimulate (or activate) these receptors, much as the natural brain chemical (called the ligand) does (dopamine is the natural ligand for dopamine receptors) (Figure 7.4). These drugs are useful supplements for situations in which the natural ligand is in low supply or is missing.

Antagonist drugs are sometimes called 'blockers' (e.g. the dopamine antagonist **chlorpromazine**). Antagonists bind to specific receptors (chlorpromazine binds to dopamine receptors) and block them without stimulating them. As a result, the ligand is prevented from binding. This reduces the activity of the ligand on the receptors significantly, and antagonists are used when activity of these receptors is excessive and therefore causing symptoms (Figure 7.5).

Competitive antagonists are two or more drugs that compete for the same binding site. Each drug usually has a 50% chance of binding, so the therapeutic outcome may be less certain. Because of this, prescribing two drugs at the same time which are competitive antagonists is usually unjustified and would be better avoided.

Partial agonists are drugs that bind to the receptor and activate the receptor but not to the same extent that a full agonist or the ligand would do. A simple way of looking at this is to say that if the ligand or the full agonist drug activates the receptor 100%, the partial

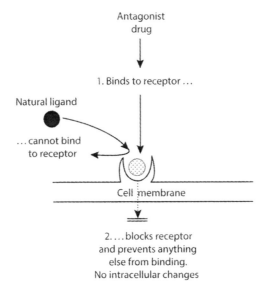

Figure 7.5 An antagonist drug is one that bind to a receptor and blocks it. It does not activate the receptor and prevents the natural ligand from binding to that receptor. Antagonists are often called 'blockers'.

agonist may only activate the receptor 70%. This has the effect of not switching the receptor off totally but reducing its activity. In some respects, partial agonists act in a similar way to antagonists because by preventing the ligand from binding they reduce ligand activity in the brain, just as antagonists do.

Drugs acting on ion channels

Ion channels exist in nearly all neuronal membranes and when these channels are open they allow for the passage of an ion in or out of the cell. Ion channels (especially Na^+ and K^+ channels) are particularly important during nerve impulse (**action potential**) transmission along an **axon** (Chapter 3).

A range of drugs act on ion channels in the brain to control events such as action potential transmission. Many of the drugs are **channel blockers**, i.e. they prevent the passage of the ion through the channel. Typical of this kind of drug are anticonvulsants such as sodium or calcium channel blockers.

Drugs acting on transport pumps

Some drugs work by blocking (or inhibiting) the action of **pumps** in the cell membrane. Some cell activities rely on the transportation of substances, such as neurotransmitters, across the membrane, and this process can be interrupted to change the balance of these substances in the brain and thus affect brain cell activity. A good example of this is the use of certain antidepressant drugs that inhibit the membrane pumps at the neuron terminus and therefore increase neurotransmitter in the synapse (Chapter 11).

Pharmacotherapeutics

Pharmacotherapeutics is the study of how drugs are used in clinical practice, including prescription, dose calculation, means of administration, patient assessment for reactions and side effects, drug storage, and many other aspects.

Drugs come in several different forms (see also Table 7.1):

- **Tablets** and **capsules** are probably the most common form of drugs and are taken orally (Table 7.2).
- **Syrups**, **elixirs**, **solutions**, **colloids**, and **suspensions** are liquid medications (Table 7.3).
- **Injectable solutions** are **intravenous (IV)**, **intramuscular (IM)**, **subcutaneous (SC)**, or **intrathecal** (via a **lumbar puncture**). Injectable drugs are absorbed quicker than oral drugs and are used for emergencies, and to avoid digestion and first pass metabolism. Intrathecal injections are much more efficient at reaching the central nervous system than any other route.
- **Inhalations** are sprayed and inhaled directly into the lungs, mostly to treat a respiratory condition.
- **Suppositories** are lubricated and inserted into the rectum, mostly to treat a rectal condition.
- **Creams**, **lotions**, **ointments**, and **patches** are applied directly to the skin, either for the treatment of skin conditions (**topical** applications) or systemic conditions (e.g. patches).

Biosimilar medications are those that are being developed to be very similar to natural medications (i.e. those derived from a natural organic source and referred to as the '**reference**' or '**originator medicine**'). The biosimilar drugs are clinically equivalent to the reference medicine, i.e. they act in the same way, and are increasingly replacing the original drugs.

Therapeutic window

The therapeutic window is the dose range that exists from the lowest effective dose of a drug up to a dose where there are more harmful effects than beneficial effects. Below the lowest dose of the window the drug is ineffective and useless. Above the highest dose of the

Table 7.2 Different types of dry oral medication

Tablets and **powders**	Most commonly prescribed format for medication, each tablet contains a single dose of the drug. Tablets may be **enteric coated** (a coating that allows the medication to survive gastric conditions and be absorbed further into the digestive tract and also to reduce gastric irritation). Others may be soluble in water before drinking (including **powders**). Each sachet of powder contains a single dose of the drug. **Modified-release** tablets contain special inert substances used to modify the rate, the site, or the time of release of the active drug.
Capsules	Medication, often in granular format, contained within a soft dissolvable shell. Different granules may have variable time delays in absorption, so an even absorption rate is achieved over several hours (modified release).
Gum	Chewable medication in a gum, the drug is released in the mouth during chewing.
Melts	Medication made in a solid form that dissolves (melts) in the mouth, mainly for oral absorption.

Table 7.3 Different types of liquid medication

Solutions	A **homogeneous** (i.e. uniform throughout) mixture of two or more substances. One substance is the solvent (often water) and the other is a solute (an agent dissolved in the solvent), e.g. a sodium chloride solution (used in medical practice as **normal saline**, a 0.9% solution of sodium chloride in water).
Colloids	Very small solids (particles that do not dissolve) that remain dispersed in a liquid for a long time due to their small size (less than 1 mm) and their electrical charges. These particles take a very long time to settle because their very small masses have extremely low gravitational force. Some colloids are given intravenously as **plasma expanders**, to boost plasma volume following blood loss.
Suspensions (usually for oral use) and **lotions** (for external use only).	A **heterogeneous** (i.e. made from non-uniform dissimilar components) mixture with relatively large undissolved particles dispersed throughout a liquid. Larger particle size results in settlement of the particles quickly when left to stand. Therefore suspensions must be shaken before use to disperse the particles. An example is a pediatric suspension of paracetamol, a pain-relieving drug. Lotions are aqueous preparations containing a very fine particle insoluble substance. They are for external use only. They often have 'Shake well' and 'External use only' labels. An example is calamine lotion.
Elixirs and **syrups**	The active drug is mixed and dissolved in a liquid, either a concentrated sucrose solution (as in syrups) or an aromatic, sweetened hydroalcoholic solution (as in elixirs).

window the drug becomes a threat to health, with the potential for severe side effects and a risk of overdose. Some drugs have a narrow therapeutic window and must be prescribed and administered with caution because it would not be difficult to go above the therapeutic window and cause toxicity.

Drugs are normally given a dose range that falls within this window. Generally, patients are prescribed the lowest dosage within this range at first, and this can then be raised safely at a later time if necessary.

Drug names

All drugs have three types of name:

- A **chemical name**, based on the chemical structure, used only in science, and never used in clinical practice (i.e. not used on prescriptions). An example is **7-chloro-1,3-dihydro-1-methyl-5-phenyl-2H-1,4-benzodiazepin-2-one**.
- An **official**, **approved**, **generic** or **nonproprietary** name, used in clinical practice on prescriptions. *Nonproprietary* means there is no legal protection by means of a trademark, patent, or copyright on this drug name. As such, this name identifies the drug but it does not belong to any particular drug company (see the next point below). The generic name for the example chemical above is **diazepam**.

- A **trade**, **brand** or **proprietary** name, given to the drug by a specific pharmaceutical company who produces it. *Proprietary* means the drug name is legally protected by a copyright, trademark, or patent. Different companies in different countries will give the same drug different trade names. The result is a large collection of trade names worldwide for each separate agent. In the UK, the best-known trade name for Diazepam is **Valium**. Trade names are not used on UK NHS prescriptions because of cost implications.

Drug administration

Before any drug is prescribed (other than in an emergency), a patient assessment is required. The purpose of this assessment is to determine whether drugs are necessary, what drugs would be most beneficial to the patient, and to check if the patient is able to comply with the treatment regime. The assessment consists of a medical and drug history (including an appraisal of the patient's current medication, if any), an examination of the main physical parameters by clinical observations (especially pulse, blood pressure, and respiration), a psychological evaluation to determine the patient's ability to comply with a drug regime safely, and an assessment of the patient's social and cultural background (e.g. the patient may be part of a drug addiction culture, or may have social problems that could interfere with safe drug administration). A treatment plan is drawn up that sets out not just the pharmacological therapy, but other therapies considered beneficial to the patient. The patient's family members are probably in the best position to help to ensure compliance to the treatment plan, and are usually eager to help. It is therefore very important to involve the family whenever possible, with the patient's knowledge and agreement, in the planning of a treatment regime. Information on the drugs prescribed, dosage, administration routine, effects, and side effects is shared with the patient and the family. In the community, monitoring consists of checking daily or weekly to see if the patient is taking the drugs correctly and what improvements or side effects have occurred. The family can assist by giving a progress report and by reporting any problems. In hospital, with 24-hour care, it should be easier to check drug compliance and the wanted and unwanted affects of the drugs. For patients on long-term drug regimes, healthcare professionals maintain a liaison role with the patient and their family on all matters concerning the drug therapy.

When administering drugs, it is vital to ensure that:

- the correct drug is given, according to the prescription;
- the correct dose is given, according to the prescription;
- the drug is given to the correct patient;
- the drug is given at the correct time, according to the prescription;
- the drug is given via the correct route.

In addition, it is necessary to check these factors with another healthcare professional where possible, as this reduces the error risk, and to record the administration on the appropriate documentation.

Drugs are kept safe by:

- preventing children and confused patients from having access to them;
- preventing drug abusers from gaining access to prohibited drugs;
- ensuring they are stored correctly according to the law (in the case of controlled drugs) and according to the instructions given with the medication to prevent deterioration;

- keeping drugs only while in date;
- disposing of unwanted and out-of-date drugs safely, usually by returning them to any pharmacy.

Disposal of unwanted medical preparations (**DUMP**) campaigns are sometimes carried out to encourage people to stop the storage of unwanted drugs at home. In one such campaign, one-third of a million tablets and capsules were returned to pharmacies, and over 70% of these were more than a year out of date. On another occasion, in one UK city alone, two-and-a-quarter tons of out of date medications were returned! Worse than storing these unwanted drugs is flushing them down the sink or toilet. This should never happen – especially with antibiotics, which must *never* be released into the environment.

Dose calculations

It is so important to calculate the correct dosage of medications to prevent potentially dangerous drug errors. Olsen et al. (2010) state that there are four elements to calculating drug dosage accurately:

- common sense;
- the ability to carry out mental arithmetic;
- the ability to check the answers with a calculator;
- understanding the correct formula.

For tablets, the formula for calculation is:

Dose prescribed ÷ stock dose

Here are two simple examples:

1   Six milligrams (6 mg) of the drug is prescribed, but the tablets kept in stock are 2 mg each. The number of tablets to be given is: $6 \div 2 = 3$ tablets.
2   One gram (1 g) of the drug is prescribed, but the tablets are 500 mg each.

First convert grams to milligrams (1 g = 1000 mg) so that you are working in the same units throughout the calculation (in this case milligrams). Never work in mixed units, because this makes the answer to the calculation meaningless. The number of tablets to be given is:

$1000 \div 500 = 2$ tablets.

For liquids, the formula for calculation is:

(Dose prescribed ÷ stock dose) × stock volume

Two simple examples:

1   Fifteen milligrams (15 mg) of the liquid drug is prescribed; the stock syrup is 10 mg per 2 millilitres (2 ml). The volume of syrup to be given is:

$(15 \div 10) \times 2$.

Always do the bracket part of the calculation first, which in this case is (1.5), then remove the brackets to complete the calculation, e.g.

1.5 × 2 = 3 ml.

[A quick check of accuracy is possible: in this case 2 ml is too little (only 10 mg), but 4 ml is too much (20 mg), so the answer falls between 2 ml and 4 ml, i.e. 3 ml].

2   Prescribed: 250 mg; stock dose is 100 mg per 1 ml. The volume of syrup to be given is:

(250 ÷ 100) × 1

Doing the bracket part first gives:

2.5 × 1 = 2.5 ml

[Quick check, 250 mg to give: 1 ml of syrup is 100 mg (not enough);

2 ml = 200 mg (still not enough); 3 ml = 300 mg (too much); so the result must be between 2 ml and 3 ml, i.e. 2.5 ml].

Always state the units in the answer (i.e. mg or ml). Simply giving a number with no units could mean anything, and is therefore potentially dangerous and confusing.

Polypharmacy and drugs in the elderly

Polypharmacy means that multiple different types of drugs are prescribed at the same time. Generally, it is better to prescribe as few types of drugs together as possible, and to leave a time gap, often several days, when switching from one drug to another. This time gap allows the body an opportunity to fully excrete the first drug before starting the second. Unfortunately this is not always possible, and it is not unusual to find two, three or more drugs prescribed together. It should be remembered that polypharmacy also occurs when a single drug is prescribed but the patient decides to take additional drugs for themselves, such as a headache remedy or even drugs of addiction. Polypharmacy increases the risk of drug interactions and side effects, and this is why it is better avoided when possible. Also, with polypharmacy, some patients may get drugs muddled up and start taking the wrong drug at the wrong time, increasing the risk of serious drug errors. Since the elderly are prescribed more drugs than any other age group, and they can get confused more often than younger people, they carry the biggest risk of serious drug errors, side effects, and interactions. Multiple drugs may also be stored badly, labelled poorly or not at all, and even in some cases mixed up in a single container. When this happens, multiple drugs stored together makes it easier to forget individual drug administration times and also often means drugs are kept long after their expiry dates. With some patients, drug compliance is a problem when only one drug is involved, so the problem of compliance is compounded by the prescription of several drugs together. All this turns safe administration of drugs into a nightmare.

The incidence of drug reactions and interactions, and drug-related mortalities, increases with age. About 10% of UK elderly admissions to hospital are due to drug reactions, and the most common drug groups involved are cardiac drugs (e.g. digoxin) and drugs for the central nervous system (e.g. antidepressants). The elderly don't always provide an accurate drug history during examination and rely on relatives to fill in any gaps in their memory. A confused and poor drug history makes diagnosis difficult. Confusion can be a side effect of the some drugs, so it may be prudent to stop the drugs and wait until they have been eliminated before examination, diagnosis, and further prescription.

Drug reactions in the elderly are usually due to:

- overprescription, some patients accumulating 10 or more different drugs;
- inadequate review of long-term medication;
- inadequate clinical assessment;
- altered pharmacokinetics due to age and disease;
- complicated drug regimes leading to impaired drug compliance.

Poor compliance in the elderly is a big problem. About 75% of elderly patients make mistakes in drug administration. Some 25% of these mistakes are dangerous, life-threatening errors. The reasons for poor drug compliance are as follows.

- As symptoms improve the patient stops taking the drug as they feel it is not required anymore. This is a big problem, especially with antibiotics, because the course of medication must be completed.
- Poor eyesight means they cannot read the labels and they may resort to guessing, or stopping the drug.
- Inadequate explanation given about taking the drug when it's first prescribed (e.g. a significant number of elderly patients fail to remove the wrapper from suppositories before use). It may be beneficial for this information to be written down and displayed in a prominent position.
- Drugs may be difficult to swallow or taste bitter, or they cause unpleasant side effects, and these problems may cause the patient to stop taking them.
- Some drug containers are child proof, and as a result are often elderly proof as well, especially for a patient with arthritic fingers.
- Some patients will always simply forget to take their medication.

Preplanning and discussion with the patient and their relatives is required when drugs are prescribed, to ensure the patient is fully aware of the nature of the drug and its potential side effects. A series of drug reviews should be scheduled at regular time periods (e.g. weekly) to enable the patient to get the greatest benefit from the prescribed medication. The following is a guide to safer drug administration in the elderly:

- Prescribe the smallest number of drugs as possible at any one time – generally no more than three – and at the lowest effective dose. The starting dose should be kept at a minimum at first, but can be increased later if necessary when it can be confirmed that the patient is not reacting to the drug (Labbate et al. 2010).
- Don't add any more drugs to the original prescription at a later date unless they are essential, and if another drug is required, consider which drug to stop first in order to keep to the maximum of three.
- Monitor the drugs weekly, checking particularly for drug compliance and side effects.
- Patients and relatives should be aware of potential side effects, so they can check daily, and that they know what to do about them.
- Ensure the administration details are easily readable and displayed in a relevant place, e.g. in large print, and maybe fixed to the front of the drugs cabinet.

Changes in the body as we get older affect the pharmacokinetics of drugs, so these changes must be allowed for when prescribing medication. The elderly have increased gastric pH (i.e. less acid), less gut movement (reduced motility), and lower blood flow to the stomach. These changes affect the absorption of drugs given by mouth. However, despite these changes the elderly generally tolerate oral drugs well. Diseases or disturbance of the gastrointestinal system, including vomiting and diarrhoea, may seriously disturb drug absorption rates. Diarrhoea often involves an increased in gut transit time, i.e. the bowel contents are propelled through the gut faster. This includes any oral medication, much of which may be eliminated before it is absorbed. Changes in the structural tissues of the body result in an overall reduction in body weight, and this also includes a reduction in the total body water content. Water-soluble drugs are eliminated quicker because of this reduced water content, and these drugs will then have a shorter half-life. Stored lipids in adipose tissue increases with age, and this changes the lean to fat ratio, which has implications for drug storage in the tissues.

There are variations in this ratio between the sexes, with females generally storing more adipose than males. Increased storage of fat-soluble drugs in adipose delays excretion and lengthens the drug half-life. Plasma albumin falls with age, and this reduces the protein binding of drugs and increases the bioavailability due to increased amounts of free drug in circulation. Lower cardiac output in the elderly slightly delays drug distribution, and this favours an increase in plasma drug levels. Reduced liver mass and less blood flow through the liver with increasing age causes slower enzyme activity and reduced drug metabolism (increasing the drug half-life). The overall effect of all these changes is generally to increase the amount of active drug in the blood. These are the normal changes expected with growing old, but if you add disease states to this picture the changes become truly significant. With increased active drug in the body, taking additional doses creates a serious risk of drug accumulation in the body.

Renal elimination of drugs is reduced as renal function declines. Reduced glomerular filtration will increase the drug half-life because the drugs and metabolites are then retained in circulation. If multiple drugs are prescribed, some of these drugs may compete for excretion through tubular secretion (the third stage of urine production) and those that lose this competition are delayed in their elimination, further lengthening their half-lives.

Drug interactions

Drug interactions are unwanted effects caused by one drug acting against another when more than one drug is administered. Interactions occur not only between prescribed drugs, but also when only one drug is prescribed but the patient decides also to take an *over-the-counter* medication. A typical scenario may be a patient who takes their prescribed medication then shortly after decides to take an aspirin for headache. The self-prescribed aspirin may interact with the prescribed medication. Also, drug interactions can occur between a prescribed or self-prescribed drug and substances consumed on a regular basis, such as nicotine, alcohol, or caffeine. It is common for patients to smoke and to drink alcohol or coffee, and this introduces more drugs into the system, which can then interact with the prescribed drugs. It is often the case that prescribed medication information leaflets warn patients not to drink while taking the medicines. In the case of drug abuse, patients run a high risk of interaction if they continue to abuse drugs while taking prescribed or over-the-counter medication.

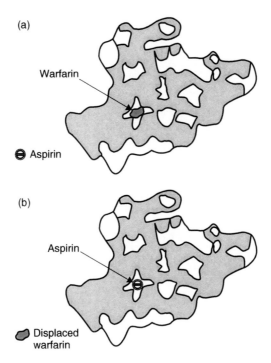

Figure 7.6 Pharmacokinetic interaction involving competitive binding during distribution. Here the stylised albumin molecule in (a) binds the drug warfarin. Aspirin has arrived in the circulation. In (b) the aspirin has displaced and replaced the warfarin, which is now unbound. Each free drug molecule increases the activity of the medication (in this case the warfarin), but in practice this activity increase is minimal, given that free drug is excreted quickly, and that it is diluted rapidly because it is distributed throughout the circulation.

Drug interactions fall into two main categories: those that occur during pharmacokinetics, and those that occur during pharmacodynamics.

Pharmacokinetic interactions

These interactions occur during absorption, distribution, metabolism, or elimination of drugs. During absorption, competition between drugs for absorption sites may mean that one medication is delayed in absorption, and this will affect its activity in the body. During distribution, one drug may compete for protein binding with another drug, and so one may displace the other drug from its binding site. This increases the activity of the displaced drug (because it is now free) but delays the activity of the competing drug (because it is now protein bound) (Figure 7.6).

The greatest risk of interactions occurs during metabolism. Drugs may compete for the enzyme systems that process them. If the enzyme system is busy processing one drug (call it drug A), a second drug (call it drug B) may have to wait its turn to be processed. This lengthens the half-life of drug B and it will continue to perform its functions longer than expected. If then a second dose of drug B is administered, this overlap in dosage could

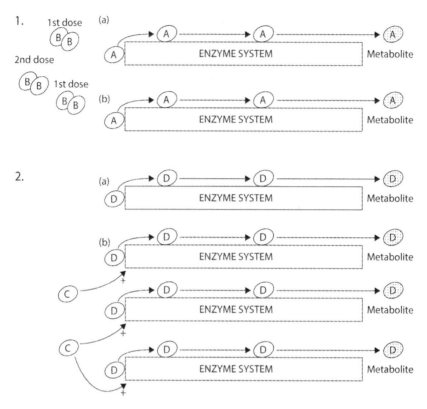

Figure 7.7 Drug interaction in the liver by enzyme occupation and induction. In 1(a), drug A is being metabolised by the enzyme system, while drug B metabolism is delayed, which prolongs drug B's half-life. In 1(b), a second dose of drug B causes the potential for an overdose. In 2(a), drug D is occupying a minimal amount of enzyme system. In 2(b), the arrival of drug C activates further enzyme systems, which increases the metabolism of drug D, thus shortening its half-life.

raise the blood level to the maximum of the therapeutic window or above, and cause an accidental overdose. Many drugs activate enzymes (in a process called enzyme induction) or increase or reduce enzyme activity in the liver. Either way, one drug (call it drug C) may significantly influence the metabolism of another drug (call it drug D) by the process of enzyme induction, causing changes in the activity, half-life, and excretion of drug D (Figure 7.7).

Pharmacodynamic interactions

Drugs may compete with each other for the same receptor binding sites at the point of activity. Competitive antagonists are an example of this (Figure 7.8).

Two competing agonists would enhance each other's activity and therefore give a greater effect than expected, possibly to the point of toxicity. Two drugs with the opposite effects to each other may just cancel each other out and become ineffectual. A few pharmacodynamic

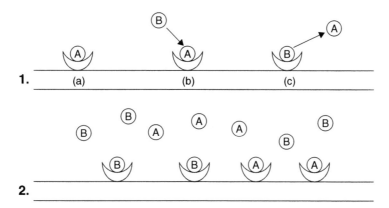

Figure 7.8 Pharmacodynamic interactions at a receptor. In 1, drug A occupies the receptor. In 1(b), drug B challenges drug A for receptor occupancy. In 1(c), drug B has replaced drug A at the receptor, shortening the active period of drug A. In 2, a mix of drugs A and B, both being equal competitors for the receptors, results in some receptors being occupied with drug A, others with drug B. The result could be a doubling of the effect (if they both had similar activity) or a cancellation of the effect (if they both had opposing actions).

drug interactions are beneficial, but by far the majority cancel each other out at best, and can be harmful or even fatal at worst.

Toxicology and side effects

Toxicology is the scientific study of the effects of toxic chemical agents (poisons) on the human body. Toxicology covers not just drugs but any chemical agent taken into the body, e.g. the accidental ingestion of a detergent or bleach by children. The toxic effects of drugs are known as **pharmacotoxicology**. Drugs are most likely to cause toxic effects in the upper range of their therapeutic window and in **overdose** (dosages above the therapeutic window), but any dose of a drug can cause a rapid and unexpected toxic effect in susceptible people. The term *side effects* is used to describe unwanted, unpleasant adverse symptoms occurring as a result of drug consumption at normal dosage. They are usually mild and mostly cause no lasting harm. However, toxic effects (or toxic reactions) are sudden, serious effects on the body, usually as a result of high dosage, which are potentially harmful or even life-threatening.

Side effects are the result of the drug acting on parts of the body it was not intended for it to act on. An example of this is the dopamine antagonist chlorpromazine. Ideally this drug should block receptors in the brain pathways known as the **mesocortical** and **mesolimbic** pathways, but unfortunately it also blocks receptors in the **nigrostriatal** pathway, and this causes unwanted side effects involving difficulties with movement (Chapter 10).

Side effects may be the reason for patient noncompliance, and this should be considered when patients refuse to take their medication. Side effects are often mild, and they may reduce in severity over a period of time without any need for intervention. If they are unpleasant enough, the patient should seek medical advice so the drug dose may be safely reduced, or another drug substituted. There should be no need to put up with unpleasant side effects.

With toxic reactions the drug must be stopped immediately and urgent medical intervention obtained. Very severe reactions may require life-support measures, and investigations may be necessary to determine the liver and renal function. Overdose from ingested drugs often requires measures to be taken to recover as much drug from the body as possible, e.g. a **gastric lavage**, also known as a 'stomach washout'. The action of some drugs can be reversed by giving a second drug, e.g. the effects of morphine can be reversed with the drug **naloxone**.

A full account of drug side effects, interactions, and allergies can be found in Blows (2012, Chapter 14).

Tolerance, dependence, addiction, and withdrawal

Tolerance means that over a period of time on a specific drug the effects of this drug gradually diminish, and the patient finds the need to slightly increase the dosage, every so often, to get the same beneficial effect. Of course, increasing the dosage means a higher risk of side effects and a step closer to achieving a toxic dose. Tolerance may be due to changes in the cell surface receptors that bind the drug. Over a period of time of taking the same drug, the surface receptors decrease in number (in a process called **downregulation**), so with fewer receptors the cell binds less drug. One course of action, which may prove better than increasing the dose, is to stop the drug altogether for a few days whenever possible (sometimes known as a '**drug holiday**'). The exceptions to this are antibiotics, where it is important to complete the course. A few days without the drug encourages the cells to replace the receptors (called **upregulation**).

Dependence occurs over a long period of time when the drug becomes an everyday part of normal life, because stopping the drug would mean that withdrawal symptoms then occur. **Withdrawal** symptoms are usually very unpleasant (e.g. headache, vomiting, sometimes fits) and the drugs are taken to avoid these, i.e. taken just to feel normal. Sometimes you hear people say 'I can't do anything in the morning until I have had my cup of coffee'. This is a form of caffeine dependence.

Addiction is when drugs are taken repeatedly for the purpose of mental pleasure and euphoria. One such experience promotes a repeat of this experience. After a number of repeated doses, failure to take the drug results in an unpleasant low state of mind, akin to depression, which the addict tries to avoid by taking more drugs. Therefore, both dependence and addiction promote legal or illegal drug-seeking behaviour but for different reasons. Occurrence of addiction varies according to different drugs (some cause addiction faster than others), but generally addiction occurs over a shorter time span than dependence.

Pharmacogenetics

Pharmacogenetics is the study of how genetic variation between people causes different responses to drugs. It has been known for many years that no two people respond alike to the same dose of the same drug, but it has always been difficult to explain why. Now, recent advances in genetics have revealed that because everyone has a unique set of genes they respond to drugs in a unique manner. This applies to any one individual and to any race. There are clinical implications attached to this research because is shows that no single drug, even at identical dosage, will have the same impact on everyone. Drug treatments should be tailormade for each individual if possible, with the drugs and dosage that are best for them. This indicates that careful assessments combined with a sound knowledge of drugs are critical prerequisites for prescribing drugs.

Key Points

Pharmacokinetics

- Pharmacokinetics is the study of the way drugs pass through the body from the point of entry to the point of exit.
- First pass metabolism reduces the dose of many drugs given by mouth but does not affect drugs given by injection.
- The bioavailablity is the amount of drug arriving in general circulation after first pass metabolism.
- The half-life is the time it takes to reduce the blood concentration of a drug by 50% over each successive half-life period.
- Most drugs are metabolised by the liver and excreted through the kidneys.
- Liver and renal disease will affect drug half-lives.

Pharmacodynamics

- Pharmacodynamics is the study of the way drugs act in the body.
- An agonist is a drug that binds to a receptor and activates that receptor.
- An antagonist (or 'blocker') is a drug that binds to a receptor but does not activate that receptor. Instead, it prevents the natural ligand from activating that receptor.

Pharmacotherapeutics

- It is so important to calculate the correct dosage of medications to prevent dangerous drug errors.
- Dosage may be affected by the lean to fat ratio, which can change with age, and by liver or kidney disease.
- The therapeutic window is the dose range from the lowest effective dose of a drug up to the dose where there are more harmful effects than beneficial effects.
- Patients should be warned of the most common side effects and given information on what to do if side effects occur.
- Drugs should never be kept or used after the 'use by' date, and should be disposed of safely by returning them to the pharmacy.
- Weekly or monthly drug reviews should be part of the standard care.
- As few drugs as possible, and certainly no more than three drugs, should be given at a time, to prevent drug interactions.

Pharmacogenetics

- The study of how genetic variation between people causes different responses to drugs.

Note

1 The *hepatic vein* and *hepatic portal vein* are easily muddled. The hepatic portal vein provides a passage, or portal, between the digestive system and the liver and is not part of the general circulation. Blood flows from the gut to the liver. The hepatic vein drains blood from the liver back to the general circulation, i.e. it is part of the general circulation.

References

Blows, W. T. (2012) *The Biological Basis of Clinical Observations* (2nd edition). Routledge, Abingdon, Oxon.

Labbate, L. A., Fava, M., Rosenbaum, J. F., and Arana, G. W. (2010) *Handbook of Psychiatric Drug Therapy*. Lippincott Williams and Wilkins, Philadelphia, PA.

Olsen, J. L., Giangrasso, A. P., Shrimpton, D. M., Dillon, P. M., and Cunningham, S. (2010) *Dosage Calculations for Nurses*. Pearson Education, Harlow, UK.

Sadock, B. J. and Sadock, V. A. (2008) *Kaplan and Sadock's Concise Textbook of Clinical Psychiatry* (3rd edition). Lippincott, Williams and Wilkins, Baltimore, MD.

8 Drug abuse

- The reward pathways of the brain
- The opiate drugs
- Cocaine
- Amphetamines and other dopamine-enhancing drugs
- Cannabis
- Alcohol
- Nicotine
- Caffeine
- The hallucinogenic drugs
- Potential for drugs of addiction now used in medicine
- Key points

The reward pathways of the brain

One of the major quests in brain research has been to identify the neurological areas involved in euphoria and pleasure. This endeavour has met with some success and has resulted in the identification of some areas of the brain involved in drug addiction. As with many other functions of the brain, the so-called **reward centres** are not one or two isolated areas but rather appear to be several centres linked by reward pathways involving mostly dopamine as the neurotransmitter (see Chapter 1, Table 1.2).

Important areas stand out as reward centres: in particular the **medial forebrain bundle (MFB)**, which links the **ventral tegmental area (VTA)** of the midbrain with the **nucleus accumbens (NA)** (Figure 8.1). This pathway forms part of a system called the **mesotelen-cephalic dopamine system** (Figure 8.1a and c). Cells bodies of this system within the VTA give rise to axons that become the MFB. These then pass to the NA. The system also serves other nuclei, notably the **septum** and the **prefrontal cortex** and two other important areas of the brain, the **limbic cortex** and **amygdala** (Chapter 1). This dopamine pathway is strongly implicated in many self-administered stimulatory drug effects including those of the opiates and amphetamines, and is therefore of great importance in drug abuse research. The VTA is involved in behavioural arousal, and activation of this centre causes dopamine to be released from the synapses at the end of the medial forebrain bundle. This dopamine binds to receptors in the NA, causing activity of the NA. One such receptor is the **A1 receptor**,

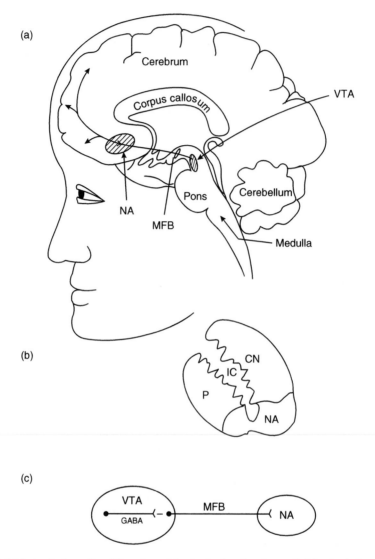

Figure 8.1 (a) Lateral view of a mid-section of the brain showing the medial forebrain bundle (MFB) extending from the ventral tegmental area (VTA) to the nucleus accumbens (NA). (b) The nucleus accumbens in association with the caudate nucleus (CN), internal capsule (IC) and the putamen (P). (c) The mesotelencephalic doperminergic system in schematic view.

a variation of the normal dopamine 2 receptor. If this variation is present, it increases the risk of addiction, especially to alcohol. Like all receptors, its presence or absence depends on inheritance: the gene that codes for the A1 receptor variation can be passed between generations of the same family, or may be absent entirely from a family. Alcoholic fathers who have the gene can pass it to their children, who may therefore develop a higher than average risk of alcoholism.

Other brain areas involved in the reward mechanisms, and therefore reinforcing pleasure-seeking activity, are the septum (a site of sexual pleasure, optimism, euphoria, and happiness), the temporal lobes of the cerebrum, and parts of the hypothalamus (Figure 8.2). The septum as well as the NA also receives input from the VTA via the medial forebrain bundle. This bundle also carries connections linking the substantia nigra (in the midbrain) with the NA (Figure 8.2). All of these connections are dopaminergic, and stimulation of either the VTA or parts of the substantia nigra causes an increase in dopamine levels in the NA during a sensation of euphoria or pleasure. It should not be a surprise, therefore, to find that many stimulant and addictive drugs are those that cause high dopamine levels to occur in the brain, and in the NA in particular. The medial forebrain bundle is normally inhibited by a GABA inhibitory pathway within the VTA, so the MFB is not active all the time.

Drug addiction, especially alcoholism, has become the subject of increasing genetic research. Interest grew in this area mainly because of the individual variations shown by people in response to drugs, a phenomenon that is most likely to have a genetic basis. But it appears that epigenetics are involved as well (see Chapter 6). Activation of the dopaminergic MFB appears to create reward memories, i.e. memories of what gives pleasure. This memory process is thought to be part of the reason for repeated drug use and drug-seeking behaviour. The mechanism behind this memory formation involves the expression of two genes, *Egr 1* and *Fos*, within the VTA. The epigenetic **methylation** of genes (adding a **methyl group**, or **CH$_3$**), and **demethylation** of genes (removing the methyl group) can act as genetic on–off switches (Chapter 6). Methylation and demethylation can cause expression of these two genes during pleasure-seeking activity. This may ultimately lead to therapies being available that reduce memory of the pleasure and thus change drug-seeking activity (Day et al. 2013).

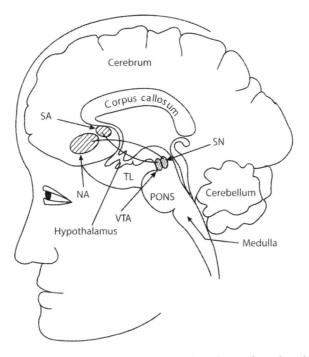

Figure 8.2 Same view as in Figure 8.1(a), showing the main pathways from the substantia nigra (SN) to the nucleus accumbens (NA), and from the ventral tegmental area (VTA) to the septal area (SA). TL is the temporal lobe.

Studying the hereditary nature of drug abuse suggests that genes which contribute to the habit are being passed from one generation to the next. But genes are not the only part of developing behaviour patterns such as drug abuse. The experience provided by the environment within which the offspring are raised is of great importance. Children born to parents who are drug abusers are eight times more susceptible to become drug abusers themselves than children born to non-drug abusers. Part of the answer to this was the discovery that children born in drug-abuser families had significant brain changes when compared with children from non-abuser families. These brain changes were abnormal connections between brain areas involved in control, reward, and motivation, which appear to be present from an early age. In addition, they also showed larger than normal **putamen** and **medial temporal lobes**. These areas are involved in habit forming, memory, and learning. Some drug abuse, such as parents smoking, could be regarded as a learnt behaviour by the children exposed to it. Another brain area, the **orbitofrontal cortex**, was smaller than average in offspring of drug abusers, and this reduction in size may contribute to the difficulty in stopping the habit (Ersche et al. 2012). In a similar study, individuals with a smaller than normal **amygdala** and **medial prefrontal cortex** (i.e. reduced grey matter volume) were more likely to escalate their stimulant drug habit from occasional use to regular and prolonged use (Becker et al. 2015). Brain changes like these may be useful in early prediction of drug misuse behaviour and therefore identify those who would benefit from intervention therapy. Such therapies could, in the future, include vaccines given to addicts to prevent the euphoria when drugs are self-administered. As with vaccines given to prevent infectious diseases, drug-abuse vaccines would stimulate the presence of **antibodies**, which would target the addictive drug and prevent its activity in the brain. Drug abusers who relapse from the treatment programme into further drug taking would benefit from the antibody effect of blocking the drug. In this way, their return to drug abuse would be thwarted by the vaccine, and they would therefore be more likely to return to therapy. Antibodies can last for years in the blood, allowing the abuser to stay clean from their drugs for a long time.

It appears that there is some discrepancy between the sexes with regards to addiction. Women appear to be more vulnerable to drug abuse than men because the female hormone **oestrogen** increases the euphoric state. The hormone boosts the level of dopamine release into the nucleus accumbens. Oestrogen rises and falls naturally over the 28-day **ovarian cycle**, with highest levels occurring just prior to ovulation (mid-cycle, about day 13 or 14), so the effect of the drugs rises and falls in relation to this cycle. **Progestrerone**, the other female hormone, counteracts the oestrogenic effect to some degree, and therefore reduces the risk of addiction (Anthes 2010).

The opiate drugs

These drugs are derived from **opium**, a resin obtained from the opium poppy. The best-known examples of the opiate derivatives are **morphine, heroin, pethidine,** and **methadone**. They are all potentially addictive and dangerous; morphine and heroin together killed 754 people in the UK in 1999 and 897 people in 2008.

Opiates (opiate drugs) act on specific opioid receptors (*opioid* = 'like opium', the word refers to the endogenous neurotransmitters), which occur mostly in the upper parts of the spinal cord and the brain stem. These receptors are called **mu (μ), delta (δ)** and **kappa (κ)**. Opioid receptors are metabotropic, involving the activation of the secondary messenger **cyclic adenosine monophosphate (cAMP)** via a **G-protein coupling** mechanism.

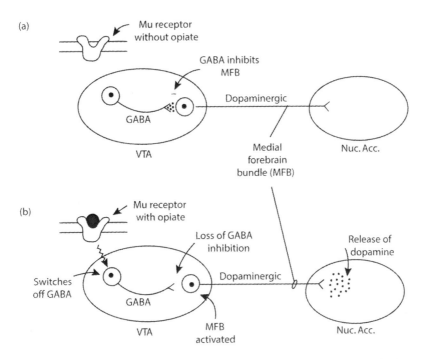

Figure 8.3 (a) The mu receptor without opiate binding has no influence over the GABA neurons of the ventral tegmental area (VTA). These neurons therefore inhibit the dopaminergic neurons of the medial forebrain bundle (MFB), which pass from the VTA to the nucleus accumbens (Nuc. Acc.). (b) Opiates binding to mu receptors switch off the GABA neurons, thus removing the GABA inhibition, and the MFB becomes activated, causing release of dopamine in the nucleus accumbens.

Opiate drugs cause a number of different effects on both the body and the mind, including analgesia, euphoria, sedation, and depressant effects. The effect of most importance in drug addiction is the euphoria and the feeling of well-being these drugs induce, as this is the reason that people take them. The complete mechanism by which this effect is achieved is gradually becoming better known, and it appears to be mediated through binding primarily to the mu receptor at the VTA. At the same time, activity on this receptor in several brain stem areas causes the classic analgesic effects and reinforces drug-seeking behaviour. This mu receptor binding at the VTA causes release of dopamine into the NA. Dopaminergic neurons of the medial forebrain bundle are inhibited by a GABA-mediated system within the VTA (Figure 8.1c). Opiate drugs acting in the mu receptor reduce this inhibition, allowing the MFB to become active, and this causes dopamine to be released in the NA (Figure 8.3). **Morphine** binds mostly to the mu receptor and least of all to the delta receptor, while **pethidine** also has its greatest activity on the mu receptor. **Heroin (diamorphine)** is made from morphine but is more lipid-soluble and more potent than its parent molecule.

Morphine binding to the mu receptor at the VTA also causes reduction in a chemical called **brain-derived neurotrophic factor (BDNF)**, and this reduction is necessary for the reward effect. It is possible that the BDNF stimulates the GABA system, which then fails to work when BDNF is low, thus allowing the MFB to become active. Morphine activity directly

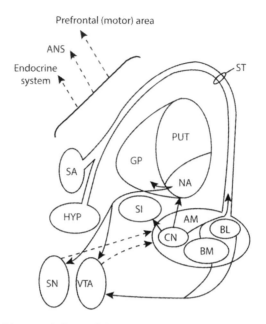

Figure 8.4 Pathways of the extended amygdala. The amygdala (AM) main nuclei are the central nucleus (CN), the basolateral nucleus (BL) and the basomedial nucleus (BM). Part of the stria terminalis (ST), which links the amygdala with the septal area (SA) and the hypothalamus (HYP), is involved, along with the sublenticular substantia innominata (SI), the nucleus accumbens (NA), the substantia nigra (SN), the ventral tegmental area (VTA), and the globus pallidus (GP). This system influences the prefrontal motor area (motor planning), the autonomic nervous system (ANS), and the endocrine system, the last two through the hypothalamus. PUT is the putamen.

on the NA has become better understood. The expression of two genes, *sox11* (involved in embryonic development) and *gadd45g* (involved in sexual development, brain development, and the cell's stress response) prevent any reward activity by morphine within the NA. There are many long-term physical effects of chronic use of morphine and heroin, in particular damage to the immune system, making addicts more susceptible to infections.

Opiate addiction, as with other drugs, leads to two problems encountered by the addict. One is **withdrawal**, a set of unpleasant symptoms that occurs within hours of abstinence from the drug and can last three or more days. Symptoms include hot and cold flushes, loss of appetite, muscle cramps, tremor, nausea, vomiting, insomnia, increased heart rate, high blood pressure, raised respiration rate, and high body temperature. While drugs are sought and taken initially for their euphoric effect (*positive reinforcement*), drug-seeking behaviour is promoted by the need to avoid the unpleasant effects of withdrawal (*negative reinforcement*). This change from *nondependent* drug seeking for pleasure to *dependent* drug seeking for prevention of withdrawal could be the result of a shift in the activation of different parts of the brain. While the neurological basis of euphoria appears to be located primarily within the mesotelencephalic dopamine system, the neurological basis of withdrawal appears to be the result of activity of another pathway, the '**extended amygdala**'. This consists of the **amygdala central medial nucleus**, part of the **stria terminalis**, part of the nucleus accumbens and the

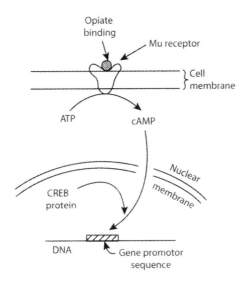

Figure 8.5 Opiate binding to the mu receptor. This creates cyclic adenosine monophosphate (cAMP) from adenosine triphosphate (ATP) inside the cell. cAMP influences gene expression inside the chromosomes of the nucleus by binding with CREB (cyclic AMP-responsive element-binding) protein.

sublenticular substantia innominata (Figure 8.4). This system has connections with other parts of the brain through inputs (afferents) and outputs (efferents), as shown in Figure 8.4. Studies of the neurochemistry during withdrawal have indicated reduced levels of both dopamine and serotonin in the brain, i.e. *downregulation* of these systems, and increased levels (*upregulation*) of **corticotrophin releasing factor (CRF)** (Koob 2000). CRF is probably best known as the hormone from the hypothalamus that enters the pituitary gland and controls the release of one of the anterior pituitary hormones called **adrenocorticotropic hormone (ACTH)**. It is also, however, a neurotransmitter of the limbic system and is involved in emotions and stress (see Chapter 9), and in withdrawal from drugs (Carlson 2012). The mechanism involving CRF in drug craving during withdrawal is not fully known, but part of the withdrawal effect appears to involve the activation of CRF systems within the central medial nucleus of the amygdala, part of the extended amygdala circuit (Koob 2000).

The second problem for the addict is that of **tolerance**, the state in which over time increasing doses of the drug become necessary to achieve anything like the original feelings of euphoria. It appears that the opioid receptors become less sensitive to the drug, a process of *downregulation* of sensitivity, although the receptor numbers remain constant. This may be due in part to the action of a protein called **cyclic AMP-responsive element-binding protein (CREB)**. When opiates bind to the mu receptor, cAMP is produced, and this passes to the nucleus and interacts with CREB (Figure 8.5). The role of CREB is one of gene regulation, and the way in which the binding of cAMP influences this role is little understood. CREB is a major link in the chain from receptor to gene, and evidence suggests it may be involved in opiate tolerance and the effects of drug withdrawal (Carlson 2012). Other proteins are undoubtedly important in drug addiction. A gene called **activator of G protein signalling 3 (*AGPS3*)** has been discovered that codes for a protein involved in euphoria. This protein is a vital component in the pathway that leads from the brain's release of **beta-endorphins** (Chapter 4) to the sensation of euphoria or pleasure that these endorphins produce. Blocking the gene (dubbed the *pleasure gene*) reduces the amount of protein produced, causing loss of the euphoric state. It is thought that the same mechanism will probably also be effective in reducing the euphoric (and thus addictive) effects of opiate drugs such as morphine and heroin. In the future, drugs designed to block the production of the protein may help heroin addicts to withdraw from their addiction more easily, with fewer or less intense side effects. The analgesic qualities of these drugs do not appear to be affected when this gene is blocked.

Some important *drug interactions* involving opiates with other drugs occur and are shown in Tables 8.1 and 8.2.

Table 8.1 Some drug interactions with opiates

Other drug	Opiate drug interaction and notes
Chlorpromazine	May react with heroin, giving uncontrolled limb jerks
Clozapine (antipsychotic)	May react with heroin, causing drowsiness. Increased hypotension and sedation generally with antipsychotics.
Fluoxetine (antidepressant)	May react with heroin, causing fits
MAOI (antidepressant)	Reacts with pethidine, potentially fatal
Barbiturates	Increases the metabolism of all opiate drugs
Alcohol	Increased sedation and hypotension
Antiepileptics	Changes in either the opiate or antiepileptic drug concentrations in the blood possible.

Table 8.2 Some drug interactions with methadone

Other drug	Methadone interaction and notes
Phenobarbitone	Phenobarbitone blocks the action of methadone, causing opioid withdrawal symptoms
Diazepam, and other benzodiazepine drugs	Inhibits methadone metabolism causing increased methadone blood levels
Tricyclic antidepressants	Methadone blocks the metabolism of the antidepressant, increasing the blood level of the antidepressant
Hypnotics (e.g. zopiclone and chlormethiazole)	Increased sedative effect with methadone
SSRI antidepressants	Increased levels of methadone in the blood
Disulfiram (anti-alcohol drug)	Some methadone products contain alcohol; a reaction with these products can be alarming and unpleasant
Other opiate drugs	Increased sedation and respiratory depression
Naloxone (opiate antagonist)	Blocks methadone action, causing withdrawal
Alcohol	Increased sedation and respiratory depression; increased liver toxicity
Nevirapine, zidovudine, and ritonavir (anti-HIV drugs)	Nevirapine causes increased methadone metabolism, i.e. lower blood methadone levels. Methadone raises blood level of zidovudine. Ritonavir may raise blood methadone levels by blocking methadone metabolism

An important drug used as a treatment of abuse of the so-called 'hard' drugs (usually heroin and pethidine) is **methadone**. Although methadone itself is addictive and harmful, it is considered to cause fewer problems than the hard drugs and for this reason has been used as a substitute for them for many years. It is hoped that by replacing heroin and pethidine with methadone not only will the need for the hard drug be removed, but at the same time the effects of its withdrawal will be reduced. However, the potential dangers of methadone are demonstrated by the 298 deaths it caused in the UK in 1999, and 378 deaths in 2008.

Because of methadone's place in opiate addiction therapy, a separate drug interaction table for methadone is given in Table 8.2. Anti-HIV drugs are included in Table 8.2 because of the increased risks of HIV infection due to the dangerous habit of needle-sharing by drug-abusing patients.

Cocaine

Cocaine is produced from the leaf of the coca bush and had been used for many years as a local anaesthetic. When inhaled through the nose or swallowed (e.g. as *crack cocaine*, a very potent form), cocaine will reach the brain quickly, giving a peak effect in 30 minutes and lasting between 1 and 3 hours. If injected by the intravenous route, the effects occur within seconds and last between 15 and 30 minutes. This drug causes a sense of well-being, euphoria, alertness, excitement, and increased energy; the person taking it becomes extraverted, restless, and talkative. It also causes a reduction in food intake and pain perception. It can cause delusions of grandeur called *cocainomania*. At high dosages users become unable to sleep and have tremors, nausea, unstable emotions, restlessness, irritability, muscle twitches, and psychotic outbursts (hallucinations, delusions, mood disturbance, paranoia, and bizarre behaviour; the so-called *cocaine psychosis*). Fits and unconsciousness may follow, with a corresponding risk of death. The lethal dose varies between individuals and their circumstances, being as little as 20 mg in some cases up to 800 mg or more in others. Cocaine is extremely addictive, partly owing to its rapid transportation to the brain and fast onset of effects. It promotes further drug-seeking behaviour beyond anything considered normal or reasonable.

Cocaine blocks the reuptake of monoamines, especially dopamine and noradrenaline, into the presynaptic bulb by inhibiting the transporters in the presynaptic membrane (Figure 8.6). These neurotransmitters then accumulate in the cleft, exerting a greater than normal effect on the receptors. Areas of the brain affected include the basal ganglia (putamen and caudate nucleus), the amygdala, and the cerebral cortex. However, the nucleus accumbens is particularly affected; the reuptake of dopamine is prevented at the terminal synapses of the medial forebrain bundle. Long-term changes occur in this area following exposure to the drug. These changes involve an increase in the density of dopamine receptors, notably D_3, and this can cause a rapid return to psychotic symptoms on re-exposure to the drug even after quite some time without it.

A single dose of cocaine has been shown to cause major changes in the brain, resulting in memory loss and addiction, due to its prolonged neuroleptic action of about a week's duration (Ungless et al. 2001). This action interferes with the normal process of memory and renders the brain vulnerable to successive doses, leading to rapid addiction. Users 'remember' the euphoria, and this reinforces further drug abuse. Cocaine is also responsible for a quarter of the nonfatal heart attacks found in those younger than 45 years of age. The drug causes cardiac spasms and induces the immune system to destroy cardiac muscle cells. Deaths from cocaine use in the UK increased sevenfold in the 6 years from 1993 to

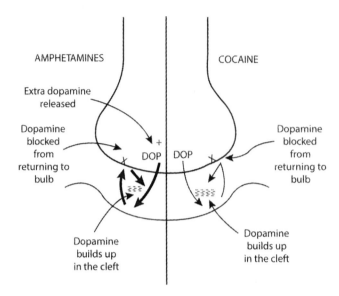

Figure 8.6 The action of amphetamines (left) and cocaine (right) at the dopaminergic synapse. Dopamine (DOP) is blocked from reabsorption back into the presynaptic bulb by both drugs, thus increasing the quantity of dopamine within the synaptic cleft. In addition, amphetamines increase the quantity of dopamine released from the bulb.

1999, i.e. 12 deaths in 1993 compared with 87 deaths in 1999. The deaths associated with the drug continued to rise, causing 235 deaths in 2008. Cocaine also causes premature ageing of the brain, with grey matter losses occurring in the prefrontal cortex (notably the dorsolateral, ventrolateral, and orbitofrontal cortex) and parts of the temporal cortex at the faster rate of 3.1 ml per annum compared with 1.7 ml per annum in nonusers. This impairs the user's abilities, in particular decision-making and self-control. Regular users experience cognitive decline and brain atrophy much earlier than nonusers.

The teenage brain is more vulnerable to the effects of cocaine than the fully adult brain, due to its immaturity. At the first exposure to cocaine, the teenager's brain will begin a strong defence against the effects of the drug, and this response is genetically regulated. This means that cocaine abuse during the teen years is more likely to cause addiction than starting the drug later in life. The first exposure to the drug changes the shape of neurons and their synapses, and this process is regulated by the gene *integrin beta 1*. The products from this gene work though a pathway that involves the enzyme **Arg Kinase** to cause changes in the cell cytoskeleton, the protein internal framework of the cell. The cytoskeleton is responsible for numerous functions, including cell shape and support, and is evolving as part of the teenage development of the nervous system. How bad or how mild the addiction becomes in teenagers may be due, in part, to the activity of the *integrin beta 1* gene in response to the drug (Gourley et al. 2012).

One possible way of treating cocaine addiction in the future may be with a cocaine vaccine. The vaccine stimulates production of antibodies, which lock onto cocaine, forming a complex that is too large to cross the blood–brain barrier and thus preventing cocaine from entering the brain. As with all drug-abuse vaccines (including the vaccine for nicotine) they are still in the developmental stages and may not be available for a few years yet.

Table 8.3 Some drug interactions with cocaine

Other drug	Interaction with cocaine
Alcohol	Increased euphoric effect. Increased heart rate and blood cortisol levels
Heroin	Increased euphoria
Lithium	Decreases the effect of the cocaine
MAOI antidepressant	High temperature, muscle rigidity and tremor, coma
Antipsychotics	Increase in the positive (psychotic) symptoms of cocaine (see *cocaine psychosis*)
Calcium-channel blockers (anti-epileptic)	Reduce the cardiac effects of cocaine, but may increase the risk of fits
Beta-adrenergic blockers (cardiac drugs)	Increased risk of cocaine-induced constriction of the coronary artery (i.e. risk of myocardial ischemia)

Some important *drug interactions* involving cocaine with other drugs occur and are shown in Table 8.3.

Amphetamines and other dopamine-enhancing drugs

Amphetamines are a large group of compounds that act in a way similar to cocaine, i.e. they increase dopamine (and noradrenaline) levels within the synapses by blocking their reuptake, but they also have the additional effect of increasing dopamine release from the presynaptic bulb (Figure 8.6). Amphetamines were responsible for 79 deaths in the UK in 1999 and 99 deaths in 2008. Two important members of this group of drugs, MDMA and crystal meth are discussed here.

Ecstasy (3,4-methylenedioxymethamphetamine, or MDMA) is one of a group of related amphetamine-associated drugs. MDMA is converted in the body to the active metabolite **4-hydroxy-3-methoxymethamphetamine (HMMA)**. Ecstasy increases the release of dopamine and noradrenaline, and this release of dopamine into nucleus accumbens is responsible for the euphoric state. It also gives the abuser strong feelings of friendliness, loving, and bonding with others, i.e. **prosocial effects**. It moves the user's attention away from negative feelings to being more positive. This is probably due to MDMA stimulating the **ventral striatum**, a brain area involved in reward expectation. It may also be attributed to MDMA's ability to raise the blood **oxytocin** level, a hormone involved in bonding (see Chapter 5). It also affects memories; reducing negative or bad memories while making positive or happy memories more vivid. However, it also has a strong affinity for serotonin neurons. It increases serotonin in the synapses of the serotonergic diffuse modulatory system (see Chapter 11) by causing the transporters that normally facilitate serotonin reuptake to reverse the flow into the synapse. The larger amounts of serotonin released in this way increases the 'high' that users experience (Concar 2002). However, some time later the levels of available serotonin will be low, partly due to inhibition by MDMA of the enzyme **tryptophan hydroxylase**, the enzyme that normally produces serotonin (see Chapter 4). This period of low serotonin can last longer that the original increase, causing the so-called 'hangover' effects, including tiredness, irritability, and muddled thinking. HMMA is associated with an increased release of the pituitary hormone **antidiuretic hormone (ADH, or vasopressin)** (Figure 8.7). This hormone causes retention of water in the blood from the kidney, preventing its loss in the urine. The extra water in the blood dilutes the plasma electrolytes, especially sodium, causing low plasma sodium due to the blood dilution (a **hyponatremia**). The change in plasma salts level affects neurons, which

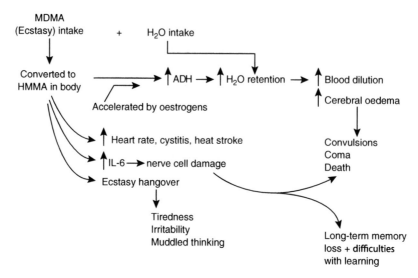

Figure 8.7 Ecstasy intake and the events that follow. ADH = antidiuretic hormone, H_2O = water, IL-6 = interleukin-6.

are sensitive to electrolyte levels in their extracellular fluid. The increased water content of the blood puts a strain on the heart, which then risks failure (**cardiac failure**). The brain becomes swollen with water (**cerebral oedema**), and drinking more water accelerates the harmful effects. Women are particularly vulnerable to this effect, as the female hormone **oestrogen** speeds up the process (see The reward pathways of the brain, on page 144). High levels of circulating oestrogen occur just prior to ovulation, about midway through the ovarian cycle, and women at this point may already be suffering some disturbance in cerebral sodium levels, putting them more at risk from the effects of ecstasy. They also risk increasing the body temperature (**hyperthermia**) leading to **heat stroke** (i.e. a state of collapse due to uncontrolled body temperature above 40°C). If the drug is taken at a party, the risk of hyperthermia is increased by dancing in a crowd. The brain reacts to the MDMA-induced excess water and hyperthermia with convulsions and coma, possibly leading to death within a few hours or days. Deaths from MDMA in the whole UK total 202 from 1996 to 2002, from 5 in 1998 rising to 44 in 2008. However, there was a worrying sharp increase in deaths reported for 2001 (England and Wales alone recorded 43 deaths) despite the media coverage highlighting the dangers. The deaths occur mostly in the under-30 age range. The cause of death was mainly hyperthermia, hyponatremia, and cardiac failure. The risks vary between individuals because of sexual and genetic differences (see Oestrogen, page 144).

For the majority of ecstasy takers who survive, other physical changes take place including increased heart rate, cystitis, and heavy periods in women, heatstroke (Blows 1998; Concar 2002) and possible **cerebral infarcts** if blood capillaries become blocked in the brain. MDMA also interferes with the immune system by raising the levels of a chemical called **interleukin-6 (IL-6)**, which at higher than normal levels can damage nerve cells, particularly the serotonergic neurons. This also puts the user at a higher risk of infections. In the brain, the **default brain network** (see Chapter 1) becomes functionally disconnected from the rest of the brain under MDMA. This causes a reduction in negative feelings and allows the state of euphoria to dominate. MDMA seriously affects the serotonin pathways (**serotonergic toxicity**), causing damage to areas of the cerebral cortex and hippocampus. This damage can occur quickly, within 4 days of ecstasy use, and is permanent, causing memory losses and difficulties with learning for years. Long-term widespread use of the drug could result in a whole generation of people with memory problems who will have difficulty in carrying out simple mental tasks. As many as 500,000 ecstasy users in the UK and 20 million people worldwide could be affected in this way. It has been estimated that between 2.5 and 5 million ecstasy tablets are taken in the UK every month!

Crystal methamphetamine (crystal meth) is a potent stimulant form of **methamphetamine (*N*-methyl-alpha-methylphenethylamine)**. Crystal meth is highly addictive, sometimes even after just one use. It causes elevated mood and alertness, increased energy, euphoria, and increased sexual desire. In high dosage it can cause psychosis, paranoia, confusion, and strokes (cerebral hemorrhage). Withdrawal from crystal meth is extremely difficult; the drug drives the user constantly towards obtaining and taking more. Symptoms suffered during withdrawal (**post-acute-withdrawal syndrome**) can last for months and includes depression, anxiety, and hypersomnia (see Chapter 16). In the long term, permanent damage to the serotonergic and dopaminergic systems occur, and it can cause weight loss, malnutrition, and '**meth mouth**', i.e. excessive drying of the mouth, which ultimately results in tooth losses.

Some important *drug interactions* involving amphetamines with other drugs occur and are shown in Table 8.4.

Cannabis

Marihuana (cannabis) comes from the dried leaves of the Indian hemp plant *Cannabis sativa*. The active ingredients consist of between 80 and 100 **cannabinoids**, many of which are probably psychoactive. The most potent of these is **delta-9-tetrahydrocannabinol (delta-9-THC or δ9-THC**, now usually called **THC**). Another substance often present is **cannabidiol (CBD)** (Figure 8.8), one of the many cannabinoids, but this one appears to have some beneficial effects. For example, it is claimed that cannabidiol can reduce some of the bad effects of THC. However, not all forms of cannabis have cannabidiol present. Two main forms of cannabis exist: so-called '**skunk**', which has high concentration of THC, but no cannabidiol; and so-called '**hash**', which has low concentration of THC and contains cannabidiol. Figures suggest that 80% of users take skunk, with the other 20% taking hash. Other beneficial claims for cannabidiol involve relief of psychoses, anxiety, and alcohol-induced brain damage.

Table 8.4 Drug interactions with amphetamines

Other drug	Interaction with amphetamines
MAOI antidepressants	Dangerous interaction: risk of hypertensive crisis due to raised sympathetic nervous system activity (i.e. sympathomimetic); plus nausea, cardiac arrhythmias, and chest pain
Opiates	Increased analgesic effect of the opiate
Chlorpromazine (antipsychotic)	Both drugs are reduced in their efficiency causing an increase in psychotic symptoms
Lithium	Reduces the amphetamine euphoria

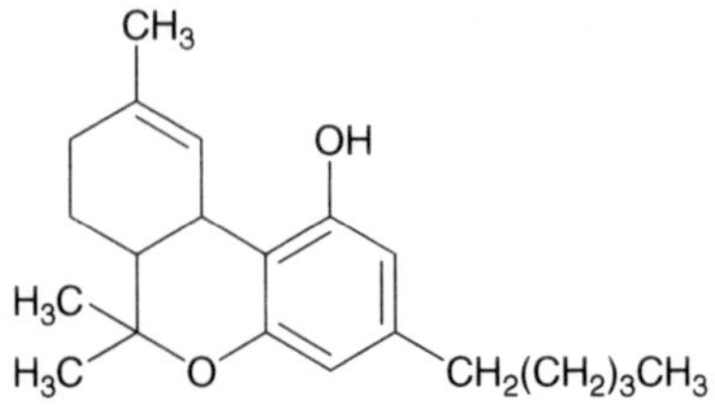

CH₃

$$CH_3$$

Figure 8.8 The chemical structure of cannabidiol.

The main psychoactive ingredient, THC, binds to cannabinoid receptors in several parts of the brain, notably the basal ganglia, the hippocampus, the cerebellum, and the frontal lobe of the cerebrum. The effects of taking cannabinoids in sufficient dosage are changes in cognition, euphoria, and other mood and emotional effects. A sense of unreality with sensory distortion, slurred speech, analgesia (without respiratory depression), sedation, and suppression of the immune system have all been reported. THC also causes **paranoia**, demonstrated by a 270% increase in paranoia associated with taking skunk, and 170% increase with taking hash. The reason for taking the drug – that is, the euphoric effect produced – is probably due to its ability to release dopamine within the NA. This is achieved because the MFB does not have receptors that can bind THC, but the GABA inhibitory system within the VTA that normally shuts down the MFB does have THC receptors. THC therefore binds to the GABA system, causing the GABA to shut down, and the MFB then becomes active and releases dopamine in the NA (Figure 8.9). Deaths recorded from cannabis for the UK in 2008 were 19.

Cannabinoid receptors occur in at least two known subtypes, **CB₁** and **CB₂**. CB₁ is the major cannabinoid receptor subtype of the central nervous system (CNS), with CB₂ in the brain limited to possibly only the cerebellum (it occurs more in other organs). The hippocampus has particularly high numbers of CB₁ cannabinoid receptors, and therefore the drug may act especially here, resulting not only in impairment of short-term memory but also

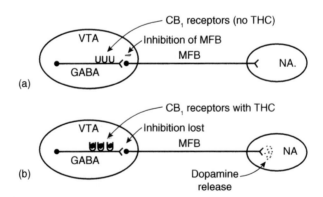

Figure 8.9 Cannabis causes dopamine release in the NA by binding to the GABA inhibitory system within the VTA. This inhibits the GABA system, in a process called disinhibition, i.e. one inhibitor (here it is CB₁) inhibiting another inhibitor (here it is GABA). With GABA shut down due to THC binding to CB₁, the MFB becomes active and releases dopamine in the NA. The MFB does not have CB₁ receptors.

in disruption of release of cortisol, a hormone involved in mood regulation. (An important function of the hippocampus is regulation of some hormones, including cortisol.) The drug also acts on CB_1 receptors in the basal ganglia, and this can cause loss of control of voluntary movements, the addition of involuntary movements, and **akinesia** (a loss of initiating a movement). CB_1 receptors are especially predominant in the **globus pallidus**, the **substantia nigra (pars reticulata)**, and the **caudate** and **putamen**. In the **limbic system**, there are significant concentrations of CB_1 receptors in the **amygdala**, an area central to the control of emotional responses, and in the **hypothalamus**, the control centre of body temperature. The **cerebellum** has some areas with dense concentrations of CB_1 receptors, enough to cause disturbance to motor function and balance given sufficient dosage of the drug. The concentrations of CB_1 receptors in the **brain stem** and **spinal cord** are lower than most other brain areas. Astrocytes (part of the neuroglia set of cells; see Chapter 3) also have CB_1 receptors, and THC binds to these receptors. This is particularly significant with astrocytes in the hippocampus, where THC acting on these astrocytes disrupts **working memory**, i.e. the short-term memory of information useful for comprehension and learning. It would appear that astrocytes have a modulating role on hippocampal memory functions, a role disrupted by cannabis. THC therefore has a double action on disrupting memory, one acting on the hippocampal neurons directly, and the other acting on astrocytes that regulate the neuronal activity. People smoking cannabis between 5 and 20 times per month have a 10% increase in memory loss, and those smoking more than 20 times per month have a 20% increase in memory loss.

The presence of natural receptors for cannabinoids suggests that the nervous system must produce its own endogenous cannabinoid substances (called **endocannabinoids**). Two such substances have been discovered: the better-known **anandamide**, an unsaturated fatty acid, and the lesser known **2-AG**. Anandamide, produced by neurons of the cortex and parts of the basal ganglia, binds to CB_1 receptors, producing analgesia, reduced levels of movement, and hypothermia (a hypothalamic effect). Its duration of action is short owing to its rapid breakdown to arachidonic acid in neurons and astrocytes. The major role of endocannabinoids in the brain is to regulate synaptic release of neurotransmitters (see Chapter 3). They are released into the synaptic cleft from the postsynaptic membrane when the neurotransmitter binds, and they feedback to the presynaptic bulb, via CB_1 receptors on the bulb, to inhibit any further neurotransmitter release. This is a system of chemical signalling across the synaptic gap in the opposite direction to the neurotransmitter. Prolonged use of cannabis leads to a reduction in the amount of anandamide naturally produced by the brain, but this recovers after stopping the drug. Cannabidiol helps to increase the amount of anandamide secreted. Cannabidiol therapy may be useful in treating those who wish to stop the habit.

It has been questioned many times whether cannabis use leads to the onset of schizophrenia, especially if the drug is used during the teenage years. It is certainly known that high doses of cannabis can lead to psychotic symptoms (e.g. hallucinations and delusions; the so-called 'cannabis psychosis'). The extra strong 'skunk' form of the drug is claimed to be responsible for a quarter of all psychotic states in the UK, i.e. around 60,000 people, despite a 40% fall in the overall use of cannabis between 2005 and 2015. It is now been shown than THC use during adolescence interacts with the *COMT* gene at locus 22q11.21. This gene codes for the enzyme **catechol-O-methyltransferase**, which breaks down the neurotransmitters dopamine and noradrenaline in dopaminergic and noradrenergic pathways in the brain. The *COMT* gene has been linked to schizophrenia (see Chapter 10), and the indication that cannabis affects this gene provides a potential biological basis for the assumption that cannabis during adolescence can contribute to the development of schizophrenia. THC may also trigger early onset of schizophrenia in those with a genetic predisposition to the disease.

THC can have effects similar to those of the so-called 'hard' drugs, heroin in particular (Wiedemann 2010). This has led to further speculation and controversy about whether the use of cannabis can lead to addiction to hard drugs like heroin. The risk of addiction to cannabis itself has always been considered to be low, usually because it is only used occasionally and because users give up smoking the drug in their thirties or forties. Recently, however, there have been indications that cannabis is as potentially addictive as heroin or morphine (Wiedemann 2010).

A brain system called the **salient network** (see Chapter 1) becomes disrupted by skunk, and this results in **amotivation** ('lacking motivation'), a state of low desire to do anything. The salient network consists of two main areas of the brain working together, the **anterior cingulate cortex** and the **insula**. The functions of the salient network include a mechanism for switching between the **default mode network** (Chapter 1) and task-orientated activity. If THC does reduce the function of the salient network, this could prevent the brain entering task-orientated activity (i.e. amotivation).

Cannabis causes an increase in appetite, so users may eat more food. Special brain cells called **pro-opiomelanocortin** (**POMC**) neurons can release either a hormone that suppresses appetite, or a different hormone that stimulates appetite. Which hormone is released by the POMC neuron is dependent on a protein derived from the cell's mitochondria. When THC activates the CB_1 receptors, the mitochondrial protein induces POMC to switch to stimulating appetite (Figure 8.10).

Some medical uses of cannabinoids are becoming better recognised. Their anti-emetic quality has been used for some time in the drug **nabilone** to prevent nausea and sickness in patients having chemotherapy in cancer treatment. Some cannabinoids have been shown to reduce fits, dilate the bronchus in **asthma**, and improve the eye disease **glaucoma**. Now the beneficial qualities of cannabinoids are becoming available in the UK to **multiple sclerosis** sufferers. **Cannabis extract** can be prescribed by specialists in the form of an oromucosal spray called **sativex**, which contains **dronabinol (delta-9-tetrahydrocannabinol)** and cannabidiol. This is to act as a muscle relaxant as part of the treatment for moderate to severe spasticity in multiple sclerosis.

Some important *drug interactions* involving cannabinoids with other drugs occur and are shown in Table 8.5. An important interaction to note is the combination of THC with

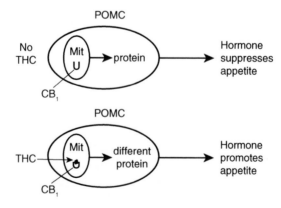

Figure 8.10 POMC neurons and appetite. Mit = mitochondrium.

Table 8.5 Drug interactions with cannabinoids

Other drugs	Interactions with cannabinoids
Fluoxetine (SSRI antidepressant)	Increased energy and sexuality
Tricyclic antidepressant	Tachycardia and restlessness, orthostatic hypotension, sedation, and unstable body temperature
Lithium	Increased blood levels of lithium, which in turn may reduce the effect of the cannabinoid
Opiates	Increased heart rate and respiratory depression
Cocaine	Raised blood levels of cocaine, causing increased cocaine activity
Amphetamines	Increased and sustained heart rate
Propranolol (cardiac drug)	Blocks the increased heart rate and blood pressure associated with cannabinoids

alcohol. This is a common combination of drugs, but the effects were poorly understood until recently. The result of taking cannabis with alcohol is to significantly increase the blood level concentration of both THC and its metabolite **11-hydroxy-THC (11-OH-THC)**, with corresponding increased impairment of task performance. This is an important finding, particularly with regards to the cause of road accidents when drivers have been found to be taking drug combinations (Hartman et al. 2015).

Alcohol

Alcohol (ethyl alcohol or **ethanol)** is a psychoactive drug with a small molecular size and therefore reaches all parts of the body quickly after absorption. At low dose it acts as a *mild stimulant*, giving a feeling of well-being, due to the release of small amounts of dopamine into the NA. This is the reason for the *social* drinking of alcohol. However, if too much alcohol is taken it becomes a *depressant*, shutting down many areas of brain activity, from front to back. Alcohol acts at the **GABA$_A$** receptor site and promotes GABA to open the chloride channels (see Figure 4.17 in Chapter 4). This increases the inhibitory effect of the GABA synapses by reducing the firing rate of neurons. At the same time, alcohol reduces the excitation of glutamate NMDA receptors. The problem is that this depressant level of alcohol can be quickly and easily reached. Such depressive effects include cognitive impairment (i.e. distorted thinking, judgement, and reasoning), slowed reaction times (one good reason for not driving after drinking), verbal impairment (slurring of speech), and motor impairment (inability to stand up or walk in a straight line). Very high doses (i.e. a blood level greater than 0.5% or 5 mg/dl) can cause unconsciousness and a risk of death from respiratory suppression. One in every eight young male deaths in the UK each year is caused by alcohol, either directly or indirectly, through alcohol-related accidents, violence, and inhalation of vomit. In 2007, recorded alcohol-related deaths reached 8724 in the UK. Some 12.8% of British men aged 15–29 years, and 8.3% of British women of equivalent age die from alcohol-related causes each year (Harrington-Dobinson and Blows 2006, 2007a and 2007b).

Alcohol also has a dilatory effect on peripheral blood vessels, taking blood from the core towards the skin (the 'red nose effect'). Blood flushing the skin makes the skin *feel* warmer, but actually this blood moves more heat out from the body's core and that actually cools down the body temperature. It seems at odds with the way they *feel* to say that alcohol makes the person colder. However, in this situation, the brandy barrel carried by the rescue dog is not the best thing a very cold person needs when trapped in snow. Alcohol abuse over time causes both tolerance (the individual can consume more and more without undue effect) and dependence (the person needs alcohol in order to get through the day without symptoms). Quick withdrawal from a long-term drinking habit causes nausea, vomiting, headache, and tremors, as well as **alcohol withdrawal delirium** (previously known as **delirium tremens**, or **DTs**), a collection of symptoms including agitation, confusion, tachycardia, hallucinations, and delusions. The person in withdrawal can also become **hyperthermic** (i.e. have a raised body temperature) because in the absence of alcohol it is no longer available to promote heat loss.

Korsakoff's syndrome is a chronic state of **amnesia** (memory loss) and **Wernicke's encephalopathy** is a state of intellectual impairment. These often occur together in a patient with a history of long-term alcohol abuse. Both syndromes are thought to be due to a combination of factors, notably the deficiency of the vitamin called **thiamine** (vitamin B_1), alcohol neurotoxicity, and hepatic dysfunction (Nolen-Hoeksema 2007). Distinguishing one syndrome from the other in chronic alcoholic patients is not always easy. Many alcoholics lack nutrients as they tend not to eat properly, and chronic alcohol abuse results in gastritis and gastric damage, which impedes the absorption of vitamins, particularly thiamine. These factors lead to a degeneration of the brain stem (**periaquaductal grey**), the hypothalamus (**mammillary bodies**), and the thalamus (**dorsomedial nucleus**). Korsakoff's syndrome is characterised by a loss of short-term memory, inability to learn new skills, disorientation, and confabulation to fill in missing gaps in memory and knowledge. The features of Wernicke's encephalopathy are rapid eye movements with double vision (**diplopia**), reduced muscle coordination, and a decline in mental ability that may be of any degree from mild to severe. Some recovery may be possible provided the damage is not severe, the patient abstains from alcohol for at least 6 months, and ensures an adequate intake of thiamine.

People have varying responses to alcohol, and not every drinker is equally at risk of becoming alcoholic. Two basic types of drinkers have been identified: the *steady drinker* and the *binge drinker*. Steady drinking has a strong genetic basis, a case of 'like father like son'. If the father has a history of alcohol abuse as a steady drinker, the son has a seven times greater risk of abusing alcohol than the son of a non-drinker. They also have a greater than average risk of developing a personality disorder. The daughters of steady drinking fathers do not show the same degree of slide into alcoholism as the sons, but they do tend to complain more about physical symptoms for which pathology cannot be found; a condition known as **somatisation disorder**. The offspring of alcoholic mothers also show three to five times more risk of developing a psychopathology, e.g. depression, anxiety, misconduct, or **attention deficit hyperactivity disorder** (**ADHD**), compared with age-matched low-risk children from non-alcoholic mothers.

Steady drinking starts early in life and is associated with many kinds of antisocial behaviour, such as fighting, impulsive actions, and lack of remorse. Binging alcohol abuse has a greater environmental than genetic cause. The father-to-child hereditary pattern is only activated in an environment in which the child is exposed to bouts of heavy drinking. Bingers start drinking later in life and can be of either sex. They show increased emotional states and anxiety, become rigid in their outlook, fearful of any changes, cautious, and sensitive to social cues.

Alcohol causes an acute rise in testosterone in women, about five times greater than normal. This is a concentration of male hormone the female brain is not used to, and this raises the women's sexual desire and aggression, as portrayed by drunk women in the streets outside clubs late at night. In men, the testosterone is actually reduced by about 30% because alcohol aids the conversion of testosterone to the female hormone oestrogen. So intoxicated women have too much testosterone, and intoxicated men have too much oestrogen. Persistent drinking causes a chronic decline in testosterone in men, resulting in smaller testes, low sperm count, and male breast development (**gynaecomastia**). Males have more of an enzyme called **alcohol dehydrogenase**, in the stomach than women do. This enzyme is the first reaction in the break-down of alcohol, reducing the amount of alcohol entering the blood in men by about 20% compared with that in women. This is one reason men can tolerate alcohol more than women. The normal metabolism of alcohol changes in alcoholics. The second reaction in the metabolic pathway is reduced. This is the enzyme **aldehyde dehydrogenase**, which converts acetaldehyde (derived from the alcohol) to acetate. The reduction of this reaction allows acetaldehyde to accumulate in the brain, causing sedation and reduced motor control.

Drinking alcohol during pregnancy can cause problems with the infant called **fetal alcohol syndrome (FAS)** (see Chapter 15). Alcohol crosses the placenta and has serious effects on the unborn child at a time when the brain is developing rapidly. Errors in brain development due to teratogens such as alcohol cause brain damage, which cannot then be corrected. **Teratogens** are substances such as drugs that cross via the placenta from mother to child and cause harm to the unborn infant. The effects of FAS include many physical defects, but the mental defects are particularly troubling for the child and family alike. After birth, FAS causes hyperactivity, impulsive behaviour, cognitive deficits, visuospacial and thinking problems, and lack of understanding of their own behaviour and normal social protocol. The only completely safe amount of alcohol to drink during pregnancy is none (Chapter 15).

The genetic basis of alcoholism has become the subject of greater interest with the sequencing of the human genome. It became particularly important with the discovery of the *A1* **allele** on chromosome 11. This particular allele is a variation of the gene that codes for the dopamine receptor known as D_2, and its presence increases the risk of alcohol abuse. Of all severe alcoholics, 56.3% have the *A1* allele compared with only 25.7% of a control population. Given that dopamine is involved in the reward pathways of the brain, it may be that the *A1* allele is also linked to increased risk of abuse of other drugs. Other genes are becoming more important in alcohol research. The gene *CYP2E1* codes for one of the **cytochrome P450** enzymes, which carry out metabolic reactions in the liver and elsewhere. It is important in alcohol metabolism, and the enzyme can be induced (activated) by alcohol. It is thought that between 10% and 20% of people may have a variation of this gene that codes for an enzyme that breaks down alcohol quicker than normal, and this may have bearing on how much these individuals can drink before becoming intoxicated.

Some important *drug interactions* involving alcohol with other drugs occur and are shown in Table 8.6. Healthcare professionals need to be aware of these interactions because of the common social nature of alcohol consumption, but particularly because of the risks with known alcoholic patients taking other medication.

Nicotine

The two biggest health problems of this century are **human immunodeficiency virus (HIV, the causative agent of acquired immunodeficiency syndrome, or AIDS)** and **tobacco smoking**. Both problems are increasing globally. Any individual in the Western world who can avoid both HIV and tobacco has a life expectancy of 70 years at least, and often more. Both these problems are relevant to the subject of drug abuse because HIV infection is a major risk to intravenous drug abusers who share contaminated needles, and tobacco contains the commonly used addictive drug nicotine.

Table 8.6 Some drug interactions with alcohol

Other drug	Interaction with alcohol
Barbiturates; warfarin; phenytoin; rifampicin	Interaction varies according to how much alcohol is consumed. Heavy drinking increases at least one liver enzyme activity, withdrawal decreases that activity
Paracetamol	Alcohol increases activity of the liver enzyme that acts on paracetamol, causing increased toxicity of paracetamol at normally nontoxic dose. Overdose of paracetamol with alcohol can cause lethal liver failure
Opiates; benzodiazepines	Alcohol adds to the depressive effect of the drugs on the brain
Tricyclic antidepressants	Unexpected reactions and behavioural changes. Lower blood levels of the tricyclic reduces clinical effects
SSRI antidepressants	No known interaction
MAOI antidepressants	Risk of hypertension, especially if tyromine is present in the alcoholic drink. Modern reversible MAOI may not be such a problem
Antipsychotics	Poor psychomotor skills and impaired nervous system function
Disulfiram (anti-alcohol)	Flushing, hypotension, nausea, increased heart rate, some reactions could be fatal
Nonsteroidal anti-inflammatory drugs	Increased risk of gastrointestinal bleeds since alcohol is a gastric irritant
Insulin	Too much alcohol causes severe and prolonged hypoglycaemia in diabetic patients, following lowering of stored liver glycogen
Antihypertensive drugs	Increased risk of postural hypotension

Nicotine addiction is a major hazard, causing the deaths of about *300 people per day* in the UK alone from smoking-related diseases. In 2008, diseases caused by smoking claimed the lives of more than 100,000 people in the UK. This is a massive death toll, but one that is entirely avoidable, simply by choosing not to smoke. Unfortunately, however, the health message is not reaching young people, as more and more take up the habit. Smoking in young women in particular is increasing alarmingly.

Nicotine addiction must not be underestimated. Addiction to this drug prevents many people who want to give up smoking from doing so. Only about 20% of people attempting to stop smoking are still nonsmokers 2 years after abstaining from cigarettes, and this 80% failure rate still occurs even when they are faced with serious health problems, or even death. Nicotine is probably the worse addiction problem facing society today. Vaccines against nicotine are now in an advanced stage of development. About 99% of nicotine in tobacco smoke is of the 'left-handed' molecular version, with 1% being the 'right-handed' version. Vaccines developed to respond to both varieties had poor results, but more recent vaccines developed to respond only to the left-handed variety were met with greater success. Now a second generation of vaccines is in trials, those based on only the left-handed variety.

Nicotine binds to nicotinic **acetylcholine** receptors (see Chapter 4) on the VTA, and this increases the level of dopamine in the NA but also raises the activity levels of many dopaminergic neurons. By binding to nicotinic receptors, nicotine also causes the opening of sodium channels and increases cellular excitation. Another (as yet unidentified) substance in tobacco smoke causes inhibition of the enzyme **monoamine oxidase B (MAO-B)**, which normally breaks down dopamine. Inhibition of this enzyme results in accumulation of dopamine in the NA. Smokers have between 30% and 40% less MAO-B in their brain than nonsmokers. Nicotine peaks in the blood within 10 minutes of inhalation, but it wears off quickly, therefore requiring further inhalations of the drug multiple times per day. Typically, a smoker will use

Table 8.7 The effects of inhaling nicotine on nonsmokers and smokers

Nonsmokers	Smokers
Various combinations of nausea, vomiting, coughing, sweating, dizziness, flushing of the face, even abdominal cramps and diarrhoea	Relaxation, alertness, reduced hunger

Table 8.8 Some drug interactions with nicotine

Other drugs	Interactions with nicotine
Benzodiazepines	Increased activity of the liver enzymes that metabolise the benzodiazepines, causing reduced efficiency of these drugs
Analgesics	Mixed reactions, mostly result in lower plasma levels and reduced analgesic efficiency
Diazepam	Reduced efficiency of the diazepam
Imiprimine	Faster removal from the body

up to 30 cigarettes a day, with 10 puffs per cigarette. That's 300 nicotine 'hits' per day in order to maintain the drug in the brain, and this contributes to the rapid addiction. After a period of smoking abstinence, e.g. during a night's sleep, the drop in nicotine in the brain causes cholinergic (acetylcholine) activity to be raised above normal. This makes the smoker agitated and uncomfortable until they smoke another cigarette, which restores the nicotine receptor blockade and they become more relaxed. They feel that they 'need' the cigarette to calm down, but it is only because they have themselves artificially pushed up their cholinergic activity by blocking the nicotinic receptors with nicotine in the first place.

Evidence is now pointing towards smoking tobacco as an important cause of anxiety states, depression, and perhaps other mental health disorders, due in part to the increased dopaminergic activity that nicotine causes in the brain (Petit-Zeman 2002). Table 8.7 demonstrates the effects of inhaling nicotine on both nonsmokers and smokers. Given these differences, it becomes obvious how tolerance to nicotine changes a person's perception of the drug and how intolerable passive smoking is to the nonsmoker.

A few *drug interactions* involving nicotine with other drugs are shown in Table 8.8. Other interactions probably do occur, but they remain unstudied. Smoking is a common habit, not least among those under treatment for mental health disorders. Combinations of prescribed drugs with nicotine may be a problem that healthcare professionals should be aware of.

Caffeine

Caffeine is another widely used drug mainly consumed in the form of coffee, but present in a wide range of beverages, including soft drinks, especially those advertised to boost energy levels. It causes release of dopamine in the NA, thus promoting a state of well-being. But caffeine is best known as a drug that promotes wakefulness. This is achieved by binding to **adenosine receptors** in the brain, in particular the **A2a adenosine receptor**. **Adenosine** is a central nervous system modulator, and by binding to adenosine receptors this neurotransmitter slows neural activity and induces sleep. Caffeine is an adenosine receptor antagonist, and by blocking the receptor it prevents adenosine from binding. This causes wakefulness and alertness, clearer thinking, and better physical coordination. In children (drinking caffeine mostly in soft drinks) the caffeine can reach high dosage quite quickly, and causes an increase in alertness, anxiety, nervousness, agitation, recurrent headaches, twitching, and stomach upsets. Caffeine has another role: that of increasing the release of adrenaline and noradrenaline (epinephrine and norepinephrine) from the adrenal cortex. Adrenaline can also increase the alertness of the brain by as much as 40%. In high doses, caffeine has a wide range of psychological and physiological effects, including increased respiration, tremors, fits, cardiac arrhythmias, gastric irritation, and raised blood pressure. Caffeine dependency can occur if enough is consumed on a regular basis, and in such cases stopping the drug quickly may cause withdrawal symptoms such as headache, nausea, and persistent drowsiness.

The hallucinogenic drugs

One of the most potent hallucinogenic agents is **lysergic acid diethylamide (LSD)** (Figure 8.11), which is derived from a fungal disease of grasses called **ergot**. The fungus has the scientific name ***Claviceps purpurea***. LSD produces a dream-like state with heightened senses and a strange blending of senses such that, for example, visual images can cause sounds or weird smells. During the early stages of LSD administration, the effect is of witnessing abstract coloured geometric shapes, such as parallel stripes, hexagons, and checkers. This is followed by the appearance of four specific forms: tunnels, spirals, cobwebs, and honeycomb patterns. This phenomenon is similar to hallucinations, and the study of these effects may give clues to the origin of psychotic hallucinations. Under the influence of LSD, neurons in the visual sensory area of the brain (area VI, Brodmann 17, in the occipital lobe) fire even when there is no stimulus on the retina to see (Mackenzie 2001).

Although the exact mechanism of action of LSD in the brain is not fully understood, the chemical structure of LSD is very similar to that of serotonin, and it binds to the serotonergic 5-HT2A receptor, so it seems likely to work on the serotonergic pathways. The major serotonergic system involves the raphe nuclei of the brain stem, which are the starting point for the serotonergic diffuse modulatory system (see Chapter 4). LSD causes the raphe nuclei to reduce their firing rate, which means the serotonergic system activity is significantly reduced and the brain loses serotonin's modulatory control. This serotonin system usually has an inhibitory function on multiple brain areas and LSD removes this inhibition, so the brain becomes more active. It also binds to the D_2 receptor and therefore exerts some of its effects on the dopaminergic systems. 'Bad trips' on LSD may produce unpleasant hallucinations, dreadful thoughts, nightmares, and acute anxiety. In a few cases, LSD (and perhaps other psychedelic drugs) can cause **hallucinogen persisting perception disorder (HPPD)**, a state in which the 'trip' does not appear to end, and involves incessant distortions of visual stimuli, shimmering lights, and multiple coloured dots. Physical symptoms of LSD use include sweating, nausea, tremors, dry mouth, feelings of numbness, fits, loss of consciousness, anorexia, high blood pressure, and dizziness.

Phencyclidine (PCP, or **1-phenylcyclohexylpiperidine)** is a synthetic hallucinogen causing euphoria, excitement, agitation, delirium, distorted body image, poor concentration and coordination, disordered thinking, bizarre behaviour, memory loss, and mixed, disorganised sensory perception. It is an NMDA glutamate receptor antagonist and causes the blocking of dopamine reuptake so that dopamine accumulates in the synaptic cleft. It also acts as a partial agonist on the D_2 dopamine receptor.

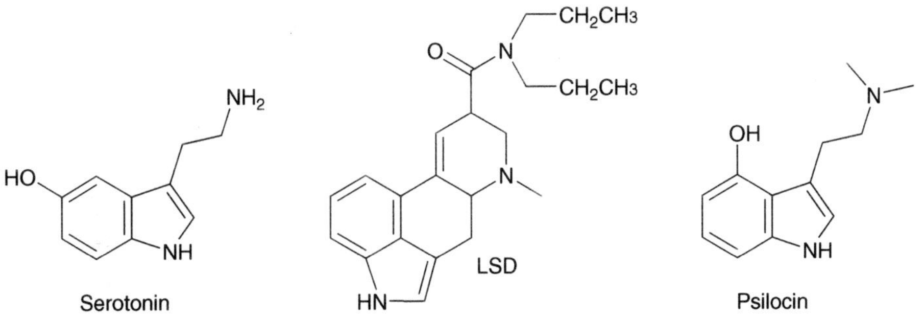

Figure 8.11 Molecular structure of serotonin, LSD, and psilocin.

Another less potent NMDA receptor antagonist is **ketamine**, which is an anaesthetic at high dose, but a hallucinogenic at subanaesthetic doses. It can cause dream-like states, vivid hallucinations, and a sense of detachment from the body (**depersonalisation**) and from reality (**derealisation**). It not only works by blocking the NMDA receptor, but it also acts on opioid receptors and the transport proteins that move dopamine, serotonin, and noradrenaline back into the presynaptic bulb (reuptake; see Chapter 4). The hallucinogenic effects last for about 60 minutes when inhaled or injected, and for about 2 hours if ingested (see also Chapter 11).

Psilocybin is the drug found in so-called 'magic mushrooms', a group of psychedelic mushrooms including the genus *Psilocybe*. The drug causes euphoria, altered thinking and time perception, **synesthesia** (i.e. stimulation of one sense, e.g. hearing, causes involuntary stimulation of a second sense, e.g. vision), and spiritual experiences. Psilocybin is a prodrug, i.e. it requires metabolism within the body to become active. It is converted to **psilocin** (Figure 8.11), a molecule similar in structure to serotonin. It is a partial agonist on several serotonin receptors, with a high affinity for the 5-HT2A receptor. It has some dopaminergic activity, and it is this plus the serotonergic activity on 5-HT2A that are the main cause of its effects.

N, N-dimethyltryptamine (**DMT**) is found in many plants but is also produced naturally in the mammalian body, even in humans (known as 'endogenous DMT'). It binds as an agonist to several serotonin receptors as well as the dopamine D_1 receptor and the adrenergic **alpha 1** (**α1**) and **alpha 2** (**α2**) receptors. It causes euphoria and hallucinations. The hallucinations associated with DMT are often centred on seeing small humanoids (sometimes called '*machine elves*'), and strange humanoid-looking creatures. It has been suggested that perhaps 'alien abductions', i.e. people claiming to have been captured by small aliens in space ships, may actually be the result of these people suffering from the effects of their own endogenous DMT.

Solvents and some gases also have hallucinatory and intoxicating effects. The common factor is that they are inhaled, often by young people of secondary school age, perhaps using a plastic bag to concentrate the vapour. Many are **volatile hydrocarbons**, compounds based on carbon and hydrogen and mostly derived from petroleum. As a liquid, these hydrocarbons evaporate rapidly at room temperature and are used as a wide range of solvents in glue, paint thinners, nail polish and its remover, aerosol propellants, lighter fluid, varnish, and many other products. They include such chemicals as **benzene**, **toluene**, and **butane**, and most are highly flammable. **Carbon tetrachloride**, based on carbon and chloride, has hallucinatory toxic effects on the body when inhaled. It was used in the dry cleaning industry until a safer alternative was introduced. Gases include **nitrous oxide (N_2O)**, which is used in medicine both as an anaesthetic and as an analgesic at subanaesthetic dose. It is also produced ready mixed with oxygen (50% each of gas and oxygen), and this is often used at the scene of an accident or in emergency obstetric situations. Inhalation of gases and solvent vapours causes a drunk-like state with the possibility of hallucinations, emotional disturbance, and distortions of perception. They enter the blood and move quickly to the brain and liver. In the brain they have an initial euphoric effect, causing a 'high' that is probably due to dopamine release. However, this is followed by disorientation, auditory hallucinations, slurred speech, double vision, possible loss of consciousness and fits, nausea and vomiting, headache that may last for days, and a depressant effect that slows respiration and heart rate, and reduces mental activity. In sufficient doses, the heart may go into fibrillation. Long-term use may cause weight loss, nose bleeds, mouth and nasal sores, memory loss, fatigue, depression, and paranoia. Liver, kidney, and brain damage have all been reported in long-term abusers of solvents.

These agents are slow to be excreted from the body and therefore the effects can last for days. Death can occur from **asphyxia** (cessation of breathing) due to obstructing the airway when using a plastic bag, respiratory or heart failure, or sudden cardiac arrest. Solvent abuse caused 50 deaths in the UK during 2008, mostly of young people. Solvents also cause tolerance and addiction, and withdrawal causes symptoms similar to alcohol withdrawal.

Bromo-benzodifuranil-isopropylamine is better known as **Bromo-DragonFly (BDF)**, a potent hallucinogen only slightly less potent than LSD. It has a very long period of activity in the brain, causing hallucinogenic symptoms for up to 72 hours. It can cause distortion of visual perception, a loss of the sense of time, vomiting of blood, and dreadful nightmares.

Potential for drugs of addiction now used in medicine

The potential for the use of these drugs in the treatment of medical conditions, in particular mental health disorders, is gradually becoming realised after years of minimal research due to legal restrictions. The growing use of cannabis as a medication has been mentioned earlier, as well as the potential for the use of cannabidiol as a treatment of multiples conditions. Cannabis may prove useful in managing attention deficit hyperactivity disorder (ADHD; see Chapter 15) and insomnia (see Chapter 16). MDMA's ability to reduce bad memories and enhance happy memories may be a useful adjunct in the treatment of post-traumatic stress disorder (PTSD, see Chapter 9). It may also find a place in the treatment of Parkinson's disease (see Chapter 13). LSD could become part of the therapy for anxiety disorders (see Chapter 9) and alcoholism. Psilocybin could become available to treat obsessive-compulsive disorder (OCD), anxiety states, and PTSD (see Chapter 9). Ketamine is already a general anaesthetic, but it may also be very useful in treating depression, especially bipolar disorder, having produced good antidepressant effects within hours of administration (see Chapter 11). Of course, the medical use of these drugs would have to be strictly controlled, and the dosage carefully worked out, in order to minimise the risk of addiction.

Key points

The reward pathways

- The medial forebrain bundle links the ventral tegmental area of the midbrain with the nucleus accumbens. This pathway forms part of the mesotelencephalic dopamine system.
- This dopamine pathway is strongly implicated in the activities of many self-administered stimulatory drugs.
- Many stimulant and addictive drugs are those that cause high dopamine levels to occur in the brain, and in the nucleus accumbens in particular.

Opiate drugs

- Opiate drugs cause analgesia, euphoria, and sedatory and depressant effects.
- The mechanism that leads to euphoria and the feeling of well-being appears to be mediated through the mu (μ) receptor, which also reinforces drug-seeking behaviour.
- Withdrawal from drugs is associated with reduced levels of both dopamine and serotonin in the brain, and increased levels of corticotropin-releasing factor (CRF).
- Tolerance appears to result from receptors becoming less sensitive to the drug, which may involve a protein called cyclic AMP-responsive element-binding protein (CREB).

Cocaine

- Cocaine blocks the reuptake of dopamine into the presynaptic bulb by inhibiting dopamine pumps in the synaptic membrane.
- Dopamine accumulates within the synaptic clefts of the nucleus accumbens.

Amphetamines

- Amphetamines block the reuptake of dopamine into the presynaptic bulb by inhibiting dopamine pumps in the synaptic membrane.
- Amphetamines also increase dopamine and noradrenaline levels within the synapses by increasing dopamine release from the presynaptic bulb.
- Ecstasy (MDMA) is converted in the body to an active metabolite (HMMA), which causes increased antidiuretic hormone (ADH or vasopressin).
- ADH increases water in the blood, and this extra water dilutes the electrolytes around the neurons. The brain becomes swollen and suffers convulsions and coma, with a potential to cause death.

Cannabinoids

- Marihuana comes from the dried leaves of the Indian hemp plant *Cannabis sativa*.
- The psychoactive ingredients are cannabinoids.
- The most potent is delta-9-tetrahydrocannabinol (THC), which binds to cannabinoid receptors in the brain, notably the basal ganglia, the hippocampus, the cerebellum, and the frontal lobe of the cerebrum.
- Cannabinoids cause not only dopamine release in the nucleus accumbens but also high levels of CRF release during withdrawal.

Alcohol

- Alcohol is a psychoactive drug that in low dosage acts as a mild stimulant, giving a feeling of well-being.
- In higher doses, alcohol is a depressant to many parts of the brain. Depressive effects include cognitive impairment, slowed reaction times, and verbal and motor impairment.
- Very high doses of alcohol can cause unconsciousness and death.
- Rapid withdrawal from alcohol causes nausea, vomiting, headache, and tremors, as well as alcohol withdrawal delirium, i.e. agitation, confusion, tachycardia, hallucinations, and delusions.
- Korsakoff's syndrome is a chronic state of amnesia with confabulation and Wernicke's encephalopathy is a state of intellectual impairment; these occur often together in a patient with long-term alcohol abuse.
- There are two basic types of drinkers: the steady drinkers and the bingers.
- Steady drinking has a strong genetic basis, starting early in life, and is associated with antisocial behaviour.
- Binging alcohol abuse is more environmental than genetic in origin. It starts later in life and affects both sexes.

Nicotine and caffeine

- Nicotine causes major problems of addiction, and tobacco smoking causes about 300 deaths per day in the UK alone.
- Nicotine and caffeine both increase the level of dopamine in the nucleus accumbens.

Hallucinogenic drugs

- These drugs are vapours and gases, which are inhaled.
- Many of the vapours are hydrocarbons based on petroleum.
- They cause intoxication, dreamlike states, and hallucinations.
- They cause long-term addiction and brain damage and have the potential to kill the user by heart or respiratory failure.

References

Anthes, E. (2010) She's hooked. *Scientific American Mind*, **21**, 14–15. DOI:10.1038/scientificamericanmind0510-14.

Becker, B., Wagner, D., Koester, P., Tittgemeyer, M., Mercer-Chalmers-Bender, K., Hurlemann, R., Zhang, J., Gouzoulis-Mayfrank, E., Kendrick, K. M., and Daumann, J. (2015) Smaller amygdala and medial prefrontal cortex predict escalating stimulant use. *Brain, A Journal of Neurology*. DOI: 10.1093/brain/awv113.

Blows, W. T. (1998) Crowd physiology: the 'penguin effect'. *Accident and Emergency Nursing*, **6** (3): 126–129.

Carlson, N. (2012) *Physiology of Behaviour* (11th edition). Pearson Education, Harlow, UK.

Concar, D. (2002) Ecstasy on the brain. *New Scientist*, **174** (2339; 20 April): 26–33.

Day, J. J., Childs, D., Guzman-Karlsson, M. C., Kibe, M., Moulden, J., Song, E., Tahir, A., and Sweatt, D. (2013) DNA methylation regulates associative reward learning. *Nature Neuroscience*, **16**: 1445–1452. DOI: 10.1038/nn.3504.

Ersche, K. D., Jones, P. S., Williams, G. B., Turton, A. J., Robbins, T. W., and Bullmore, E. T. (2012) Abnormal brain structure implicated in stimulant drug addiction. *Science*, **335**: 601–604.

Gourley, S., Olevska, A., Warren, S., Taylor, J. R., and Koleske, A. (2012) ArgKinase regulates prefrontal dendritic spine refinement and cocaine-induced plasticity. *Journal of Neuroscience*, **32** (7): 2314–2323.

Harrington-Dobinson, A. and Blows, W. T. (2006) Part 1: nurses' guide to alcohol and promoting healthy lifestyle changes. *British Journal of Nursing*, **15** (22): 1217–1219 (14th December 2006).

Harrington-Dobinson, A. and Blows, W. T. (2007a) Part 2: nurses' guide to the impact of alcohol on health and wellbeing. *British Journal of Nursing*, **16** (1): 47–51 (11th January 2007).

Harrington-Dobinson, A. and Blows, W. T. (2007b) Part 3: nurses' guide to alcohol and promoting healthy lifestyle changes. *British Journal of Nursing*, **16** (2): 106–110 (25th January 2007).

Hartman, R. L., Brown, T. L., Milavetz, G., Spurgin, A., Gorelick, D. A., Gaffney, G., and Huestis M. A. (2015) Controlled cannabis vaporiser administration: blood and plasma cannabinoids with and without alcohol. *Clinical Chemistry*, May 2015. DOI: 10.1373/clinchem.2015.238287.

Koob, G. F. (2000) Opiate tolerance and dependence. *Science and Medicine*, **7** (2): 28–37.

MacKenzie, D. (2001) Secrets of an acid head. *New Scientist*, **170** (2296; 23 June): 26–30.

Nolen-Hoeksema, S. (2007) *Abnormal Psychology*. McGraw-Hill, Boston, MA.

Petit-Zeman S. (2002) Smoke gets in your mind. *New Scientist*, **174** (2338; 13 April): 30–33.

Ungless, M. A., Whistler, J. L., Malenka, R. C., and Bonci, A. (2001) Single cocaine exposure *in vivo* induces long-term potentiation in dopamine neurons. *Nature*, **411** (31 May): 583–587.

Wiedemann, C. (2010) Addiction: cannabis against heroin? *Nature Reviews Neuroscience*, **11**: 3.

9   Stress, emotions, anxiety, and fear

- The limbic system and the biology of emotions
- The biology of stress
- The emotions of life experiences
- Anxiety disorders
- Fear and phobias
- Eating disorders
- Anxiety-related personality disorders
- The anxiolytic drugs
- Key points

The limbic system and the biology of emotions

The limbic system is a series of centres collectively involved in *preservation of the individual* (i.e. *self-preservation*) and *preservation of the species*. It governs behaviour essential to the survival of the individual, ensuring, for example, that we seek food or respond to threats, and also promotes reproductive behaviour to ensure survival of the species. The major components of the limbic system (Figure 9.1) are the **amygdala**; the **mammillary bodies** of the **hypothalamus**; the **anterior and dorsal nuclei of the thalamus**; several deep nuclei; and the **septal area**. The **orbitofrontal cortex** of the cerebrum, several other areas of the cortex, such as the **hippocampus**, the **parahippocampal gyrus,** and parts of the **temporal lobe** are together known as the **limbic association cortex** because of their close association with the functions of the limbic system.

The limbic system has the following functions:

- It is the centre for the control of emotions, including fear and aggression.
- It controls reproductive and other survival behaviours.
- It influences memory, because the hippocampus stores short-term memory.
- Through the hypothalamus, it influences hormonal release and the autonomic nervous system.

The whole system is set in a ring structure (*limbic* = 'bordering' or 'ringing') deep in the brain (see Chapter 1, and Figures 1.4, 1.5, and 9.1).

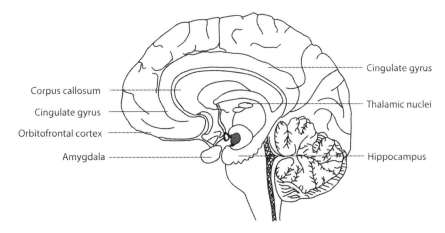

Figure 9.1 The main components of the limbic system.

The **amygdala** (Figure 9.2) is a pea-sized collection of nuclei situated within the limbic system inside the temporal lobes, below the level of the cortex. It sits at the end of the tail of the caudate nucleus (see Figure 1.4 on page 8). The important nuclei of the amygdala and their functions are listed below.

1   The **corticomedial group** is very small and not well defined in humans. It plays a role in inhibiting aggressive behaviour.
2   The **basolateral group** relays sensory information from the primary sensory cortex of the cerebrum (Brodmann 1, 2, and 3), the sensory association cortex (Brodmann 40) and the thalamus to the central nucleus.
3   The **central nucleus** receives the information from the basolateral group and has its output to the brain stem and the hypothalamus (see Figure 7.3 in Chapter 7). The output to the brain stem is to various nuclei that carry out different functions in relation to emotional reactions. The output to the hypothalamus causes physical responses by influencing hypothalamic control of both the sympathetic nervous system (neuro response) and the pituitary hormones (endocrine response), collectively known as a **neuroendocrine response**.

The amygdala receives input from several sources, as listed in point 2 above, with slightly delayed time intervals. The following text should be read in conjunction with Figure 9.2.

Primary amygdala input. The primary input to the amygdala is the direct automatic input of sensory stimuli from the thalamus, just as they are received from the environment. This unprocessed (or *raw*) data is the first to arrive at the amygdala and for a brief moment it is all the structure has to work on to determine the emotional response. As a result there is a rapid, but not always appropriate, response. The amygdala simply gives the individual the best option for survival, responding in a protective manner that may turn out to be unnecessary. Impulsive reactions and behaviour can be seen as *acting without thinking* or, in the case of the amygdala, acting on unconsidered, and therefore unprocessed, stimuli (note here an interesting correlation with murderers, see page 90). It should not be surprising that impulsive

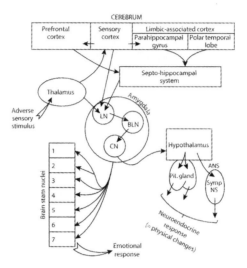

Figure 9.2 Inputs and outputs of the amygdala. Sensory information coming into the thalamus is passed to the sensory cortex, but also directly to the **lateral nucleus (LN)** of the amygdala. The sensory cortex passes the information to the prefrontal cortex to produce an action plan, which is passed to the septo-hippocampal system. Information identifying the sensory information passes through the limbic-associated cortex to the septo-hippocampal system. From here, input to the amygdala is via the lateral nucleus, to the **basolateral nucleus (BLN)**, and on to the **central nucleus (CN)**. The central nucleus has outputs to the brain stem nuclei (for emotional response), and the hypothalamus (for physical response).

behaviour of this kind is often seen in children, as a child's limbic system is immature. The processing and consideration of sensory stimuli requires sophisticated and complex neural systems, coupled with extensive memory stores, both of which the young brain has not had time to develop fully.

Not only has the sensory stimulus gone from the thalamus to the amygdala, but the thalamus has also passed the raw stimulus on to the primary sensory cortex of the cerebrum (if the stimulus comes from the body) or to one of the specialist sensory areas such as hearing or vision. Here the task of interpretation takes place to determine what the stimulus actually is. This involves comparing the new stimulus with memories of previous stimuli to find a match. The cerebrum adds a conscious element to the stimulus, so the individual is aware of the stimulus and can add a degree of reason to the response.

Secondary amygdala input. The secondary input to the amygdala comes from the cerebral cortex. This cerebral output also passes to the **limbic-associated cortex**, which is made up of the **parahippocampal gyrus** and the **polar temporal lobe cortex**. The limbic-associated cortex consists of those areas of the cerebral cortex that work with the limbic system in the determination of stimuli. It should not be surprising to find the cerebrum and limbic system working together on emotions, as the limbic system does not have extensive memory banks to use in the identification and evaluation of stimuli. Most of the memory banks for this are found in the sensory association areas of the cerebrum. Thus it is in the limbic association cortex that interpretations and evaluation of the stimulus are mostly made. The polar temporal lobe cortex evaluates the stimulus for potential danger to the individual. The sensory cortex also sends the stimulus to the **prefrontal cortex**, where an action plan is formulated in response to the stimulus. The prefrontal cortex is close to the main motor cortex that activates skeletal muscle, so any action plan, such as running away or fighting, can be rapidly implemented. The outputs from the prefrontal cortex and the limbic-associated cortex are passed to the **septo-hippocampal system**, consisting of the **septum** and the **hippocampus**. Here integration of the action plan with the interpretation and evaluation of danger can take place, with input from short-term memory and perhaps aggression control if needed, as these are both functions of the hippocampus.

Tertiary amygdala input. The tertiary input to the amygdala is the final output from the septo-hippocampal system. The amygdala now has all the relevant information necessary to determine an appropriate emotional response.

We can put all this together in a simple scenario. Your friend decides to play a joke on you. She hides behind the door with the intention of jumping out and surprising you. As you enter the room she does just that, springing out and making a loud noise. The *primary and secondary amygdala inputs* would occur so close together that they would appear to be simultaneous. You would become aware of the sudden appearance of someone jumping out at the same time as hearing a loud noise. This could be anyone or anything, a potential threat to safety. In a purely automatic defensive strategy, you are likely to attempt to move out of danger and perhaps lash out physically. This may be coupled with a scream, or some brisk language, and very rapid changes in physiology – for example, the cardiovascular system would show a dramatic rise in the pulse rate and blood pressure. But very quickly the *tertiary amygdala input*, hot on the heels of the previous two inputs, will allow you to recognise this person as a friend and their intentions were simply to play a joke. Your response to the outburst would then be modified once this tertiary input has established the true nature of the surprise.

The outputs from the amygdala (Figure 9.3) can activate:

1   Various nuclei of the **brain stem** responsible for the following *emotional reactions*:

- the **trigeminal** (cranial nerve V) and **facial** (cranial nerve VII) nuclei, which control the muscles of facial expression during emotions such as fear;
- the nuclei of the **periaqueductal grey** (**PAG**) area, which cause four main responses, those of *freeze reaction* (i.e. behavioural arrest), *defensive* and *predatory aggression*, and *flight from danger*, depending on which part is stimulated;
- the **nucleus reticularis pontis caudalis**, which causes a startled response;
- the **dorsal lateral tegmental** nucleus, which activates the higher centres of the cortex onto full alert;
- the **locus coeruleus** nucleus, which increases cortical vigilance through noradrenergic pathways;
- the nuclei of the **ventral tegmental area**, which increases behavioural arousal through dopaminergic pathways and mediates for offensive aggression.

2   Various nuclei of the **hypothalamus** responsible for the following *physical responses*:

- the **periventricular group** of nuclei, which causes increased *sympathetic nervous system* activity;
- various nuclei that together influence the release of stress-related *hormones* into the blood.

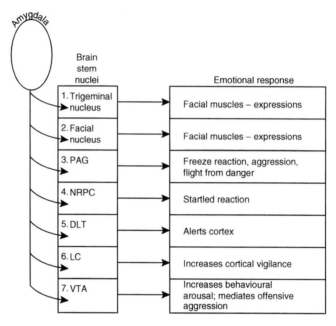

Figure 9.3 The brain stem nuclei are influenced by the amygdala to achieve various emotional responses, depending on which nucleus is activated. DLT = dorsal lateral tegmental nucleus, LC = locus coeruleus, NRPC = nucleus reticularis pontis caudalis, PAG = periaqueductal grey, VTA = ventral tegmental area.

The neurobiology of emotions is now becoming clearer as research unpicks the delicate nerve networks that link the various components of the brain.

The biology of stress

As a subject, stress is assuming much importance in everyday life, with many articles being published on aspects such as stress in the workplace and **post-traumatic stress disorder**. Stress is both a physical and a mental phenomenon, and an examination of the physiological processes it causes emphasises the harm that excessive or long-term stress can do.

Stressors – adverse environmental factors causing stress – cause undesirable stimuli to enter the thalamus of the brain via the sensory nervous system. Using the emotional pathways shown in Figures 9.2 and 9.3, the stress stimuli pass through the amygdala and on to the hypothalamus. The hypothalamic **neuroendocrine response** (Figure 9.4) occurs, causing a number of physical changes:

- The autonomic nervous system switches to *sympathetic* activation and this causes the heart rate, blood pressure and blood sugar to rise. The hormone **adrenaline** is secreted into the blood from the **adrenal medulla** by direct stimulation from the sympathetic nervous system. This has the effect of augmenting the sympathetic activity, pushing up the blood pressure and heart rate further. The other hormone released into the blood from the adrenal medulla is **noradrenaline**, which diverts blood away from the skin to supply to the brain and muscles. This may be essential for a quick retreat from the stressor.

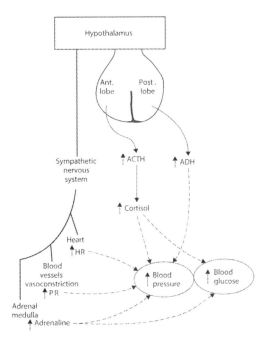

Figure 9.4 The neuroendocrine response to stress.

- The endocrine component of the hypothalamus releases **corticotropin-releasing factor or hormone (CRF or CRH)**, which causes the release of **adrenocorticotropic hormone (ACTH)** from the anterior lobe of the pituitary gland into the general circulation. This in turn causes the release of **cortisol** from the adrenal cortex. The blood concentration of cortisol then increases, a well-known physical response to stress. In fact, the rise in blood cortisol concentration is significant in stress, and it has been suggested that measurement of blood cortisol concentrations could be a way of measuring stress itself.

Cortisol binds to receptors in the cytoplasm of many neurons and causes **gene transcription** (activation of genes) leading to **protein synthesis**. The production of proteins is, in the short term, protective to nerve cells. One effect is to increase the influx of calcium (Ca^{2+}) into the neurons, and this improves neuronal function. Cortisol also activates the brain so that it can cope better with new experiences in the short term. It causes increased blood glucose concentrations by counteracting the action of **insulin**. In the long term, as in chronic stress, high cortisol concentrations appear to inhibit **GLUT3**, one of several **glucose transport molecules** found in cells. GLUT3 is widely found in neurons and is responsible for the passage of glucose into neurons. Long-term inhibition of GLUT3 may cause cellular damage due to reduced glucose energy supply. The hippocampus (and thus short-term memory) is particularly affected in this way. High concentrations of cortisol in stressed children can damage their mental ability, causing them to become upset easily and adopt withdrawn, shy behaviour. They also show increased physical ill health. The hippocampus has the ability to produce new neurons after birth, but excessive cortisol during stress inhibits this normal process. The result is to increase negative effects such as anxiety, fear, and aggression. **Brain-derived neurotrophic factor (BDNF)**, a molecule produced to help develop healthy brain tissue, reverses these negative effects.

CRF is itself generating a lot of interest among researchers because high or low CRF concentrations are now implicated in a number of neuropsychiatric conditions, including anorexia nervosa, anxiety, and depression (see Chapter 11). A low CRF concentration is also involved in neurodegenerative disorders such as Alzheimer's disease (see Chapter 14). Two CRF metabotropic receptors have been isolated, **CRF1** and **CRF2**, which bind the hormone in the pituitary gland, in several parts of the brain and, somewhat surprisingly, in the gut and spleen. Stress normally causes a downregulation of the number of CRF receptors in the anterior pituitary. In chronic stress, this downregulation may be insufficient or simply fail, and a future generation of drugs designed to block CRF receptors is under development to help relieve the symptoms of chronic stress.

Components of the immune system become involved in the stress response, in a process studied under the title **psychoneuroimmunology** (meaning *mind, nervous system and immune system*). Stress causes changes to the immune system, in particular **immunosuppression**, a reduction in the immune response that increases the risk of infection. **Natural killer (NK) cells** (those that kill virally infected and malignant cells), **lymphocytes** (the main cells of the immune system), and an antibody called **immunoglobulin A (IgA)** are all significantly reduced in stress. These responses suggest that brain neuromodulators released during stress have a wide influence over body functions both inside and outside of the nervous system (Kaye et al. 2000).

A protein called **lipocalin-2** is only produced in the hippocampus during stress, and this changes the shape of dendritic spines, i.e. minute spines on the dendrites of neurons where memories are stored. 'Thin' spines are changing connections until they store a memory, then they become mushroom-shaped, and their connections become stable and more permanent. Lipocalin-2 removes or prevents the mushroom-shaped memory spines from forming during stress, and this protects the brain when subjected to future stress by reducing the stress memories. In this way, the protein stops the acute response to future stress, allowing the individual to cope better with stress (Mucha et al. 2011).

The symptoms of stress are pallor, raised pulse rate and blood pressure, deeper respiration, sweating, raised blood sugar concentrations, dilated pupils, nausea, frequency of urination, and restlessness. Many of these can be recognised as 'side effects' of the neuroendocrine response; the sweating, for example, is due to increased sympathetic activity, and this combined with adrenaline also drives up the blood pressure and increases the heart rate. The release of cortisol helps to drive up the blood glucose concentrations. These **compensatory mechanisms** are brought into play by the body to correct the initial physiological changes, which would otherwise cause the body harm during the period of stress.

In the long term, when stress is persistent for months or years, the result is different. The body tries to compensate for the effects of stress for as long as possible, but eventually fails. When this happens, the individual suffers symptoms of ill health, both physically and mentally. Three distinct phases are recognised in the **General adaptation syndrome (GAS)** (Figure 9.5) (Nolen-Hoeksema 2007). Phase 1 (**alarm phase**) occurs soon after exposure to the stressor. Physiological factors such as blood pressure and blood glucose concentrations fall, but the neuroendocrine response then compensates to restore the blood pressure and blood glucose concentrations. Phase 2 (**resistance phase**) is the period during which compensation is able to continue. How long this lasts depends on the severity and the time duration of the stressor. Phase 3 (**exhaustion phase**) is marked by the collapse of the neuroendocrine response and the return of symptoms. If the exhaustion phase is prolonged, or the stressor is particularly severe, ill health will follow. Chronic stress causes many complications, including possible premature

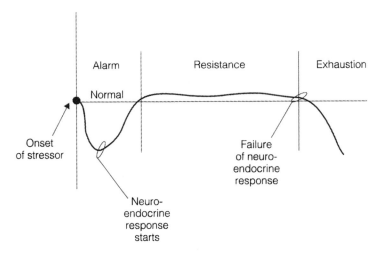

Figure 9.5 The general adaptation syndrome (GAS) with phase 1 (alarm), phase 2 (resistance), and phase 3 (exhaustion). See text for explanation.

ageing of the brain with neuronal losses. The hippocampus is the most likely candidate for cellular losses due to chronic stress. Other long-term effects of chronic cortisol release during stress include **hypertension** (high blood pressure), **peptic ulceration** (ulcers of the stomach and duodenum), depression, substance abuse, and anxiety.

It may one day be possible to harness the effects of a natural stress reduction system in the brain called the **nociceptin system**. Nociceptin is a naturally produced compound related to the endogenous opioids (see Chapter 4), but binds to its own receptor called the **NOP** (or **kappa-type 3 opioid**) receptor. *Nociception* is a word that means 'generating pain', and this system does make pain worse. It also blocks the reward effects of taking morphine and heroin. As such, then, it is an anti-opioid. But in the amygdala it has a stress reduction role that activates automatically under stress conditions as concentrations of CRF rise. In the future, it may be possible to design a drug that makes use of this system to great effect in stress relief.

Strategies for stress relief

Much is written about drug-free methods of reducing stress and anxiety, and therefore increasing longevity. How effective they are may vary between individuals. These are the main techniques:

- Social networking and a good circle of family and friends is shown to give a 50% higher chance of outliving those with little or poor social relationships. But the facts point to quality rather than quantity, so thousands of so-called 'friends' on social media websites count for little. What matters is the closeness of the friendships and relationships, including marriage. Don't bottle up the stress or guilt, but find ways of expressing these with others. Use counselling or confide in family or friends. 'A problem shared is a problem halved' is actually very close to the truth.

- Meditation and yoga are proving to be valuable tools in calming the mind. Eight weeks of meditation appears to shrink the amygdala, the emotional and fear centre of the brain, and the prefrontal cortex increases in volume. As a result, automatic fear and anxiety responses are reduced and more reasoned thought is improved. It also reduces pain perception, so physical pain is less. Yoga has similar stress and pain relief effects as meditation, but also has the physical benefits of improved cardiovascular health, reduction of obesity, and improvement of the blood lipid profile.
- An optimistic, positive outlook on life, coupled with fun and laughter are powerful medicines, apparently. Stress relief is instantaneous and this approach also reduces incidence of depression. Stress may still happen, but it is important to view the stress positively, rather than negatively.
- Getting back to nature is also important, especially when combined with fresh air and exercise. Walking in the countryside, or by the sea, reduces activity in the **subgenial prefrontal cortex**, an area involved in self-reflective inward thinking and withdrawal from the individual's surroundings. There are also claims of benefits from close proximity with animals, e.g. dogs, cats, and other similar animals are said to reduce stress. The physical and mental benefits of exercise are now well known. Just about every body system is better off after exercise, and for the brain this means improved cognitive functions such as planning and attention levels. The benefits apply even if the exercise is gentle and easy. The guideline for full fitness is 150 minutes of moderate exercise per week, but those achieving only a fraction of this can still lower their risk of premature death by 20%.

Stress and child abuse

Stress occurring during childhood causes 'a cascade of molecular and neuro-biological effects that irreversibly alter neural development' (Teicher 2002). Such stress is the result of child abuse, either active (physical beatings or sexual abuse) or passive (neglect or isolation). In each case the brain is exposed to extensive fear, and permanent damage often results from this type of stress. The damage includes:

- irregularities in the function of the left frontal and temporal lobes of the cerebrum;
- reduced size of the hippocampus and amygdala, again most often seen on the left side of the brain;
- abnormalities within the cerebellar vermis.

The hippocampus continues its development beyond birth, well into childhood, and is one of the few areas of the brain in which neurons continue to grow after birth. New neurons form new synaptic connections, and it is these neurons and their connections that are disrupted permanently when children are subjected to the extreme fear of abuse. In the amygdala, the $GABA_A$ receptor is significantly altered by the fear accompanying abuse, causing a loss of its inhibitory function. The result is excessive stimulation of the limbic system (called **limbic irritability**), i.e. abnormal excessive activity of the area that governs emotions.

The cerebellar vermis (the central ridge between the cerebellar hemispheres) is another area that continues growing and developing new neurons after birth. The vermis has some control over noradrenaline and dopamine release within the brain stem. Vermis abnormalities (now being linked to several mental disorders, including depression, schizophrenia, and autism) may push these neurotransmitters into imbalance. Activation and dominance of the dopamine system is linked with increased attention in the *left* hemisphere; activation and dominance of the noradrenaline system is linked with increased attention in the *right* hemisphere. Developmental abnormalities occurring in the vermis after birth as a result of the stress from child abuse may be the cause of the left lateral defects observed in the cerebral and limbic areas. The results of such damage are depression, withdrawal, suicidal tendencies, anxiety, anger, aggression, delinquency, unstable relationships, and personality disorders, any of which can occur at any point later in life. Teicher (2002) summarised the studies by saying:

> Society reaps what it sows in the way it nurtures its children. Stress sculpts the brain to exhibit various antisocial . . . behaviours. . . . Stress can permanently wire a child's brain to cope with a malevolent world. . . . Our stark conclusion is that we see the need to do much more to ensure that child abuse does not happen in the first place, because once these key brain alterations occur, there may be no going back. (Teicher 2002)

Rather bizarrely, some children become emotionally attached to their abusers, rather than do everything they can to leave the relationship. This situation is akin to **Stockholm syndrome** in which hostages become emotionally attached to their kidnappers and do what they can to help them, rather than punish them for their crime. In the case of abused children, the 'emotional' attachment to the abuser is thought to be an adaptive response caused by the child's need for care, despite the poor quality of that care. Neurobiologists have pinned down this phenomenon to low concentrations of dopamine in the child's amygdala (Westly 2010).

The emotions of life experiences

Human emotions fall into five basic categories, which are, in themselves, independent of religious, cultural, or social groups, and therefore likely to be the product of innate neurological activity. The five categories are sadness, happiness, fear, anger, and disgust. The neuroanatomy and physiology of these, and many other possible human emotions have fascinated neuroscientists for a long time. Here, we consider some of these emotions and what we know of their neurological basis.

Humour

Humour is both a pleasant emotion and one that is said to be beneficial to our health and well-being. It is often considered as a 'medicine' for stress and anxiety and other mental and physical conditions. Imaging techniques have highlighted several areas of the brain involved in understanding a joke and responding to it with laughter. The brain areas most active in this process are the **left posterior temporal gyrus**, the **left inferior frontal gyrus**, and the **temporoparietal junction**. Humour requires language appreciation, learning, and decision-making skills, and these areas are involved in these functions. Activity also takes place in the **ventral striatum** of the limbic system, the emotional area of the brain. Here, the level of activity corresponds well with our recognition of how funny the humour is. The **hypothalamus** and **periaqueductal grey** are involved in laughter, and **dopamine** is released in the reward centres (i.e. the **nucleus accumbens**; see Chapter 8) during the viewing of comedy films. Variations between the sexes also occur, e.g. women show greater activity in the prefrontal cortex and a greater response to funny situations from the limbic system than men do. This suggests that women undergo more in-depth executive and language processing than males when getting to grips with a joke, although the reasons for these differences are not clear. So-called 'extroverts' appear to have greater activity in their reward circuits of the brain, including the ventral striatum, during humorous situations than do 'neurotic' or 'introverted' individuals (Elkan 2010).

Religious experiences

Religious experiences occur when a subject becomes aware of a sense of an almighty power in their presence, which they usually call God, and may sometimes experience what they call Heaven. In some people this has changed their lives and they have become ministers of various churches and preach or administer healing powers to others. Neuroscientists go to some lengths to point out that while they have no wish to attempt to disprove the existence of God, they have found that specific types of stimulation of the **temporal lobes** of the cerebrum (especially the right temporal lobe) and the limbic system can generate what can be an overwhelming religious feeling. This is usually coupled with a release of endogenous opiates, which intensifies the experience. It is interesting that some people suffer overwhelming religious feelings when first visiting the holy city of Jerusalem. The so-called **Jerusalem syndrome** causes previously unaffected individuals to re-enact scenes from the bible, in full biblical dress, at the sites in Jerusalem where they originally took place. During this time they are overwhelmed with emotion, bordering on psychosis. This sounds like a joke, but in 1999 more than 50 people with no previous mental health problems needed emergency psychiatric care while visiting the city.

Love

Love is an experience most people go through at some point in their lives. Scans of the brains of volunteers taken during the intensified mental emotions of love reveal four main areas of increased brain activity: the **anterior cingulate cortex** (see Figure 9.6, and Figure 10.1 in Chapter 10), the **medial insula** (part of the cerebral cortex hidden from the surface), and two areas of the **corpus striatum** (part of the basal ganglia) (Figure 9.6) (Phillips 2000a). But love is not confined to the emotions experienced between two people. It is common to love abstract concepts such as music or art, or to express love of a place of great beauty. **Stendhal syndrome** (also known as **Florence syndrome**) is a feeling of palpitations, dizziness, fainting, confusion, and even hallucinations when coming face to face with a piece of great art, or overwhelming amounts of great art. Florence syndrome is named after the city of Florence in Italy where substantial numbers of visitors have become overwhelmed by the city's beautiful art and architecture, and have needed treatment. There have been discussions concerning the possibility of stationing ambulances at regular intervals in the streets of Florence because of the number of visitors falling emotionally ill when confronted with the beauty of the city!

Music

Music has attracted much interest from neuroscientists for several reasons. Notably, musical ability is often associated with being a genius, and what makes a genius is of great interest

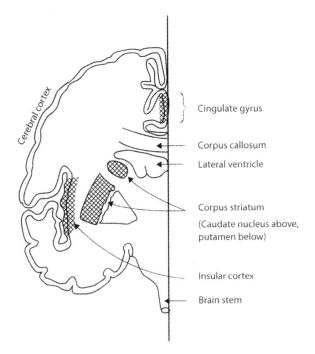

Figure 9.6 The brain areas of love. The areas shaded are activated during the emotional feelings of love.

to many people. Music has therapeutic properties and for many years has been used as a psychological therapy (*music therapy*). More research needs to be done before we can fully explain why music therapy is good for the disturbed mind. Also, learning to play an instrument as a child is now recognised as beneficial in improving attention, giving better control over anxiety and emotions, increasing memory, greater language and reading skills, and better engagement in social activity. Musical children usually achieve above average at school. These benefits are caused by thickening and improving the cortical structures of the brain in areas involved in music processing at the time when the brain is still developing; benefits that will last a lifetime.

Music generates some of the most intense emotions in some people, anything from excitement to depression, and the question is *Why?* We still do not have all the answers to this question, but some interesting concepts point the way. Music has a lot to do with *motion*, and motion has a lot to do with *emotion* (the two words have a common origin, i.e. *motum* = 'movement'). Indeed, the separate sections of a symphony are called movements, and when experiencing emotion from the music the listener may describe the experience as 'moving'. Specific emotions, such as love or fear, have definite signs that we can identify in each other and can respond to. Tonal music also has specific signatures that we can pick out and relate to, like a rhythm or a tune, and music is rarely static, it is constantly driving forward. So music and emotions have very similar components. Just as one angry or laughing person can make others angry or laugh, so music performed by one person can engender emotional moods in an audience.

The parts of the brain involved in music appreciation are slowly being revealed (Figure 9.7):

- The **auditory cortex** (temporal lobe) processes the main elements of music, i.e. pitch and volume, and relays the components of music to multiple areas of the brain. The surrounding area includes the **auditory association area,** which processes harmony and rhythm.
- The right **insula** processes aesthetic experiences from all the senses together. The insula is involved in love (above) and therefore is involved in the love and appreciation of music.
- The **anterior cingulate cortex (ACC)** is where emotions, reward and cognition interact, e.g. the **dorsal ACC (dACC)** processes reward and connects directly with the nucleus accumbens and the caudate nucleus (part of the striatum). The ACC updates cognitive decisions in relation to emotional cues such as music. The ACC has two directional connections with the insula, and this together with the ACC and the hypothalamus control the physiological response to music through the **autonomic nervous system (ANS)**.
- The **prefrontal cortex** assesses the value of the music and, like the ACC, also has connections with the nucleus accumbens and caudate nucleus.
- As seen in Chapter 8, the **nucleus accumbens** is a major site for pleasure and reward. Dopamine and endogenous opioids released into the brain, notably dopamine released into the nucleus accumbens and the striatum during music, causes a 'feel good' situation.
- Music creates a state of arousal in the **amygdala**, and this heightens the emotional qualities of music. Connections with the amygdala and hypothalamus provide simultaneous emotional and physiological response.
- The **caudate nucleus** (part of the striatum) adds additional qualities to the music experience, qualities such as sequencing the sounds, creating and heightening expectancy within the music, and anticipating the musical outcome. Dopamine is released into the caudate nucleus in anticipation of the pleasure music will bring. The caudate nucleus has connections with the prefrontal cortex, midbrain (part of the brain stem), and the ACC. Connections between the striatum and the auditory cortex are very busy during the perception of music.
- The speech centre, **Wernicke's area**, becomes active in the presence of music, particularly if the music involves singing words.
- **Motor areas** also get involved, including the **cerebellum**, which coordinates movement.

Clearly, these areas are especially active when dancing to music. Since sound is one of the earliest experiences we have, even while still in the uterus, the sounds of pitch and rhythm affect our neurological development from the start of life. Neuroscientists believe that the corpus callosum is involved in the mother–child relationship, of which sound is a major part, and the corpus callosum, along with the limbic system, is associated with emotion. Another unusual observation is the appearance of bizarre musical hallucinations in patients who have had damage to the dorsal part of the **pons** (part of the brain stem). The music they hear is in keeping with the style of music that is already familiar to them, as though a musical memory is unlocked and floods out into the conscious brain. Perhaps the damage has removed certain inhibitory pathways, allowing the music to be heard.

Apart from the effects noted above, there is now some evidence that performing music has a beneficial effect at genetic level (Kanduri et al. 2015a). Classical music enhances activity of a number of genes involved in dopamine production and transportation, neurotransmission at the synapse, memory, and learning, but reduces activity in genes involved in

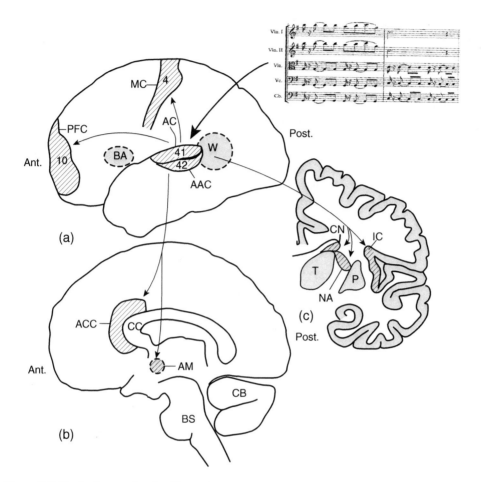

Figure 9.7 The brain areas involved in music.

neurodegeneration (Kanduri et al. 2015b). Three of these important genes that are activated by music are:

1   **Synuclein-alpha (*SNCA*)** at 4q21, which codes for the protein alpha-synuclein. This protein is found in presynaptic bulbs (see Synapses, Chapter 3) where it helps to facilitate the supply of neurotransmitter vesicles, interacts with tubulin (see Chapter 14) and may have a role in regulation of dopamine release.
2   ***FOS*** gene at 14q24.3, which is involved in the regulation of cell proliferation, differentiation, and transformation.
3   **Dual specificity phosphatase 1 (*DUSP1*)** gene, which has an important role in the cellular response to stress (Kanduri et al. 2015a,b).

A lot of speculation revolves around whether musical ability is genetic, and therefore runs in families. The composer Mozart was taught by a musical father and had a highly talented musical older sister, and other famous composers such as Bach and Johann Strauss also had musical offspring. Mendelssohn also had a highly talented musical sister who was a composer. Now scientists have identified genes that are involved in the musical ability of both parents and their offspring. An association between the variations of the **arginine vaso-pressin receptor 1A (*AVPR1A*)** gene and music has been found. Vasopressin is also known as antidiuretic hormone. It is produced in the hypothalamus and is released from the posterior pituitary gland. Vasopressin binding sites are found in the septum, thalamus, amygdala, and brain stem, all areas associated, in one way or another, with emotion. The *AVPR1A* gene had previously been linked to emotion and various social behaviours.

One or several genes are thought to control the function of a few sites in the brain that determine **pitch perception**, i.e. the ability to recognise different notes when played. Pitch and rhythm are reported as left hemisphere functions, while the right hemisphere works on melody and timbre (the tone quality of an instrument). Indeed, a part of the temporal lobe called the **planus temporale** (see also Williams syndrome, Chapter 6) is normally bigger on the left than the right, but is bigger still on the left in those persons with perfect pitch. Children with pitch control genes that are active from an early age can progress quickly with music, while others without these genes may progress more slowly or abandon music in favour of other pursuits.

Ghosts, phantoms, doppelgangers, and out of body experiences

Ghosts, phantoms, and doppelgangers may have a neurological basis. The phenomenon of **phantom limb** (i.e. the feeling that an amputated limb is still present) has been a problem for years. Certain cells in the somatic sensory cortex that receive sensations from that limb find they no longer have an input because the limb is gone. They are redundant cells, but they are still alive and may generate their own random impulses, which then trick the brain into thinking that the limb is still present.

Perhaps the **doppelgangers** (identical copies of a person, often called 'doubles', but not involving identical twins), which are seen by that same person, or by someone else, may have a similar cause; i.e. the phantom limb phenomenon may be elaborated to become the entire body. **'Out of body' experiences** and ghosts could also be phantom copies of the body generated by the cerebral cortex, 'seen' by the *mind* rather than the eye, and interpreted as an external image (Phillips 2000b). One good example of this was the case of a man driving his van to work who passed *himself* driving exactly the same van in the opposite direction. Both *he* and *himself* stared at each other in amazement as they drove past. For such an event to occur in reality is impossible, and a mental image of himself, generated by his own brain and 'seen' by the mind as an external image, is the best explanation we have at present. The fact that neither 'person' stopped, got out, or spoke to the other (i.e. the obvious thing to do) suggests that physical evidence of the other person being real was probably unobtainable, indirectly supporting the brain image theory.

Other cases of out of body experiences (also called **depersonalisation**), such as the patient who felt as though *he* (his conscious self) was about one metre in front of *himself* (his physical body) all the time, can cause a great deal of distress and may require some form of 'therapy' and very sensitive care. It is part of a collection of pathologies called **dissociative disorders**, which include the following.

- **Derealisation syndrome**, in which the patient feels that the world around them is a film they are watching, and everyone else is an actor in that film. It affects 1 or 2% of the population, although many more people are thought to experience it very briefly in their lifetime.

- **'Near death experiences'** (Kotler 2005), a type of depersonalisation in which some people have 'died' for several minutes and were then revived. Some tell of an out of body experience during this time, where they floated above their dead body.

Mild stimulation of the right temporal pole, just above the right ear, sometimes causes out of body experiences, hearing heavenly music, intense religious feelings, and hallucinations. Right temporal lobe epilepsy induces similar symptoms. Electroencephalogram (EEG) studies show that those claiming near-death experiences entered rapid-eye movement (REM) sleep later (110 minutes into sleep) than normal (60 minutes into sleep) and they needed less sleep than normal (see Chapter 16). The significance of this is not yet established.

The anaesthetic **ketamine** (see Chapter 8) can induce out of body experiences, with those taking it reporting that they have hovered over their body and looked down on it. To explain this, neuroscientists point out the **mirror neurons** (see Chapter 15) in the premotor cortex that link with the prefrontal cortex. These mirror neurons allow the individual to imitate the actions of others. The prefrontal cortex is the site of 'self' (or our conscious understanding of ourselves), and is also that part of the brain which prevents the mirror neurons from automatically copying other people. So the link between the prefrontal cortex and the mirror neurons allows you to maintain individuality while being able to interact with others. When the prefrontal cortex becomes detached from the mirror neurons (as with ketamine), a sense of detachment of the 'self' from the body can occur.

Anxiety disorders

Anxiety is a major psychological problem to which there is no easy solution. Drugs can alleviate the symptoms (see Anxiolytic drugs on page 196) and make life more tolerable for the patient, but they are not a cure, and can cause problems in the long-term. We all get anxious at times, and in certain situations that is to be expected. However, it becomes a disorder when there is no apparent cause and it disrupts the individual's life. The causes of anxiety disorders are still largely unknown, but one possibility is the parent–child relationship. Authoritarian mothers who push their children to do well, with the threats of harsh punishment, could be condemning their sons and daughters to anxiety-related problems later in life. When children make errors they produce a specific electrical pattern in their brain, called the **error-related negativity (ERN)**, which comes from their medial prefrontal cortex. The ERN appears to help correct the brain activity which resulted in that error so the problem is not repeated. Genetics has some influence over the strength of this signal, but harsh criticism and parental punishment weakens the signal significantly. This is another good example of the importance of environmental factors, both good and bad, on child brain development. Feedback from the parents should be kind and gentle, to reinforce this signal, not harsh and critical.

The psychological symptoms of anxiety include a sense of fear or apprehension, restlessness and irritability, loss of concentration, and disturbed sleep. The physical symptoms include sweating, pallor, palpitations, dry mouth, numbness, dizziness and fainting, frequency of micturition, difficulty in swallowing, shortness of breath, and tightness of the chest, perhaps with chest pain.

There are three categories of anxiety disorder: **general anxiety disorder**, **phobias**, and **panic attacks**.

General anxiety disorder (GAD)

This is a long-term state of anxiety with no obvious cause. It is characterised by uncontrollable and excessive worry and apprehension, to the extent of disrupting the daily life of the sufferer. About 2% of Europeans have GAD, and it is seen more often in women and in illicit drug users. A significant number of cases appear to have a family history of this condition, suggesting that genes may be involved.

The amygdala is expected to process all human emotions. In GAD there seems to be a failure of the amygdala to process the emotions of fear and anxiety. The basolateral complex of the amygdala receives sensory input and assesses the threat value of this input. It then communicates this to other brain areas, e.g. the medial prefrontal cortex and the sensory areas of the cerebral cortex. The central nucleus of the amygdala has the role of controlling the fear response, and it does this through connections with the brain stem, cerebellum, and hypothalamus. These connections appear to be reduced in function in GAD, and the central nucleus has more grey matter than usual. There are also fewer connections between the amygdala and the insula and cingulate than expected, and more connections between the amygdala and the prefrontal and parietal cortex (Figure 9.8). This all amounts to the amygdala not being able to process fear and anxiety properly, and also causing excessive activity in those areas that govern the response to anxiety, i.e. the prefrontal and parietal cortex. The result is a greatly exaggerated overreaction to a very minor threat, or indeed, no threat at all.

The genetic basis of anxiety is becoming better understood. Excessive activity of a gene called **Glo 1**, which codes for the enzyme **glyoxylase 1**, has been found to increase anxiety-related behaviour. This enzyme metabolises, and therefore lowers, an inhibitory substance called **methylglyoxal (MG)**, which is a waste product of **glycolysis** (glucose breakdown). Normally, MG inhibits anxiety-related behaviours, and any reduction in MG will increase these behaviours. It may be possible in the future to use drugs to reduce *Glo 1* activity, or increase the amount of MG, in order to improve the lives of anxiety sufferers (Figure 9.9).

Fear and phobias

Fear is potentially a useful attribute, as its presence is a warning that something is hazardous and should be avoided, and this can save lives. A good example of this is walking too close to the edge of a cliff; the fear of falling over the edge keeps the individual a safe distance back from the edge. But fear is a double-edged sword; it is a phenomenon that can be either exciting or destructive in people's lives. As an excitement, people seek fear for recreational purposes (rollercoaster rides or horror movies, for example); but as a destructive mechanism, fear keeps people at home and prevents them from getting on with their lives. Neuroscientists are keen to understand the anatomy and physiology of fear in order to be able to unlock the prison in which so many frightened people spend their lives.

Three brain components appear to be communicating during periods of fear brought about by a potentially threatening environmental stimulus, either real or imaginary:

- The prefrontal cortex of the frontal lobe, which, along with the tip of the temporal lobe, assesses the stimulus for its life-threatening potential. These two areas are often collectively called the **neocortex**. Part of the prefrontal cortex, known as the **ventromedial prefrontal cortex (vmPFC)**, acts to switch off fear by reducing the activity of the amygdala, a function sometimes called 'fear extinction'.

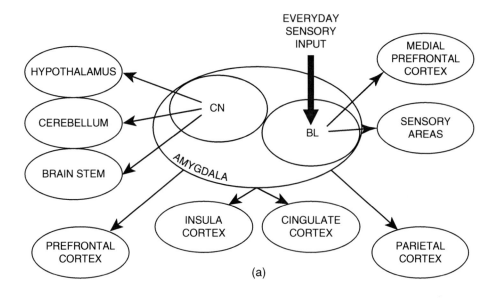

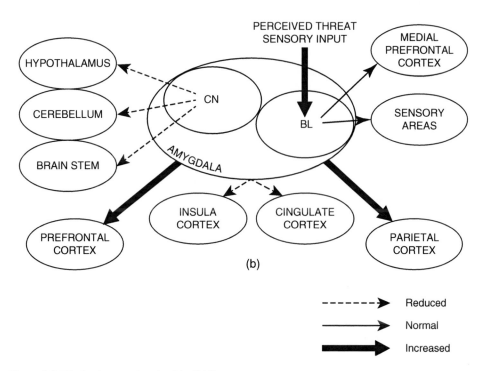

Figure 9.8 The brain areas involved in GAD.

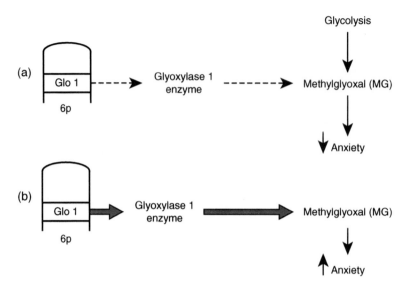

Figure 9.9 The mechanism of *Glo 1* and MG in anxiety-related behaviour.

- The amygdala, which adds the emotional dimension to the experience of fear, and is the centre of emotional memories. The amygdala has been called 'the driver of fear' as it has outputs to the brain stem and hypothalamus, which generate all the emotional and physical symptoms of fear under amygdala control.
- The hypothalamus, which sets in motion the **hypathalamo–pituitary–adrenal axis** (i.e. **HPA axis**, the CRF to ACTH to cortisol route) and autonomic nervous system (sympathetic) responses.

The importance of the temporal lobe and amygdala in the creation of fear is illustrated in the **Klüver–Bucy syndrome**. This condition is caused by a lesion of the temporal lobes, apparently extending into the amygdala below. Such a lesion may be the result of a stroke or a head injury or may be associated with epilepsy or dementia, and brings about a general blunting of emotions coupled with a profound loss of fear. Five distinct behavioural symptoms are characteristic of the disorder:

- **Psychic blindness**, an inability to recognise common objects and what they represent, despite normal vision. This means they cannot recognise any objects that are a potential threat.
- Oral tendencies, where all such objects are 'tested' by being put in the mouth. This leads to the concept that these patients eat everything, but more probably they are using the mouth as a mechanism of sensory input to aid recognition.
- **Hypermetamorphosis**, an overwhelming compulsion to explore everything in the immediate environment, despite any hazards.
- Increased sexual tendencies, including making inappropriate sexual advances to others, even inanimate objects.
- Emotional blunting (known as **flattening of affect**), with a profound loss of all sense of fear.

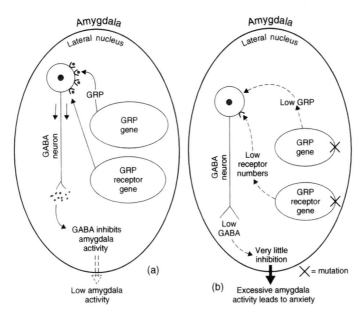

Figure 9.10 The genetic basis of fear within the amygdala. Either one gene mutation causes low GRP, or another causes few GRP receptors. Either way, the result is low inhibitory GABA, and the amygdala becomes excessively active, leading to acute anxiety or fear.

The mechanism by which the amygdala becomes overactive, thus triggering fear and anxiety, is related to the concentration of gamma-aminobutyric acid (GABA) within circuits built into the organ's lateral nucleus (Figure 9.10). GABA is a major inhibitory neurotransmitter that is vital for reduction of excessive brain activity. With low GABA in the amygdala, emotional memories can surface and generate the symptoms of acute anxiety and fear responses. Two genetic errors may be involved:

1   The gene that codes for **gastrin-releasing peptide (GRP)**, a protein that binds to GRP receptors found on neurons in the lateral nucleus of the amygdala. On binding to the receptors, GRP promotes GABA release, which then inhibits the amygdala. Failure of the gene causes low GRP and therefore low GABA response.
2   The gene that codes for GRP receptors. Errors in this gene could cause low numbers of receptors, or receptors that do not bind GRP, and therefore failure to bind adequate amounts of GRP leads to low GABA concentrations.

The hormones released during fear are basically **adrenaline** (released into the blood and circulated to all parts of the body) and **endorphins** (released into the central nervous system). These help the brain to cope with the stress that accompanies the fear; adrenaline promotes the sympathetic response and endorphins help to protect the brain from excessive stress stimuli. After the experience of fear is over, the hormone **dopamine** is released into the brain, giving the mind a sense of joy, well-being, and the satisfaction of achievement (similar to the feelings achieved by increased dopamine as a consequence of drug abuse; see Chapters 5 and 8). The *feel-good factor* created by dopamine is probably the reason why some people seek out the excitement linked to fear. The dopamine receptor D_4 appears to be involved, and this receptor is coded for by a gene on chromosome 11 (the ***D4DR*** gene). However, there appears to be two forms of this gene: *long* and *short*. Those who have inherited the slightly longer form of the gene are more resistant to dopamine, and therefore need additional dopamine to have the feel-good effect that they call a *buzz*. These people have to take extra risks to obtain more dopamine, and therefore they seek out adventurous and risky activities. For those with the shorter version of the gene the dopamine binds much better, and so less dopamine is required, making risk-taking activities unnecessary and appear foolhardy.

The hormone **oxytocin** and a compound called **brain-derived neurotrophic factor (BDNF)** have both been shown to reduce fear. As well as its more usual function in promoting bonding (as in breastfeeding), oxytocin increases activity in the prefrontal cortex (which controls fear reactions) and reduces activity in the amygdala, and this has a calming effect. People with a variation in the gene that codes for BDNF show an extended response to fear, suggesting that a lack of BDNF is responsible. Despite the fact that relatively small quantities of BDNF cross the blood–brain barrier, both oxytocin and BDNF may prove to be future options for treating fear-related disorders.

Fear can be stored as memories (called *emotional memories*) in the brain in a form unlike all other memories. These emotional memories amount to 'learnt fear', i.e. fear learnt from previous adverse experiences, and can, in susceptible people, short-circuit rational thinking and block normal behaviour even in non-fearful situations. As with other memories, an often-harmless trigger is enough to cause uncontrollable outbursts of irrational behaviour. In anxiety, emotional fear appears to dominate the personality, and emotional memories are often life-long.

Another fear-related phenomenon is **mass psychogenic illness**, where fear is spread throughout a community or family, from person to person, including from parents to their children. It can be a 'learnt behaviour' where a child copies the parents fear reaction to something (e.g. mice) and therefore learns that fear is the 'normal' reaction to mice. There may even be a genetic predisposition to learnt anxiety and fear within some families, making these families more susceptible to mass psychogenic illness. Twin studies identified about 30% of variation in anxiety states was due to genetic inheritance.

A **phobia** is an irrational and pathological fear centred on a specific situation or object, which dominates the lifestyle of the sufferer. There are many common phobias, e.g. fear of an *object* such as a spider (**arachnophobia**) or fear of a *situation* such as an enclosed space (**claustrophobia**), but there are many less common phobias, e.g. fear of phobias (**phobophobia**), and some very rare and rather bizarre phobias, e.g. the fear of becoming ill (**nosophobia** or **nosemaphobia**). Ironically, the word for 'fear of long words' is **hippopotomonstrosesquipedaliophobia**! **Agoraphobia** sufferers avoid public and unfamiliar places, especially large, open spaces where there are no hiding places. This particular disorder is responsible for keeping some sufferers 'trapped' in their homes for 40 years or more because they fear leaving their home. This is the way the patient copes with their fear, by staying in their home. The person concerned avoids the cause of the phobia as much as possible, and this allows them to continue a 'normal' life, albeit a poorer quality of life. Pathological phobic states incapacitate the patient and require medical intervention to re-establish a reasonable quality of life.

Panic attacks

Panic attacks are a sudden acute onset of intense fear or apprehension, where the sufferer thinks they are dying, under severe threat of harm, or going insane. About 7% of the population develop panic attacks every year, and between 3 and 4% will develop panic attack disorder at some point in their lives. The most common age when attacks begin is between teenage and mid-30s. Abnormal concentrations of **cholecystokinin (CCK)** appear to be involved, in particular CCK-4, which is also known to induce panic. Genetics may account for between 30 and 40% of cases. A trinucleotide repeat (see Chapter 6) on chromosome 15 is found in about 90% of families that have this disorder. There may also be some gene variations involved in the serotonin (5-HT) system of the brain, although exactly how this influences the condition is not fully known.

The neurobiology involves an area of the midbrain, the **periaqueductal grey**, which becomes active and induces a defensive response, maybe running away from danger, or a freeze reaction, during an attack. In addition, reduced frontal lobe and abnormal temporal lobe activity decreases their normal influence over the amygdala, which then acts alone and drives the panic state. The more severe the temporal lobe abnormality, the younger the age of onset of the attacks.

Post-traumatic stress disorder

Post-traumatic stress disorder (PTSD) is a stress condition that occurs in some people exposed to a severe traumatic incident, such as a train crash, either as a survivor or as a rescuer. It affects children and adults subjected to abuse, casualties or witnesses of traumatic events, soldiers in battle situations (originally called 'shell shock', 'battle fatigue', or 'combat neurosis' during the Second World War), victims of violent crime, long periods of incarceration, and those receiving bad news, such as the loss of a family member or being told about the presence of an illness with a poor prognosis. The incident that triggers the stress clearly has some major effect on brain function, involving changes in the neurochemistry. Neuroimaging has established the major problem as abnormal activity of the **ventromedial prefrontal cortex (vmPFC)**, which normally reduces fear by inhibiting the fear response from the amygdala. The vmPFC is part of a loop linking the dorsolateral prefrontal cortex with the amygdala and hippocampus (Insel 2010). The dorsolateral prefrontal cortex is important in learning to tolerate and overcome fear. Each time the vmPFC decreases its function, the link between the dorsolateral prefrontal cortex and the amygdala is diminished (or broken) and the fear shutdown activity is lost. As a result, fear response levels increase in the amygdala. This causes the sudden manifestation of symptoms of PTSD, such as **flashbacks**, in which the original events of the incident, e.g. the sights, sounds, and smells, are relived, often many times for months or years after the event. The vmPFC in PTSD sufferers is also smaller than normal, and this directly reduces this area's ability to switch off fear (Insel 2010). The pathway that links the hypothalamus to the pituitary, and on to the adrenal gland (known as the **HPA axis**; the hormones being CRF, ACTH, and cortisol, see Figure 11.5 on page 244) is severely affected, resulting in low cortisol release into the blood (the opposite of acute stress) and therefore causing a compensatory increase in cortisol receptor sensitivity. In the brain, serotonin and noradrenaline activities are increased, both of which are involved in memory retrieval, and the hippocampus is enlarged. Since the hippocampus is a site of memory function, these changes may account for the number and frequency of flashbacks these people suffer. This constant re-enactment of the incident is a trauma in itself, seriously disturbing the lifestyle of those who suffer from it. It may require several years of therapy and sensitive understanding on the part of the healthcare profession to achieve an outcome that improves the quality of life for those who suffer from this problem.

Breedlove et al. (2010) reported studies done on American Vietnam war veterans with PTSD who suffered from memory changes (e.g. **amnesia** of some traumatic events), flashbacks, and problems with short-term memory. They showed an 8% reduction in the size of the hippocampus, but no other structural abnormality. There also appeared to be a genetic susceptibility involved, making some more vulnerable to the effects of trauma than others.

Eating disorders

Several stress-related disorders that result in disturbance of normal eating patterns are discussed here. The most important of these are **obesity** (excess weight), **anorexia nervosa** (inadequate eating), and **bulimia nervosa** (loss of control of food intake). The sufferer of anorexia nervosa will eat very little, leading to severe weight loss and starvation to the point of death. In contrast, the patient with bulimia nervosa will periodically go on a 'binge-eating' episode. They will eat lots of high-calorie food and then, feeling guilty, they will cause vomiting and use laxatives to get rid of it. Despite the problems, science is now getting a better understanding of what is going wrong in these disorders.

Normal mechanism of appetite control

The biological mechanism of normal food control is very complex and as yet not fully understood. **Adipose tissue** (stored fat under the skin and around internal organs) releases a hormone called **leptin** into the blood (Figure 9.11). This hormone binds to **leptin receptors** in the **arcuate nucleus**, one of the nuclei of the hypothalamus. The binding of leptin to its receptor causes a shutdown of neurons that normally secrete a combination of two proteins, **neuropeptide Y (NPY)** and **agouti-related protein (ARP)**. Together, these two proteins normally act by binding to, and inhibiting, another receptor, the **melanocortin-4 receptor (MC-4)**. Inhibition of the MC-4 by NYP and ARP in the hypothalamus causes feeding activity, so the blocking of NYP + ARP by leptin stops the individual from feeding. This makes sense when you consider that the greater the mass of adipose tissue the larger the release of leptin; and in circumstances of large adipose mass the need for food should be less. To reinforce this effect, leptin receptors activated by the binding of leptin also stimulate other arcuate neurons, which then release two other proteins called **cocaine and amphetamine regulated transcript (CART)** and **alpha-melanocyte stimulating hormone (α-MSH)**. Together these two neuromodulators act on MC-4 receptors to inhibit feeding. So leptin causes *inhibition* of feeding behaviour by *increasing* CART+ α-MSH and *decreasing* NYP+ARP (Figure 9.11).

Insulin also inhibits ARP when it works together with leptin. A protein that is integral to both the insulin and leptin pathways is **Fox01**, and by reducing Fox01 in animal models scientists created lean animals with better glucose metabolism. If this can be applied to people with obesity, it may be a way to help solve the problem.

The neurophysiology of eating is further complicated by other control mechanisms. For example, the liver detects concentrations of blood glucose and fatty acids and signals the brain about these via the **vagus nerve** (cranial nerve X) (Figure 9.12). The signals arrive at the

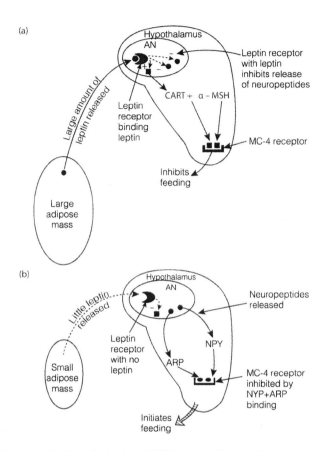

Figure 9.11 Adipose feedback to the brain. (a) With large adipose volume, more leptin is released, which binds to leptin receptors in the arcuate nucleus (AN) of the hypothalamus. This causes inhibition of neuropeptide release, but promotes the release of the cocaine and amphetamine regulated transcript (CART) and the alpha-melanocyte stimulating hormone (α-MSH). These bind to MC-4 receptors and inhibit feeding. (b) Little adipose volume releases low concentrations of leptin; the empty leptin receptor then inhibits the CART/α-MSH release but causes release of neuropeptides. When these bind to MC-4 receptors, feeding is initiated. ARP = agouti-related protein; NPY = neuropeptide Y.

nucleus of the solitary tract (NST) in the brain stem. This nucleus, in turn, relays the information to the hypothalamus. In this way the liver keeps the hypothalamus informed of nutrient concentrations in circulation. The **lateral hypothalamus** is a major player in the generation of hunger, which would be activated through this route if the blood nutrients arriving at the liver were low. The **ventromedial hypothalamus** initiates the sensation of **satiety**, i.e. the feeling of fullness, which would be activated if the blood nutrients arriving at the liver were high, as would be the case shortly after a meal. However, most researchers in this subject also acknowledge the important regulatory role played by other brain areas, notably the amygdala, the frontal cortex, the substantia nigra, and the hippocampus. **Orexins (hypocretins)** are two neuropeptide hormones, orexin A and B. They promote food intake and wakefulness. They

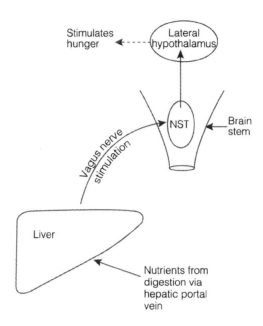

Figure 9.12 The liver control of hunger. Vagus nerve stimulation by the liver informs the hypothalamus, via the nucleus of the solitary tract (NST) in the brain stem, about the condition of nutrients in storage. Low nutrient concentrations may stimulate hunger.

are products of the lateral hypothalamus (Carlson 2012). Orexin is also active in the sleep–wake cycle (see Chapter 16). They bind to two excitatory metabotropic receptors, OX_1 and OX_2. Leptin appears to inhibit orexin production.

Ghrelin, a hormone from the stomach, promotes food intake by activating orexin production. Ghrelin binds to **ghrelin receptors (GHSR1a)**, and these are distributed throughout the brain. However, ghrelin itself is rarely found in the brain. A subset of neurons in the hypothalamus produce both GHSR1a and the dopamine receptor DRD2, and a combination (or interaction) of GHSR1a with the dopamine receptor DRD2 changes the shape of DRD2 (changing the shape is known as **allosteric modification**). This affects the binding of dopamine to DRD2, and the response to dopamine will therefore be different. An antagonistic agent that selectively blocks GHSR1a receptors prevents dopamine response from neurons that express both receptors, while neurons that express only DRD2 receptors remain unaffected. This would allow partial modification of the dopamine system (the subset of neurons only) as a potential treatment for obesity and maybe other dopamine-related disorders.

Anorexia nervosa

It appears that short-term acute stress causes the normal neuroendocrine response, resulting in raising the blood adrenaline and cortisol concentrations. This change in hormone concentrations acts to switch off ARP, just as leptin does, and therefore inhibits feeding. However, once the acute stress is over, the cortisol and adrenaline concentrations fall to normal, and ARP is activated again with feeding behaviour restored.

In **anorexia nervosa**, the stress is retained in a chronic form (although it may not be recognised as such by the patient or their family), so that higher than normal concentrations of adrenaline and cortisol are retained in the blood. In this way, ARP is continually inhibited, feeding behaviour may be chronically suppressed, and the individual will starve. One of the long-term effects of persistent starvation is that the hippocampus shrinks, causing a permanent reduction in the hippocampal role in regulating appetite. Long-term anorexia may cause the type of brain damage that is both irreparable and perpetuates the problem.

Mutations in the serotonin receptor 5-HT2A are linked to anorexia. This receptor is also involved in food intake regulation, and anorexic women appear to have double the number of 5-HT2A genetic mutations than those without anorexia.

Anorexia nervosa has also been associated with abnormally low concentrations of some immune chemicals called **interleukins (Il,** in particular **Il-6)**, and **tumour necrosis factors (TNF,** in particular **TNF-1β)**. This may increase the risk of infection. Anorexia has also been linked to disturbance of **haematopoiesis** (blood forming), a bone marrow function that normally produces the circulating red and white blood cells. Disturbance of this function leads to abnormal blood cell counts.

Bulimia nervosa

In **bulimia nervosa**, the pathophysiology is slowly getting better understood. Three types of bulimia have been described:

1 **Simple bulimia nervosa** starts in girls under 18 who were regarded as normal before they started showing symptoms. It may be triggered by an emotional upset, and dieting in this bizarre manner may be seen by the sufferer as a way of restoring self-esteem.
2 **Anorexic bulimia nervosa**, which starts with a period of anorexia first. This recovers and there is a brief time of normality before the bulimia begins. The food binging intensifies, with vomiting being introduced at part of the process. These girls often have a disturbed family background.
3 **Multi-impulsive bulimia nervosa** is a severe variation than starts similarly to simple bulimia nervosa. The girls lack control over their emotions and their eating habits, and they succumb to impulsive behavioural problems. There is often a highly disturbed family background, which offers little or no support to the patient.

Bulimia may involve disturbed serotonin concentrations in the brain, and even recovered bulimia patients often show abnormal brain concentrations of serotonin. Low serotonin causes low mood, and it may be that binging on carbohydrates (especially sugar foods) improves the serotonin concentrations. This restores their mood to normal and they feel better. Brain scans of bulimic women have shown a poor response from the dopaminergic reward pathways (see Chapter 8), and suggest that this response was linked to the cycle of binging episodes. The scans also demonstrated that the eating behaviour pattern directly affects these dopamine pathways. It then becomes a vicious circle; the behaviour disturbs the pathway, which then in turn drives the behaviour. It may be that the binge eating is a way to try and bring the reward pathway up to normal function at times when it becomes very low in dopamine. However, there appear to be environmental and social causes that contribute to this disorder.

Obesity

Obesity may be due to a reduction in the brain's *sensitivity* to leptin, rather than a reduction in the amount of leptin production. This is possible through several mechanisms:

- The gene for leptin (the **OB** gene at 7q31.3) mutates, the changed gene coding for a form of leptin that does not bind to its receptor.
- The gene for the leptin receptor (the **Db** gene at 1p31) mutates, the changed gene then coding for a form of receptor that cannot accept leptin.
- The transporter system that is essential for leptin to cross the blood–brain barrier becomes faulty and less leptin reaches the brain.
- The gene for the MC-4 receptor may develop errors and therefore MC-4 does not function normally.

Some of these genetic mechanisms have been found in humans, often occurring in families as an inherited trait. In addition, other genes may be involved in producing a state of obesity. Mutations of the **fat mass and associated obesity (FTO)** gene on chromosome 16 and its interactions with the gene **Iroquois homeobox protein 3 (IRX3)** can contribute to being overweight. If the *FTO* mutation was at one allele, this would cause the individual to be 1.2 kg heavier than those with the normal gene, while the mutation at both alleles would cause them to be 3 to 4 kg heavier. The normal gene is involved in deoxyribose nucleic acid (DNA) function. *IRX3* appears to be linked to body mass and composition, thus affecting the proportions of fat to lean in the body.

A number of proteins called **uncoupling proteins (UCPs)** are involved in cellular energy production, i.e. using stored energy such as adipose for the production of **adenosine triphosphate (ATP)**, the high energy molecule. One such protein called **UCP2** reduces the production of ATP in favour of heat production. This process is useful in newborn children to keep them warm, but becomes less important as they get older and muscles take over the role of heat production. However, UCP2 gene mutations may be linked to obesity in some adults. A plant extract substance called **genipin** blocks UCP2 function and improves insulin production. Medications based on genipin may be available in the future to help to reduce obesity and improve diabetes type 2, a condition strongly linked to obesity.

One idea is that anorexia nervosa is a *fat phobia*, and *compulsive eating* is a major cause of obesity, in which case these may be a distinct subset of anxiety-related disorders. In any case, control of body weight is important for health, as being either too thin or too fat causes severe problems for all body systems, but especially for the cardiovascular, immune, and nervous systems, and these states can cause death.

The **body mass index (BMI)** is a standard method of recording if a person is under or overweight. The BMI is:

Body weight in kilograms (kg) ÷ height in metres squared (m²)

The results for both sexes are:

- BMI below 18.5 = underweight
- BMI 18.5 to 24.9 = normal
- BMI 25 to 29.9 = overweight
- BMI 30 or more = obese

It is not uncommon for anorexic women to have a BMI of less than 17. 5.

Eating disorders in children and young people

Before birth, the developing fetus may be laying down the foundations for an eating disorder later in life. A female fetus sharing the uterus with her twin brother may be at a lower risk of developing an eating disorder than she would be if sharing the uterus with a twin sister. The presence of a twin brother exposes the girl to a higher concentration of testosterone than would be the case if they were both girls. This testosterone may cause some changes in the girls developing brain, which protects her to some extent from developing an eating disorder. More work is needed to confirm this and to establish the details.

Young children and teenagers often show some specific factors linked to the onset of an eating disorder:

- Most eating disorders start during childhood and the teenage years, mostly in young females (only 5–15% are males).
- Anorexia and bulimia may alternate or overlap in young people.
- Young females tend to have a distorted body image, i.e. they believe that they are over-weight despite being dangerously thin, and this may be one source of their stress.
- Transitional events can cause sufficient trauma to trigger an eating disorder in young people, maybe because they lack the maturity to cope with these events. Six transitional events have been shown to be the main protagonists in the causation of an eating disorder. They are:

    1   changes in school;
    2   changes in relationships;
    3   death of a family member;
    4   changes in home or starting work;
    5   prolonged illness and hospitalisation;
    6   physical or psychological abuse.

- Marijuana use has long been known to cause hunger. The reason is now known, and it's due to the **delta-9-tetrahydrocannabinol** (**THC**; see Chapter 8) in marijuana binding to CB_1 receptors, which then causes specialised cells called **pro-opiomelanocrtin** (**POMC**) neurons to switch from producing a hunger suppression hormone to a hunger promotion hormone. This may have an effect in dictating when a binging episode will occur.

Anxiety-related personality disorders

Several anxiety-related personality disorders have been identified, although the underlying biology is not yet understood in most of these. It is possible that a short version (14 **nucleotide repeats**; see Chapter 6) of the **serotonin transporter** (**SERT**) gene (i.e. the *SLC6A4* gene at 17q11.1-q12) may be responsible for some of these conditions. The long version has 16 such nucleotide repeats. SERT transports serotonin from the synaptic cleft back into the presynaptic bulb, i.e. **reuptake**. It is not clear how the short version can affect this function.

The disorders are as follows.

1   **Avoidant personality disorder** occurs when individuals avoid interactions with others because they fear criticism. They become hypersensitive, nervous, and self-restrained

when interaction with others is essential. They are very anxious about being embar-rassed and tend to lead solitary lives. They may get depressed or feel inadequate when in social settings. It probably affects anything from 1 to 7% of the population. **Social phobia** is a similar problem, the difference being that those with social phobia want to enjoy others' company but may fear specific social functions, while in avoidant person-ality disorder they do not want company with others because that would aggravate their feels of inadequacy, causing an anxiety state.

2   **Dependent personality** involves those people who depend entirely on others for many aspects of their lives. These aspects include decision-making and affection, as well as personal care and guidance. They thrive only in close relationships and they fear the break-up of those relationships that would require them taking more control of their life. This disorder makes the sufferer vulnerable to exploitation and abuse. It can affect up to 6% of the population and involves more women than men.

3   **Histrionic personality** involves individuals with rapidly shifting, intense, and flam-boyant emotions. They are often over-dependent on others and form rather unstable relationships. Their dramatic approach to life makes them the centre of attention, and this can result in a higher than average number of medical consultations. Up to 22% of the population may show evidence of histrionic personality, with the majority of affected individuals being female.

4   **Narcissistic personality** affects people with dramatic, grandiose behaviour, the purpose of which is to gain admiration and affection from others. They indulge in their own self-importance, and they see themselves as superior to others. Beneath this facade, they have shallow emotions and are poor at establishing relationships. Less than 1% of the population demonstrate narcissism, and these are largely males.

5   **Borderline personality** causes unstable people with loss of control of emotions. They form very strong attachments to others fearing abandonment. They have instability of mood, which can result in depression or anxiety, and they may act impulsively, or commit self-harm. They may describe having transient **dissociative states**, which are periods of detachment from reality, in which the individual sees the world as one would see a film, i.e. they are not actually part of it (see also **Derealisation syndrome** on page 182). It affects 1 or 2% of the population, women more than men. Families with some members diagnosed with borderline personality disorders often show increased rates of mood disorder, suggesting a possible genetic origin for this problem. There is some-times an increase in the activity of the amygdala when the individual is shown pictures of faces demonstrating emotions. There is low serotonin activity (which is linked to impulsiveness) and reduced metabolism within the prefrontal cortex.

The anxiolytic drugs

The **benzodiazepines** are a major group of anxiolytic drugs (*anxio* = 'anxiety', *lytic* = 'dissolving'), typified by **diazepam, alprazolam, chlordiazepoxide, lorazepam, clobazam,** and **oxazepam**. They are used widely to reduce levels of acute anxiety. These drugs bind to the **GABA$_A$** receptor (see Figure 4.13 in Chapter 4) and promote the function of GABA to open the chloride channel that runs through the receptor. In this respect they have a similar action to that of barbiturates and alcohol. The subsequent increase in the influx of chlo-ride into the neuronal postsynaptic membrane causes a greater degree of *resting membrane* *potential* and blocks any chance of an action potential in that cell. On a widely distributed basis throughout the brain, this drug group has a sedatory effect, i.e. it calms the brain but without inducing sleep (except in high dosage). Benzodiazepines are best used as a short-term management of severe anxiety, no longer than about 6 weeks, at the lowest effective dose. Long-term use is associated with dependence and should be avoided. These drugs are well absorbed from the digestive system and well tolerated when given orally. Onset of activity is about 5 to 10 minutes after oral ingestion, with a peak blood concentration after 60 minutes. Diazepam, alprazolam, chlordiazepoxide, and clobazam have sustained action. Diazepam and chlordiazepoxide, for example, both have long half-lives (diazepam = 20 to 100 hours, chlordiazepoxide = 6-30 hours) due to their active metabolites. Lorazepam and oxazepam are short-acting (lorazepam half-life is 4 to 25 hours), and are better suited at controlling panic attacks.

Side effects of the benzodiazepines include drowsiness, confusion, and ataxia in the elderly, amnesia, dependence, and muscle weakness. They should be avoided in patients with liver or renal impairment, and during pregnancy and beyond until breastfeeding is concluded.

The non-benzodiazepine **buspirone** is thought to act at specific serotonin (5-HT1A) receptors. Relief of symptoms may take up to 2 weeks. It is rapidly absorbed from the gut, but has extensive first pass metabolism. The half-life is between 2 and 11 hours. Dependence and abuse potential for buspirone is considered to be low, but it is still recommended for short-term use only. Side effects include nausea, dizziness, headache, nervousness, and excitement.

Key points

The limbic system

- The limbic system is a series of centres involved in self-preservation and preservation of the species.
- The major components of the limbic system are the amygdala, the mammillary bodies of the hypothalamus, the anterior and dorsal nuclei of the thalamus, several deep nuclei, the septal area, the orbitofrontal cortex of the cerebrum, the hippocampus and parahippocampal gyrus, and parts of the temporal lobe.
- The amygdala is the main site for emotions, although emotional states are moderated through several other brain areas as well, notably the frontal and temporal cortex, the hypothalamus, and the hippocampus.
- The neuroendocrine response is a normal mechanism adopted by the hypothalamus to combat the effects of stress. It consists of a neurological response via the sympathetic nervous system, and an endocrine response via certain pituitary hormones.

Stress

- Stress causes raised cortisol concentrations in the blood.
- Post-traumatic stress disorder (PTSD) is a stress condition that occurs in some people exposed to a severe traumatic incident. It causes flashbacks, which appear to be due to reduced activity of the vmPFC, which normally switches off fear.

Anxiety disorders

- Anxiety appears to involve the amygdala, where increased cholecystokinin (CCK) can cause anxiety.
- There are three categories of anxiety disorder: general anxiety disorder, panic attacks, and phobias.

Fear

- Three brain components appear to be communicating during periods of fear, the prefrontal and temporal cortex, the amygdala and the hypothalamus, involving the hypathalamo–pituitary–adrenal (HPA) axis.
- The hormones released during fear are adrenaline and endorphins and, after the experience of fear, dopamine is released.

Phobias

- A phobia is an irrational fear centred on a specific situation or object.
- Reduced frontal lobe activity is implicated in panic attacks.

Eating disorders

- The lateral hypothalamus is the main component that causes hunger, the ventromedial hypothalamus initiating the sensation of satiety.
- The most important of the eating disorders are obesity, anorexia nervosa, and bulimia nervosa.
- In anorexia nervosa, chronic stress may cause high adrenaline and cortisol to remain in the blood, inhibiting ARP and feeding, leading to starvation.
- Obesity may be due to a reduction in the brain's sensitivity to leptin.

The anxiolytic drugs

- The anxiolytics bind to the GABA$_A$ receptor and promote GABA to open the chloride channel, causing inhibition of action potentials and calming of the brain.
- They should be used for a short-term only, no longer than 6 weeks.
- The non-barbiburate buspirone is thought to act at specific serotonin (5HT1A) receptors.

References

Breedlove, S. M., Watson N. V., and Rosenzweig, M. R. (2010) *Biological Psychology: An Introduction to Behavioural, Cognitive and Clinical Neuroscience* (6th edition). Sinauer Associates, Sunderland, MA.

Carlson, N. R. (2012) *Physiology of Behaviour* (11th edition). Pearson Education, Harlow, UK.

Elkan, D. (2010) The comedy circuit. *New Scientist*, **205** (2745): 40–43.

Insel, T. R. (2010) Faulty circuits. *Scientific American*, **302** (4): 28–35.

Kanduri, C., Kuusi, T., Ahvenainen, M., Philips, A., Lahdesmaki, H., and Jarvela, I. (2015a) The effect of music performance on the transcriptome of professional musicians. *Scientific Reports*, 5. DOI: 10.1038/srep09506.

Kanduri, C., Raijas, P., Ahvenainen, M., Philips, A. K., Ukkola-Vuoti, L., Lahdesmaki, H., and Jarvela, I. (2015b) The effect of listening to music on human transcriptome. *PeerJ*, 3:e830. DOI: 10.7717/peerj.830.

Kaye, J., Morton, J., Bowcutt, M., and Maupin, D. (2000) Stress, depression and psychneuroimmunology. *Journal of Neuroscience Nursing*, **32** (2): 93–100.

Kotler, S. (2005) Extreme states. *Discover*, July 2005, 61–66.

Mucha, M., Skrzypiec, A. E., Schiavon, E., Attwood, B. K., Kucerova, E., and Pawlak, R. (2011) Lipocalin-2 controls neuronal excitability and anxiety by regulating dendritic spine formation and maturation. *Proceedings of the National Academy of Science*, October 2011, DOI: 10.1073/pnas.1107936108.

Nolen-Hoeksema S. (2007) *Abnormal Psychology* (4th edition). McGraw-Hill, Boston, MA.

Phillips, H. (2000a) So you think you're in love? *New Scientist*, 8 July: 11.

Phillips, H. (2000b) Mind phantoms. *New Scientist*, 8 July: 11.

Teicher, M. H. (2002) The neurobiology of child abuse. *Scientific American*, **286** (3; March): 54–61.

Westly, E. (2010) Abuse and attachment. *Scientific American Mind*, **21** (1): 10.

10 Schizophrenia

- Introduction
- The genetic influence in schizophrenia
- Brain pathology
- Neurodevelopment as a factor
- The biochemical changes in schizophrenia
- The possible role of environmental factors
- Schizoaffective disorder and schizoid-related personality disorders
- The antipsychotic drugs
- Key points

Introduction

The word *schizophrenia* means 'split mind', but splitting the mind is *not* what this disorder is about. However, no matter how inappropriate the name of this disease, it is so entrenched in the literature that it would be very difficult to change it. More important than the name is the fact that enormous progress has been made since the 1960s in understanding the biology of schizophrenia, due to much intense research, with new facts, insights, and theories arising almost daily. And along with these new insights comes the overriding hope that new drugs and other therapies will be available to improve the patient's quality of life.

Schizophrenia is a major psychotic illness affecting more than 21 million people worldwide. It causes a series of symptoms that rob the patient of their cognitive thought, their socialisation skills, and ultimately their personality. These symptoms fall into two categories, positive and negative (Table 10.1). These two groups of symptoms may indicate that the term *schizophrenia* is being used to describe an amalgamation of two distinct **syndromes** that can occur together. One syndrome demonstrates a predominance of *positive symptoms* (**Type I**), the other a predominance of *negative symptoms* (**Type II**) (Nolen-Hoeksema 2007). The relationship between the two syndromes is interesting. Delays in the early neurodevelopment of an individual have been correlated with the type II negative symptoms, plus disturbance of language and attention, and poor social adjustment later in life. The negative symptoms are usually resistant to all attempts to prevent them and, in young people, this indicates a poor outcome. Type I positive symptoms such as hallucinations and delusions, on the other hand, tend to occur a little later in life, as the disorder becomes more advanced. It seems

Table 10.1 The symptoms of schizophrenia

Symptom	Types	Explanation, examples
Positive symptoms (Type I)		
Those unwanted aspects that the patient would prefer to do without; possibly caused by increased dopamine activity. Usually associated with abrupt onset of the disease.		
Thought disorder *includes* **Delusions** (disorder of thought content) (Holland et al. 1999)	Ideas of reference	Ordinary items have special meaning for the patient, e.g. 'Three milk bottles delivered today means I have three days to live'.
	Concrete thinking	Everything is literal, no abstract thinking, e.g. 'I must fly' means to the patient you will grow wings and take to the air.
	Flights of ideas	Rapid, uncontrolled thoughts passing quickly from one to another
	Grandeur	False belief of great status or importance, e.g. 'I own the hospital'
	Paranoia	False belief that harm is directed to the patient, e.g. 'Next door's TV is beaming death rays at me'
	Persecution	False belief that people are against the patient, e.g. 'The doctor is killing me with drugs'
	Body	False belief that the body is changed in some way, e.g. 'My head is made of plastic'
Hallucinations (Holland et al. 1999)	Tactile	Feeling things that are not there, e.g. worms crawling over the skin
	Aural	Hearing things that are not there, notably voices talking to them
	Visual	Seeing things that are not there, notably little people
Bizarre behaviour	e.g. catatonia or inappropriate aggression	Long periods of no visible movement Violent outbursts
Negative symptoms (Type II)		
Those attributes taken away from the patient that they would prefer to keep; possibly caused by neuron losses. Usually associated with gradual onset of the disease.		
Withdrawal from reality	Isolation from the real world into an inner world of the mind	Profound loss of self-care
Loss of volition (or motivation)	The willingness to do things is lost	Remains seated all day if not motivated
Loss (or blunting) of affect	Mood and emotions are lost or inappropriate	Remains emotionless or cries (or laughs) without reason
Loss of speech (or speech content)	Speaks very little	Remains quiet all day

Table 10.2 Genetic risk of developing schizophrenia

Family relationship	Genetic risk concordance rate (%)
Monozygotic twins	40–50
Dizygotic twins	15–17
A sibling affected	10
One parent affected	15
Both parents affected	35
One parent and one sibling affected	17

that negative symptoms, language plus attention problems and social maladjustment are also symptoms seen in **affective disorder** (see Chapter 11), but if you add positive symptoms to this scenario it becomes schizophrenia. This *two-syndrome hypothesis* appears to be supported by the action of the modern antipsychotic drugs, which act on two main pathways in the brain, one pathway (the **mesocortical system**) functioning below normal levels causing the negative symptoms, and the other pathway (the **mesolimbic system**) (see Chapter 1, Table 1.2) functioning above normal causing the positive symptoms (see Antipsychotic drugs on page 219). The age of onset of symptoms is mostly later in women than in men; males usually begin showing evidence of the disease in their teens or early twenties (around 15–25 years).

Although at the moment the cause of schizophrenia is still not fully established, there is a huge and growing volume of biological data concerning the disease. It does now appear, however, that a number of genetic, environmental, and psychological factors act together to influence the onset of schizophrenia.

The genetic influence in schizophrenia

There is no doubt now that gene mutations are a major component of the cause of schizophrenia. The risk of developing schizophrenia is about 1% for the population of the world as a whole; i.e, 1 in 100 persons will develop the disease on average. This risk percentage rises within families who carry the specific gene mutations (Table 10.2 shows the concordance rate, i.e. the percentage chance of related members of the family developing the disease). If one of a set of **monozygotic twins** develops schizophrenia, the other twin has a 40–50% chance of having the disease, which is clearly much higher than the 1% general population rate. However, given that nearly all the twins' genes are the same (about 98%), it might be expected that the concordance rate would be close to 100% if it were purely genetic, i.e. if one twin acquired the disease the other definitely would. But this difference is the result of environmental factors influencing the course of events. The disease is therefore **polygenic,** i.e. several genes involved interacting with environmental factors. What these environmental factors are is a topic for discussion later in this chapter. Table 10.3 identifies the most important genes thought to influence schizophrenia and what we understand of their function. This list is not exhaustive; other genes appear in the literature from time to time, and no doubt will continue to do so.

The type of **gene errors** involved are varied (see Table 10.3). Examples include **fragile sites, nucleotide repeats sequences,** and **translocations** (see also Chapter 6). Fragile sites are points at which the DNA is particularly prone to breakage (fragile sites are especially involved in several mental health disorders, e.g. **fragile X syndrome**). Nucleotide repeat

Table 10.3 The major genes examined in schizophrenia research. See text for explanations of terms

Gene	Gene locus	Function (if known)	Gene error (if known)	Possible role in schizophrenia
KCNN3 (*SK3*)	1q21–q22	Calcium-activated potassium channel	CAG repeats	The longer gene may code for a potassium channel with subtle abnormal changes in function, altering neuron activity
DRD3	3q13.3	Codes for dopamine receptor D_3	Polymorphism	Dopamine receptors implicated in the biochemical cause of psychosis
Multiple genetic variants*	6p21.3–22.1	Major histocompatibility complex (MHC)	Single nucleotide polymorphisms (SNPs)	Increase risk of schizophrenia
ATX1 (ATX = ataxin)	6p23	Codes for the protein Ataxin 1		Possibly associated with severity of symptoms
DRD4	11p15.5	Codes for dopamine receptor D_4		Dopamine receptors implicated in the biochemical cause of psychosis
DRD2	11q23	Codes for dopamine receptor D_2	Polymorphism	Dopamine receptors implicated in the biochemical cause of psychosis
DISC1 (DISC = disrupted in schizophrenia)	1q42.1	Codes for protein that interacts with others in neuron development	Translocation t(1;11) (q42.1;q14.3)	Disruption by translocation causes failure of neurogenesis and neuromigration
5-HT2A receptor	13q14–q21	Codes for serotonin receptor 2A	Polymorphism	Receptor variation may disturb serotonin pathways from the raphe nucleus
CHRNA7	15q14	Codes for the alpha-7 subunit of the nicotinic acetylcholine receptor	Polymorphism	Nicotinic receptors are involved in the inhibition of sensory stimuli that may be reduced in schizophrenia, leading to hallucinations

(continued)

Table 10.3 (continued)

Gene	Gene locus	Function (if known)	Gene error (if known)	Possible role in schizophrenia
GNAL	18p	Codes for the G-protein alpha subunit coupled to the D_1 dopamine receptor	Nucleotide repeat sequence	Dopamine receptors implicated in the biochemical cause of psychosis
SCZD4 (SCZ = schizophrenia)	22q11–q13		Deletions within 22q11	Increases susceptibility to schizophrenia
DXYS14	X telomere		Shared alleles in affected siblings	Schizophrenic patients often have excess X chromosomes
5-HT 1A receptor gene	5q11.2–q13	Codes for serotonin receptor		Receptor variation may disturb serotonin pathways from the raphe nucleus
cPLA2 (phospholipase gene)	Chromosome 19	Controls the production of the enzyme cytosolic phospholipase	Dimorphic site	Excess enzyme may cause neuronal phospholipid breakdown in schizophrenia
Type 1 sigma receptor gene	19p13.3	Codes for sigma receptor	Polymorphism	The drug haloperidol binds to sigma receptors
MAGI1	3p14.1	Codes for protein involved in the scaffolding structure of cell to cell junctions, notably synapses	Polymorphism	Disruption of synaptic communication
MAGI2	7p21	Involved in recruitment of neurotransmitter receptors, e.g. AMPA and NMDA glutamate receptors	Polymorphism	Causes cognitive impairment in schizophrenia
Dgcr8	22q11	Required for microRNA processing	Deletion	Possibly causes auditory hallucinations
GRIN3A	9q34	Codes for the NMDA subunit called GluN3A	Single nucleotide variants	Excess in schizophrenia, stopping NMDA receptors from working

*Multiple genetic variants within the MHC at gene loci 6p21.3–22.1 have been shown, from pooling the results of three major studies, to significantly increase the risk of schizophrenia (Stefansson et al. 2009; see text for more information).

sequences are abnormal multiple copies of three nucleotide bases along the DNA, e.g. **CAG** or **CGG repeats**, in this case **cytosine–adenine–guanine** and **cytosine–guanine–guanine**, respectively. Repeat sequences are sometimes the cause of disorders of the brain (e.g. Huntington's disease, Chapter 13). **Translocations** involve swapping genetic material with another chromosome. **Dimorphism** and **polymorphism** are the existence of two (di-) and multiple (poly-) variants of the gene, respectively. A **single nucleotide polymorphism** (**SNP**) is a number of variants (or changes) of just one base (the base being either adenine, thymine, cytosine, or guanine) within the DNA sequence of a gene.

The discovery of various SNPs within the **major histocompatability complex (MHC)** region of chromosome 6 that are linked to schizophrenia raises the prospect of the cause of schizophrenia being linked to infection. MHC proteins are cell surface proteins involved in the immune response to foreign infective agents (called **antigens**). MHC proteins are crucial for the correct and adequate response to antigens. SNPs in this gene region would alter these proteins sufficiently to prevent a proper response, and an infective agent could then survive and infect body tissues, including the brain. This links in well with the growing evidence that viral infections, particularly the flu virus, may be involved in the cause of this disorder (see flu virus under environmental factors, on page 216).

Two major studies have revealed that:

1 Schizophrenia is actually *eight diseases* (according to **genetic profiling**), *not* one disease. These genetic profiles were derived from the **genotype** of many patients, and they cluster into eight subsets. Some of these subsets show a dominance of positive symptoms, whereas others show a dominance of negative symptoms, i.e. the *two syndromes Types I and II* as discussed above (see also Chapter 6 for genotype). Some of these subsets carry a greater risk of developing the disorder than others, some cause an earlier age of onset than others, and so on. Each of the genetic subsets had different features (or profiles), and this may have implications on how we diagnose and treat the disorder (Arnedo et al. 2014).

2 There are 128 gene variants linked to schizophrenia in 108 locations within the human genome. Many of these variants occur in genes found within the MHC, as noted above. Among the 128 variants implicated are mutations of both dopamine receptor and glutamate-related genes. The study also reinforced the link between schizophrenia and bipolar disorder (see Chapter 11) (SWGPGC 2014).

Some important genes

1 The discovery of the **disrupted in schizophrenia (*DISC1*)** gene on chromosome 1 is an important breakthrough, as the normal protein product of this gene is part of a vital signalling pathway (sometimes referred to as the **Wnt** signalling pathway; Figure 10.1) involved in neurogenesis and neuromigration. This pathway becomes corrupted when there is a mutation of the *DISC1* gene, as in many sufferers of this disorder. This pathway may become available as a target for drug therapy (Figure 10.1) (Ross and Margolis 2009). It has also been found that two molecules, called **Lis** and **Nudel**, bind to *DISC1* during the first 7 days after birth, and this promotes plasticity of the brain and synaptic formation throughout adult life. Failure of these molecules to bind during this critical 7-day window prevents cortical neurons from forming synapses in adulthood. This gene discovery, called the '*Rosetta Stone*' of schizophrenia, appears to be a major breakthrough in understanding how genes are involved in this disorder, and that could lead to new therapies (Greenhill et al. 2015).

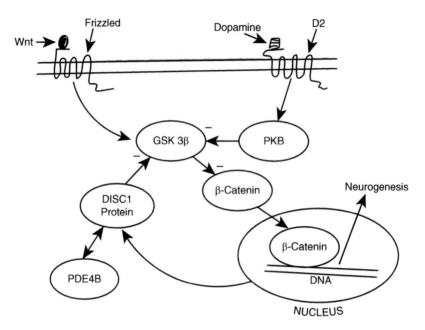

Figure 10.1 The *DISC1* gene pathway.

2   The **membrane associated guanylate kinase** genes *MAGI1* and *MAGI2* code for proteins involved in the development and function of synapses (*MAGI 1*) and neurotransmitter
receptors (*MAGI2*). Mutations of these genes, especially *MAGI1*, are linked to abnormal
synaptic connections in schizophrenia, bipolar disorder, and schizoaffective disorder.

3   The ***Dgcr8*** (**DiGeorge syndrome critical region 8**) gene is one of about 25 genes lost
in a disorder called **22q11 deletion syndrome** (22q11 is the gene locus; see Chapter 6).
In this disorder about 30% of patients develop schizophrenia. The loss of the specific
gene *Dgcr8* can now be linked to structural abnormalities of the **auditory thalamus**, i.e.
that part of the thalamus that processes sound. This may be the reason for the presence
of auditory hallucinations in schizophrenia, in particular hearing voices.

4   The **glutamate receptor ionotropic N-methyl-D-asparate 3A** (*GRIN3A*) gene codes
for a subunit (called **GluN3A**) of the NMDA receptor (see Chapter 4). The receptor
works with two **GluN1** and two **GluN2** subunits, but the addition of GluN3A prevents
glutamate from binding, so that glutamate cannot activate the receptor. The natural purpose of this subunit, which effectively stops NMDA receptors from working, is unknown.
However, in schizophrenia the levels of GluN3A subunits are high in the brain, reducing
NMDA receptor activity.

Brain pathology

The pathological changes seen in the schizophrenic patient's brain when compared with
normal brains at *postmortem* are not very obvious, but some distinct abnormalities have
been consistently reported. The most often seen abnormalities include enlarged ventricles, a

reduction in brain weight of about 5%, and a shortening of the length of the brain. Enlarged ventricles occur in some schizophrenia and bipolar depressed patients. Enlargement of the lateral ventricles requires loss of some brain tissue around the ventricle, and variations in this loss may account for some of the variations seen in schizophrenia. There may also be abnormal connections between the amygdala, hypothalamus, and the prefrontal cortex.

On close study, it can be seen that there are some reductions in the volume (i.e. neuronal losses) within the **prefrontal cortex**, the **insula cortex**, the **entorhinal cortex**, the **hippocampus**, and the **temporal lobe grey matter**. The entorhinal cortex and the anterior hippocampus both suffer losses of about 20% of their neurons. These areas of the brain also show a change in the **cytoarchitecture**, i.e. alterations in the tissue *structure*, not just numbers of cells lost.

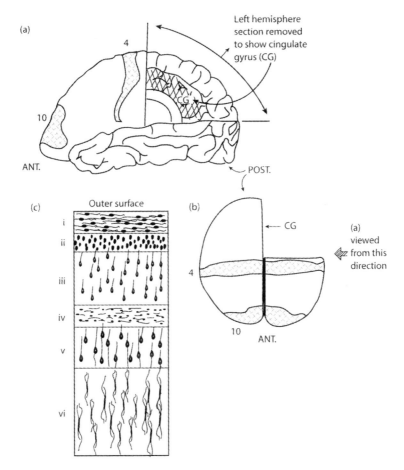

Figure 10.2 (a) Left lateral view of cerebral cortex with much of the parietal lobe removed back to the midline to show the cingulate gyrus (CG); also shows Brodmann areas 4 and 10. (b) Superior view of the same as (a). (c) Section through the cerebral cortex to show the cell layers. The areas identified in (a) and (b) all suffer a loss of cells in schizophrenia. Brodmann 4 and 10 both show cell losses in layer vi, with Brodmann 10 also showing reduced cell density in layer ii. The cingulate gyrus shows cell losses in layer v. ANT. = anterior, POST. = posterior.

The frontal cortex, like the rest of the cortex, has six cell layers, numbered **i** to **vi**. In schizophrenia, it has two large areas (Brodmann 10, the **frontopolar** area, and Brodmann 4, the **primary motor cortex**) that show changes. Brodmann 10 shows significant losses of neurons in cell layer vi, and lower than normal density of the interneurons in layer ii. Brodmann 4 shows significant cell losses in layer vi. In addition, the **cingulate gyrus** (Brodmann 24) shows notable numbers of neuronal losses in cell layer v (Figure 10.2).

Cell losses in early-onset schizophrenia have also been seen on brain scans (Thompson et al. 2001). Over the five-year period from 13 to 18 years of age, 12 schizophrenic patients who were scanned showed brain cell losses progressing from the parietal lobes to many other parts of the brain. This event, occurring in the teens, coincides with the onset of symptoms at that time, possibly triggered by an environmental agent. Those with the greatest losses of cells suffered the worst symptoms.

Much of the research on brain pathology in schizophrenia has been centred on the **entorhinal cortex** (Brodmann areas 28 and 34) and the hippocampus. These are both next to the **parahippocampal gyrus**, which in turn is part of the temporal lobe cortex (Figures 10.3 and 10.4). The **subiculum**, which blends directly into **Ammon's horn** of the hippocampus, is sometimes included as part of the hippocampus.

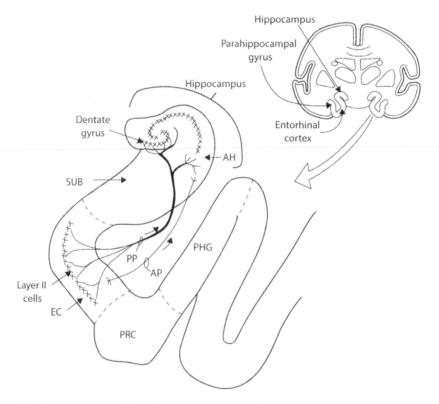

Figure 10.3 Schematic view of the hippocampal complex showing Ammon's horn (AH), subiculum (SUB), entorhinal cortex (EC), perirhinal cortex (PRC), and the parahippocampal gyrus (PHG). PP is the perforant pathway running from layer ii cells of the EC to the AH and dentate gyrus. AP is the alvear pathway running from the EC to the AH. The inset shows a section through the brain with the area involved labelled.

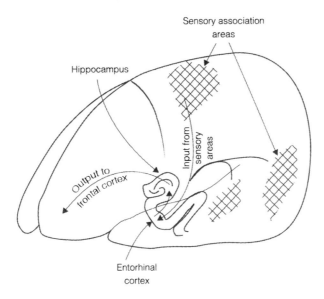

Sensory association
areas

Hippocampus

Input from
sensory
areas

Output to
frontal cortex

Entorhinal
cortex

Figure 10.4 The hippocampal complex shown within the brain (left side shown) with inputs from the
sensory association areas and output to the prefrontal area.

The entorhinal cortex receives input from all the **sensory association areas** of the cortex, i.e.
those areas of the cerebrum that process and store sensory information. It also has inputs from
the **neocortex** and **amygdala**. This is the start of a major pathway passing through the parahippocampal gyrus, the entorhinal cortex, and the hippocampus (Figure 10.5). This pathway
is vital in the production of memory, in particular recognition memory, i.e. both memorising recognised objects, people, etc., and using recognition memory to identify new sensory
stimuli. Two main pathways link the entorhinal cortex with the hippocampus: the **alvear**
pathway, which goes to **Ammon's horn**, and the **perforant** pathway, which also terminates
in Ammon's horn and the **dentate gyrus** (Ammon's horn and dentate gyrus are both parts of
the hippocampal complex) (Figure 10.3). Sensory information from the sensory association
areas is therefore channelled through the entorhinal cortex, where some sensory integration
may take place, a process necessary in order to make sense of the real world. It is then passed
on to the hippocampus, enabling it to carry out the major functions of short-term to long-term
memory and influencing thought via pathways to the prefrontal cortex. A three synaptic pathway, the '**trisynaptic circuit**' exists within the hippocampus (Figure 10.5), and although the
functions of this pathway are unclear, they may be related to short-term memory processing,
and act as a boost for information coming in from the entorhinal cortex, amygdala, and other
brain areas. The hippocampus is essential for the formation of long-term memory, i.e. any
information required to be remembered on a long-term basis must be processed through the
hippocampus first. In this context, the hippocampus has been called the 'gateway to memory'.
The entorhinal cortex, sometimes called the '*gateway to the hippocampus*', appears to be a
vital link in the chain of events that leads from the arrival of sensory impulses in the brain to
the development of a thought or idea, i.e. the *cortical sensory association areas* → *entorhinal
cortex* → *hippocampus* → *cerebral cortex* pathway (Figures 10.4 and 10.5).

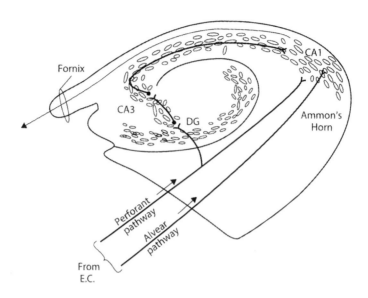

Figure 10.5 The 'trisynaptic pathway' in the hippocampus. Two pathways from the entorhinal cortex (EC) pass into the hippocampus. The perforant pathway connects with cells of the dentate gyrus (DG) (synapse 1), which connect with cells of CA3 (synapse 2), then on to cells of CA1 (synapse 3). The alvear pathway connects directly to CA1 cells. The CA1 cells connect to other areas via the fornix. This concept of three synapses forming a circuit through the hippocampus is now recognised as being more complex than this simple model suggests.

The pathophysiology of thought disorder and negative symptoms

Our thinking processes are a function of the frontal lobe of the brain. Thought is centred on our responses to sensory stimuli from the real world outside the brain, e.g. answering questions such as *What shall I eat?* or *What shall I wear?*, so correct interpretation of environmental stimuli are critical for normal thought processing. But the frontal lobe has no direct connection with the outside world, only indirectly through the sensory systems. The frontal lobe has to have a constant supply of data about the real world outside the skull supplied to it by the hippocampus. It is on this representation of the real world that the frontal lobe bases thought. But new environmental stimuli are encountered daily, so it becomes necessary for the hippocampus to be able to cope with these new experiences. The hippocampus is one of the very few parts of the brain known so far to have the ability to produce new neurons (and new synapses) after birth and throughout life. The reason is unknown, but it is possibly to do with improving the brain's ability to constantly adapt to new and changing information coming in from the environment. Because the hippocampus is also an important area for short-term memory, and thought is heavily dependent on memory, the cellular disruptions found within the hippocampus in schizophrenic patients are likely to be a cause of thought disorder. These patients often perform poorly on memory-related tasks (Fletcher 1998). Thought disorder may also be caused by the presence of a **hypofrontality** found in schizophrenic patients, i.e. a reduction in frontal lobe activity during thinking and task-related functions. The frontal lobe is a major part of the cerebral cortex innervated by the **mesocortical pathway** (which is reviewed later in this chapter; see page 214). Low dopamine in this pathway is thought to be responsible for the negative symptoms of schizophrenia, and this ties in well with the concept of hypofrontality. Further evidence for this is indicated by a reduction in the level of **phosphomonoesters (PMEs)** in the frontal lobe. PMEs are precursors of phospholipids, the molecular component of cell membranes. In addition, **phosphodiesters (PDEs)** are the breakdown products of phospholipids. A change in the PME/PDE ratio, showing a reduction in PME and higher PDE, is an indication of neuronal breakdown and losses, and is seen in both dementia and schizophrenia. Indeed, PME reduction correlates well with negative symptoms: the lower the PME, the more profound the negative symptoms in schizophrenia (Maier 1999).

Preschizophrenia

The entorhinal cortex is normally composed of six distinct cell layers, like the remaining cerebral cortex, but unlike the hippocampus, which has three cell layers. In schizophrenia, the entorhinal cortex is significantly smaller in volume than normal and shows a loss of some **layer ii** cells (Figure 10.3). There are also abnormal changes in the cytoarchitecture of the remaining cells of layer ii, including smaller cell size. This kind of structural cellular disruption can only occur during the embryological development of the brain, and therefore the individual is born with these cellular malformations already in place. It might be expected, therefore, that the individual would show the symptoms of malfunction from birth. However, the age of onset of symptoms in schizophrenia is usually in the late teens or early twenties, apparently caused by a loss of neurons at that time (Thompson et al. 2001). The question is, however, whether there are any signs during childhood.

Some of those who developed schizophrenia as an adult did show disturbed patterns of behaviour as young children, such as a poor ability to mix and socialise with friends, and were likely to underachieve at school (Carlson 2012). The size of the ventricles of the brain can now be measured during a routine prenatal scan. Those with enlarged ventricles show social, emotional, and behavioural problems for some years before the onset of the major symptoms. These early symptoms are a form of **preschizophrenia**, and enhances the notion that schizophrenia is a neurodevelopmental disorder present at birth. It would appear that in preschizophrenia the preference for social isolation, which is a major negative symptom of the fully developed disease, is present to a lesser degree in these children. Attention and language problems are also more frequent in these children. Other early symptoms seen in children who have a high risk of developing psychosis later in life are depression and anxiety in girls and aggression and serious misbehaviour, e.g. theft, in boys (Iyer et al. 2008, Gyllenberg et al. 2010). This gender difference adds weight to the growing evidence that males and females have different forms of the disease, with gender affecting the age of onset (males earlier than females), treatment outcome, and the dominance of negative symptoms. The female hormone **17β-oestradiol** is vital in the development of embryonic and fetal brain networks, and it appears to offer a degree of protection toward neurons and their networks. This protection may play a part in changing the course of the disease in females compared with males, who lack this protection.

Children born to schizophrenic parents show significant differences in their '*brain network function*' when compared with children born to non-schizophrenic parents. The brain network function is the way different parts of the brain work together, similar to a network of computers. In the children of schizophrenic parents, the communication between the different parts of the brain was found to be significantly reduced, and the network responses to different facial expressions of emotion were disrupted. This would support the concept of a neurodevelopment disorder, and provide an explanation for their lack of social interactions and the poor achievement at school.

The pathophysiology of delusions

The pathophysiology of delusional states is still under investigation, but an interesting hypothesis is now available, based on known changes in the brain. The entorhinal cortex appears to contribute toward memories centred on recognition and the individual's own bio-graphical past. The volume of the entorhinal cortex correlates well with the symptom of delusions. A large volume of the entorhinal cortex increases the likelihood of delusions, whereas a smaller volume may be too small to allow retrieval of these memories. A state of low glutamate and high dopamine activity inhibits the perforate pathway from the entorhinal cortex to the hippocampal CA1 cells, forcing the hippocampus to concentrate on the CA3/dentate gyrus cells (Figure 10.5). These CA3 cells store old memories, which are not relevant to the current (or real) environmental situation as perceived by the senses and passed though the entorhinal cortex. These old memories cannot be checked easily against the current situation, and therefore cannot be updated, resulting in false conclusions about the real world outside the brain. In particular, patients with delusions recall threatening memories, and this may be part of the CA3/dentate gyrus activity putting a paranoid perspective on reality.

Other changes seen in delusional patients when compared with non-delusional patients are:

- good preservation of the prefrontal cortex and caudate nucleus, with paranoid patients having better prefrontal function than non-paranoid patients;
- a positive correlation of the orbitofrontal volume with severity of the delusions;
- a smaller parahippocampal gyrus in delusional patients than in non-delusional patients;
- blood flow through the parahippocampal gyrus and hippocampus is increased in delusional patients, but reduced in non-delusional patients.

The pathophysiology of hallucinations

Generally, hallucinations may be produced by disturbance of the neuronal circuits in the thalamus. These circuits normally act in synchrony. Normal sensory input to the thalamus restrains (or disinhibits) this circuit activity, so the sensory input then dominates the thalamic function and is transmitted to the correct area of the brain. Hallucinations could be due to increased sensitivity of these circuits, and normal sensory input fails to restrain them. The hyperactivity then acts to interfere with the passage of the normal sensory information. In schizophrenia, these thalamic circuits are in a state of chronic oversensitivity, and the result-ing reduction of normal sensory stimuli allows background neuronal activity (or 'noise') from the rest of the brain to become dominant and produces false perceptions. A similar mechanism may act during sleep to produce dreams (see Chapter 16).

Visual hallucinations may be due to a similar **disinhibition** effect causing a reduction in the sensory input to the cortex. This would allow the cortex to generate and release its own false *endogenous* sensory stimuli (part of the brain's background 'noise'), which is then interpreted by the visual cortex as real visual stimuli. It is thought that perhaps the normal input of stimuli from the retina may have an *inhibitory* effect on the cortex, preventing any such false signals from being produced. An alternative view is that of **cerebral irritation** causing abnormally high cerebral excitation of the visual memory banks generates the false image (David and Busatto 1999). Given the integrating role of the entorhinal cortex and the hippocampus over a wide range of sensory stimuli, and the disruption of the cells in these areas in schizophrenia, it should not be difficult to see a situation in which genuine external sensory stimuli are distorted by the brain.

In schizophrenia, a small segment of the thalamus has been found to produce delta brain waves when awake. Normally these are seen as slow waves only during sleep (see Chapter 16). During waking hours, these appear to disrupt a number of normal brain activities, especially cognitive functions such as memory, and may be part of the cause of several symptoms. Delta waves were found to be generated in this thalamic region using a specific calcium channel, called a **T-type Ca channel**, and it is thought that drugs designed to block this channel may reduce the symptoms.

Auditory hallucinations may be due to the combined result of a reduction of the left superior temporal lobe gyrus function with increased right middle temporal lobe gyrus function. The temporal lobes have the sensory area for hearing (called the **auditory area**, Brodmann 41 and 42), and the left temporal lobe in particular specialises in language and speech. It is not surprising that hallucinations that involve hearing voices activate areas of the brain that process hearing. In addition, hearing voices appears to involve deletion of the *Dgcr8* gene, which affects the auditory thalamus (see *Dgcr8* gene earlier in this chapter). Clearly, memory is also involved in hallucinations, as indicated by the highly personal nature of most hallucinatory experiences, and therefore the hippocampus is likely to be part of the aetiology.

The involvement of the left temporal lobe in auditory hallucinations is consistent with the fact that the left hemisphere of the brain bears most of the pathology in this disease. This has been termed a **lateralisation**, where one side of the brain is more dominant than the other in the cause of the symptoms (David and Busatto 1999). However, pathology has also been demonstrated in the right hemisphere, although to a lesser extent. Hence schizophrenia is a disorder that is predominantly, but not exclusively, of the left side of the brain. The reason for lateralisation is possibly to do with the way the brain is put together during fetal life, i.e. it is neurodevelopmental in origin.

Neurodevelopment as a factor

The findings that the entorhinal cortex layer ii cell disruption is involved in the symptoms of schizophrenia are consistent with the theories related to the cause of thought disorder and hallucinations. Layer ii cell disruption of the entorhinal cortex could only have happened during the development of the brain in the early embryo, i.e. during neuronal development. The normal process of neuronal migration as part of neurodevelopment is described in Chapter 2.

It would appear that in schizophrenia, for reasons still poorly known, neurons of several parts of the brain, and cells of the entorhinal cortex and the hippocampus in particular, take the wrong route during migration and end up in the wrong place (therefore making wrong synaptic connections) or die (causing neuronal losses). The result is disruption of the functions of the *cortical sensory association areas* → *entorhinal cortex* → *hippocampus* → *cerebral cortex* pathway (Figure 10.4).

The migration of neuronal cells is accompanied at the same time by a similar migration of cells destined to become skin. It is these cells that form the skin patterns we recognise as fingerprints. Perhaps the disturbance of neuronal migration in the very early preschizophrenic brain is mirrored by similar disturbances in skin cell migration. Twins were used to investigate this idea, so that their finger and palm prints could be compared. In those pairs of twins in which both twins developed schizophrenia, they had identical skin patterns. However, where only one twin of the pair developed the disease, each twin had a different skin pattern. It now appears that among monozygotic (identical) twins the 48% risk of one twin developing schizophrenia if the other already has the disease is only an average figure. A closer look at these twins has identified a range of risks from 10.7% for monozygotic twins who had their own separate placentas (i.e. **dichorionic**) to 60% for monozygotic twins who shared the same placenta (i.e. **monochorionic**). The monochorionic group of twins had not only identical genes but also a virtually identical uterine environment, including the same products delivered through a common placenta. This is powerful evidence for gene and environmental interaction in the causation of schizophrenia.

It is useful to refer to the 'Big brain theory' when considering the idea that schizophrenia is a consequence of humans having a large (when compared with body size) and advanced brain. Segments of DNA called **human accelerated regions** (**HARs**) have undergone extensive evolutionary development in humans, along with the brain, but have remained unchanged in other species over millions of years. Unlike genes, HARs help to regulate neighbouring genes, and in particular many regulate genes which, if mutated, are strongly linked to schizophrenia. The evolution of HARs is crucial and beneficial to the evolution of the human brain, but their close association with mutated genes that predispose to schizophrenia puts humans at risk of the disorder. The risk of developing schizophrenia appears to be the price humans pay for developing a big brain.

The biochemical changes in schizophrenia

For many years now it has been recognised that dopamine is, in some way, involved in the production of some of the symptoms of schizophrenia. The *dopamine hypothesis* of schizophrenia was based on observations that drugs such as cocaine and the amphetamines caused schizophrenic-like psychotic events, with hallucinations and bizarre behaviour. These drugs were known to increase dopamine levels in specific synapses of the brain. In addition, it was noticed that the **phenothiazine** drugs, some of which were first used as anti-emetics, reduced psychotic symptoms in schizophrenic patients. Since these drugs block the dopamine receptors, it was postulated that excess dopaminergic transmission and receptor stimulation was involved the cause of the positive psychotic symptoms (especially involving the D_2-like receptors, i.e. D_2, D_3, and D_4 receptors), and reduced dopamine was involved in the cause of the negative symptoms.

Dopamine is the neurotransmitter within four major types of pathway in the brain (Figure 10.6) (Blows 2000):

1   The **mesocortical tracts**, passing from the brain stem to the cerebral cortex (possibly involved in the production of the *negative symptoms* of schizophrenia).
2   The **mesolimbic tracts**, passing from the brain stem to the limbic system (the system most likely to be involved in producing the *positive symptoms* of schizophrenia).
3   The **nigrostriatal tract**, passing from the substantia nigra (midbrain) to the corpus striatum (basal ganglia). This pathway produces and uses the largest amount of dopamine in the brain, but appears not to be involved in schizophrenia. It is involved in the production of extrapyramidal side effects of the drugs used to treat the disorder.
4   The **tuberoinfundibular tract**, passing between several nuclei within the hypothalamus and the pituitary stalk. This tract is not thought to be involved in schizophrenia but is involved in some drug side effects in which pituitary hormones are disturbed.

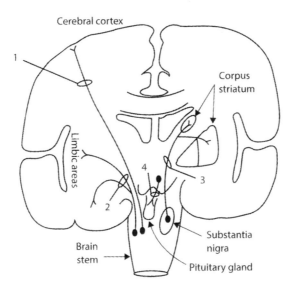

Cerebral cortex

Corpus striatum

Limbic areas

Substantia nigra

Brain stem

Pituitary gland

Figure 10.6 The four main types of dopaminergic pathway: (1) the mesocortical pathway (brain stem to cortex); (2) the mesolimbic pathway (brain stem to limbic system); (3) the nigrostriatal pathway (substantia nigra to corpus striatum); (4) the tuberoinfundibular pathway (hypothalamus to pituitary stalk).

The mesolimbic system, thought to be the pathway most involved in positive symptoms of schizophrenia, originates in the brain stem, i.e. the **ventral tegmental area** of the midbrain, and terminates in the limbic system, i.e. the **nucleus accumbens** and the **amygdala** and other associated parts (Blows 2000). The nucleus accumbens has D_4 receptors but is especially rich in D_3 receptors, and both receptor types have been found to be raised in some schizophrenics who were drug-free prior to measurement. In fact, various studies of dopamine and dopamine receptor concentrations in patients with schizophrenia have proved to be somewhat ambiguous, with relatively normal concentrations found in some patients, but disturbed concentrations found in other patients. One way of measuring dopamine is to measure the concentration of the dopamine metabolite called **homovanillic acid (HVA)**, the waste product of dopamine excreted via the cerebrospinal fluid (CSF). HVA has been found to be raised in schizophrenic patients, indicating a higher than normal rate of dopamine turnover, and in *postmortem* studies this raised concentration of HVA has been found localised to the mesocortical and mesolimbic pathways.

The dopamine hypothesis has its difficulties, indicating that a more complex picture exists. Although excessive dopamine stimulation of D_2, D_3, and possibly D_4 receptors may be the cause of *some* symptoms, especially the positive symptoms, it is clear that dopamine disturbance is *not the cause* of the disease. The dopamine hypothesis, therefore, has lost ground as a main cause of the psychoses, and is now seen as just one more small piece of a much larger jigsaw. Other neurotransmitters are involved in this disorder, in particular **serotonin, glutamate, cholecystokinin,** and **GABA**. Serotonin has a controlling effect on dopamine release, and 5-HT receptors are a target for atypical antipsychotic drugs. Glutamate is a very important neurotransmitter acting through both ionotropic and metabotropic receptors (Chapter 4). Two receptors, the metabotropic glutamate **mGluR2** receptor and the serotonegic **5-HT2A** receptor, are linked to schizophrenia, and the activity ratio between them appears to be an important factor. Healthy brains have higher activity in the glutamate receptor than the serotonin receptor, whereas in schizophrenia the ratio is the other way round. Work is in progress to find drugs that will reverse this ratio back to the healthy brain state. Glutamate and cholecystokinin are both active in layer ii of the entorhinal cortex and are thought to have an important part to play in brain cortical development. Both glutamate and cholecystokinin neurons seem to have a direct dopaminergic innervation in the brain, suggesting that dopamine disturbance could have a knock-on effect on glutamate and cholecystokinin concentrations. In addition, as an inhibitory neurotransmitter, GABA has a controlling activity over dopamine release in some pathways. In schizophrenia, reduced GABA control allows dopamine to increase in amount and activity, and also appears to be disturbed in prefrontal cortex function.

Another hypothesis suggests that problems with **glucose transport molecules 1** and **3** (**GLUT1** and **GLUT3**) may cause the early symptoms of schizophrenia by creating a situation of intraneuronal **hypoglycaemia** (low glucose uptake into the neurons from the blood). Such a low glucose uptake by the brain would result in a systemic hyperglycaemia, i.e. glucose remaining in the general circulation. This links schizophrenia with **diabetes**, although the details are complex and remain unclear.

The possible role of environmental factors

Schizophrenia is considered to be polygenic in origin and, if this is so, it should be possible to identify some environmental factors at work in its aetiology. Two particular environmental factors stand out as significant: a history of birth trauma and maternal influenza during pregnancy. Both of these factors are relevant to the period when the brain is undergoing developmental changes, e.g. maternal influenza could be detrimental to neuronal migration.

Schizophrenia shows a consistent history of higher incidence in those subjected to some form of birth trauma, such as prolonged periods of cerebral hypoxia during labour. The disorder is also higher in patients who had mothers suffering problems during pregnancy, such as **pre-eclampsia** (high blood pressure caused by pregnancy). Preterm infants subjected to perinatal trauma have a tendency to acquire enlarged ventricles (as seen in schizophrenic patients, see page 206), identified by brain scanning before and after birth. There is a link between perinatal complications and neurological abnormalities, and male infants seem to be more prone to lateral ventricular enlargement than female infants as a result of obstetric trauma. The reason is unknown; perhaps it is linked to differences in the male and female brains making the male brain more vulnerable. Such trauma may also permanently change some neural connections within the brain, which do not show symptoms until maturity.

There is also generally a 10% increase in numbers of infants destined to develop schizophrenia who were born during the late winter and early spring (February or March in the Northern hemisphere). This is a period during which viruses are particularly active (e.g. colds and influenza) and when days are short and sunlight levels are low. This lack of **ultraviolet (UV) light** can result in low **vitamin D** concentrations during a winter pregnancy (Furlow 2001). Low vitamin D concentrations during the perinatal period is now linked with schizophrenia, although the mechanism is not known. A virus may be involved in this disorder, as indicated by some studies showing a three-fold increase in the risk of schizophrenia in infants born to mothers who caught influenza during their pregnancy (3% risk compared with 1% for the general population). These findings have resulted in calls for all pregnant mothers to be vaccinated against influenza before they catch the disease. The role of the virus in this disease is the subject of much debate and research. The virus may cross the placenta as a **teratogen** (i.e. a harmful substance that passes from the maternal to fetal circulation). It then enters the child's brain and may interfere with neuronal development in genetically susceptible children. An alternative view is that the virus triggers an immune response, thus generating lots of antibodies, and some of these antibodies attack the fetal brain, causing the damage and changes seen in schizophrenia. This is an **autoimmune** response in which the individual's own antibodies are destroying their own brain tissue. These antibodies attack the NMDA receptors, and this can cause inflammation, fits, unconsciousness, and psychosis. The antibody concentrations decline after some years, but by then the damage is done. Current investigations suggest that this could account for about 6% of cases.

A similar situation may be the case with a single-celled protozoan parasite called ***Toxoplasma gondii***, which has a life cycle that involves reproduction inside the intestines of cats. It can also infect mice. Humans can get infected by contact with the parasite's eggs in the faeces of infected cats. If the hands are not cleaned thoroughly, the eggs can infect the human digestive system. The immune system reacts by producing antibodies, which may be the trigger for schizophrenia in those people already susceptible to the disorder. Those infected have twice the risk of developing schizophrenia than those not infected. *Toxoplasma* also has links with depression and suicide (see Suicide, Chapter 11).

The drug cannabis is another external factor linked with the onset of schizophrenia symptoms in teenagers. Cannabis is one drug that can cause psychotic events (see Cannabis, Chapter 8), but this is not the same as schizophrenia. However, cannabis has been seen to trigger the onset of psychotic symptoms earlier than otherwise would have been the case in those teenagers who are genetically susceptible to schizophrenia. The mechanism behind this involves a combination of cannabis with a gene called ***COMT***, which codes for an enzyme that breaks down dopamine. The combination of *COMT* and cannabis causes abnormal changes in areas of the brain linked to schizophrenia, including changes in cell size, protein concentrations, and cell density. This leads to the onset of schizophrenic symptoms and behaviour.

Smoking cigarettes appears to moderately increase the risk of developing schizophrenia, although it remains to be confirmed if this is part of the cause of the disorder in genetically susceptible people, or if it exacerbates the symptoms at an earlier age in those already within the early stages of the disease.

Environmental factors such as these appear to be one more insult in a chain of neurological insults that starts with some abnormal genes and ends with the fully developed disease. However, this chain of events is far from clear. The problem facing neurobiologists now is putting the pieces of the jigsaw together (Figure 10.7). It is not clear how the genes and environmental factors interact, or how they in turn affect the embryonic neuronal migration, or how this disturbs the biochemistry, or how these go together to cause the symptoms. There is much still to learn, but we have come a long way since the 1960s, when hardly any of the pathophysiology described above was known. With the advances being made in both neurobiology and understanding of the human genome, the prospects of solving this particular jigsaw puzzle are better now than they ever were.

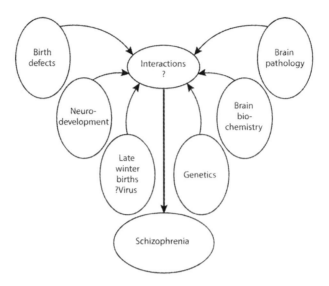

Figure 10.7 The factors affecting the cause of schizophrenia. Somehow they all contribute towards the disease, but their exact interactions, leading to the disease, are unknown.

Schizoaffective disorder and schizoid-related personality disorders

Schizoaffective disorder is the term used for those patients who suffer psychotic symptoms more or less continuously with occasional bouts of severe depression, with or without mania. It has been known for many years that very severe bipolar disorder can result in loss of contact with reality, hallucinations, and delusions, and that the two conditions, bipolar depression and schizophrenia, share common ground. It would appear that bipolar depression and schizophrenia are closer to each other in cause and effect than bipolar depression is to unipolar depression.

Various types of this disorder are seen, some more akin to schizophrenia, others more akin to depression. This may mean that it represents a comorbid state, i.e. two disorders occurring together within the same individual.

Some rare syndromes have been linked to schizophrenia.

- **Cotard's syndrome** (or **Cotard's delusion**) is where the patient is deluded in thinking that they have lost all their internal organs, or all of their blood or other body parts, with the most severely affected believing they have lost their soul and are dead. This syndrome is sometimes called '**walking corpse syndrome**', and since sufferers believe they are dead they fail to eat or care for themselves, and spend time in cemeteries. They have complete emotional detachment and loss of personal identity.
- **Capgras syndrome** causes the patient to believe their friends and family are not the original people but are *dopplegangers*, i.e. exact replicas of the originals (see Chapter 9). Even the patient's own reflection is seen as a replica of the real thing.
- **Fregoli syndrome** is similar to Capgras syndrome in that the patient believes that different people are all one person taking on various disguises.
- **Ekbom syndrome** sufferers believe that their skin is infested with invisible parasites, where in reality there is nothing there. They may even take an empty matchbox to the doctor as captured examples of the parasites.

These four syndromes appear to be different manifestations of delusions and hallucinations, i.e. false beliefs coupled with hallucinatory episodes.

Schizoid-related personality disorders fall into three types:

1   **Paranoid personality**: These individuals trust no one and are suspicious to the point at which it disrupts their normal life. They are convinced that others are trying to harm, deceive, or exploit them in some way. Paranoid personality affects about 0.5 to 5.6% of the population, with three times as many male as female sufferers.
2   **Schizoid personality**: These people are emotionally cold towards others; they prefer isolation and resist forming relationships. As with paranoid personality, schizoid personality affects three times as many men as women: about 0.4 to 1.7% of the population.
3   **Schizotypal personality**: These people seek social isolation, have odd behaviour, and are very sensitive to criticism. They have restricted emotions and show poor memory, learning skills, and recall. Their thought processes are bizarre, known as '*oddities of cognition*', e.g. they have strange beliefs, ideas of reference, and paranoia. Their speech may be vague and overelaborate. Schizotypal personality affects 0.6 to 5.2% of the population, with twice as many males as females affected. Genetics appears to be involved and there is evidence to suggest that an increase in dopamine occurs in the brain.

The antipsychotic drugs

Drugs are used to control the symptoms of schizophrenia and thereby improve the quality of life for the patient, but schizophrenia remains incurable. Many patients will require drugs for life and withdrawal from the drugs would lead to restoration of the symptoms. The antipsychotic drugs (Table 10.4, Figure 10.8) fall into several groups:

*   **first-generation drugs** i.e. the **phenothiazines** (which are further divided into three subgroups, see below), the **butyrophenones**, the **diphenylbutylpiperidines**, the **thioxanthenes**, and the **substituted benzamides**;
*   **second-generation drugs**, also known as **atypical** antipsychotics.

The main effects of these drugs are to reduce the positive symptoms of psychosis, to calm the effects of bizarre behaviour, and to improve the patient's ability to interact more with their environment. Generally they are **dopamine antagonists**, which means they block dopamine receptors and prevent dopamine from activating these receptors. This reduces dopamine activity in the brain, thus reducing positive symptoms. Some act across all the dopamine receptors (D_1 to D_5), but others are more specific for those receptors highly implicated in psychosis (D_2 and D_3), thus reducing the side effects.

The first-generation antipsychotics

Phenothiazines

Phenothiazine drugs are used as antipsychotics and sedatives, and some can be used as antiemetics. A principal member of this drug group is **chlorpromazine**, which has been said by some to have played a key role in enabling the closure of the big Victorian psychiatric hospitals in favour of community care.

Chlorpromazine (Figure 10.8a) blocks all the dopamine receptors to varying degrees, and in so doing not only reduces positive symptoms but also has the side effect of increasing the metabolism of dopamine, i.e. dopamine turnover by increasing the production and destruction of dopamine, as noted by a measurable increase in dopamine metabolites (or waste products). This may have a longer-term effect on the brain chemistry of the patient, an effect that persists beyond the duration of the drug's activity, including prolonged changes to dopamine receptor activity and sensitivity.

Chlorpromazine and the other phenothiazines are tricyclic (three-ringed) compounds (Figure 10.8a), with two outer carbon rings and a central pyridine ring. Each member of this group of drugs has different side branches in place of the chlorine (Cl) and the $CH_2.CH_2$. $CH_2.N(CH_3)_2$ chain found in chlorpromazine. The three subgroups of phenothiazines are:

- the **aliphatics (chlorpromazine, levomepromazine,** and **promazine)**, which have very good sedative effects, but moderate antimuscarinic and extrapyramidal side effects;
- the **piperidines (pericyazine)**, which have moderate sedative effects but fewer extrapyramidal side effects than the other two groups;
- the **piperazines (prochlorperazine, trifluoperazine,** and **perphenazine)**, which have fewer sedative effects and antimuscarinic side effects but more extrapyramidal side effects than the other two groups. The inclusion of prochlorperazine (*stemetil*, a valued anti-emetic medication) in this last group is a measure of the continuing importance of some of these drugs as anti-emetics as well as antipsychotics.

In terms of sedative effects (i.e. calming the patient without any loss of consciousness), the aliphatics are the most potent and the piperazines are the weakest. The main effects and side effects of the phenothiazine drugs are listed in Table 10.4.

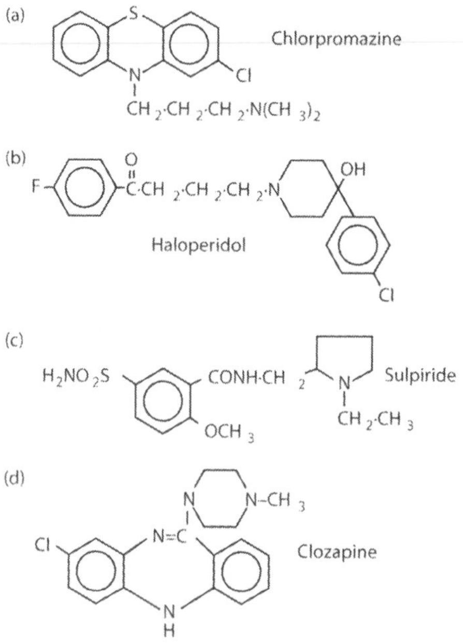

Figure 10.8 The chemical structures of some important antipsychotic drugs.

Table 10.4 The effects and side effects of the phenothiazine antipsychotic drugs

Drug	Desired effect	Main side effects
Aliphatics		
Chlorpromazine, Levomepromazine, and Promazine	Strong sedation, antipsychotic	Extrapyramidal, hypotension, hypothermia, hormonal disturbances
Piperidines		
Pericyazine	Moderate sedation, antipsychotic	Few extrapyramidal
Piperazines		
Trifluoperazine, Perphenazine, and Prochlorperazine	Weak sedation, variable anti-emetic, antipsychotic	Pronounced extrapyramidal

As dopamine antagonists, the phenothiazine drugs act on receptors within the four main dopamine pathways of the brain (Figure 10.6). In schizophrenia, the most important pathway in which to block dopamine to reduce positive symptoms is generally accepted to be the *mesolimbic* tract, but the activity of these drugs is not exclusive to dopamine receptors or to this tract. They block dopamine and other receptors also in the other tracts, and such a blockade results in unwanted side effects. These include the following:

- **Extrapyramidal side effects (EPS)** such as **parkinsonism** (tremor, stiffness of limbs, and walking difficulties), **dystonia** (abnormal movements of the face and body), **akathisia** (motor system restlessness), and late-onset **tardive dyskinesia** (abnormal repeated oral and facial movements such as lip sucking or smacking, lateral jaw movements, and flicking of the tongue, which may be irreversible). These are associated with dopamine blockade of the *nigrostriatal* pathway within the basal ganglia (Blows 2000). Parkinsonism is so named because it resembles Parkinson's disease (see Chapter 13), but unlike the disease, parkinsonism is reversible by reducing or changing the medication, or by adding anti-Parkinson drugs to the prescription.
- **Antimuscarinic side effects** occur when the drugs block the muscarinic receptor, which normally binds acetylcholine. When acetylcholine cannot bind to the muscarinic receptor it causes dry mouth, difficulty passing urine, blurred vision, dilated pupils, bradycardia (slow pulse rate), bronchoconstriction, and constipation.
- **Hypotension** (low blood pressure), due to a depressive effect on the **vasomotor centres** of the brain stem that regulate blood pressure.
- **Hypothermia** (low body temperature), especially in the elderly, due to the drugs' activity on the temperature control centre within the **hypothalamus**.
- Hormonal imbalance from the anterior pituitary gland resulting in **hyperprolactinemia**, i.e. an increase in the blood concentration of the hormone prolactin, which can stimulate breast milk production in either sex, decreased **growth hormone** and **gonadotrophins** (those hormones affecting the ovaries or testes), and variations in the concentrations of **adrenocorticotropic hormone (ACTH)** released, depending on the drug dosage. ACTH regulates the release of cortisol from the adrenal cortex, a hormone particularly important in stress. These hormone disturbances can occur because some of these drugs, such as chlorpromazine, can interfere with the balance of some hormones by blocking dopamine receptors of the tuberoinfundibular tract.

- **Neuroleptic malignant syndrome** is a very rare complication of antipsychotic drugs. The patient develops high temperature, muscle rigidity, reduced levels of consciousness, pallor, tachycardia, and urinary incontinence. It can last some days after stopping the drug and may be fatal. There is currently no effective treatment other than withdrawal of the drugs and supportive therapy.

Butyrophenones

Drugs more specific to one of the subtypes of dopamine receptor, especially D_2, would be more efficient, causing fewer side effects for the patient than the phenothiazines. A selective D_2 receptor inhibitor would, at least, avoid the complications of blocking the other receptors (especially D_1) (Blows 2000) as the phenothiazines appear to do. Such a drug is **haloperidol** (Figure 10.8b), a member of another group, the butyrophenones, which also includes **benperidol**. These are both potent antipsychotics with few sedative properties, but they can produce extrapyramidal side effects by D_2 blockade in the nigrostriatal pathway. They have a different chemical structure from the phenothiazines in that they are not tricyclic (see haloperidol structure, Figure 10.8b). Haloperidol has a one hundred times greater affinity for the D_2 receptor than for the D_1 receptor and is therefore a more selective D_2 receptor antagonist than any of the phenothiazines. Haloperidol is very useful as a treatment for acute psychotic states as it causes a quick recovery of normal behaviour. Benperidol is used to control deviant antisocial sexual behaviour, although its usefulness in this role is not yet established. **Droperidol** is a butyrophenone used in the management of postoperative vomiting.

Thioxanthenes

The thioxanthenes group contains two drugs: **flupenthixol**, which is useful in the treatment of withdrawn and apathetic patients, and **zuclopenthixol**, which should not be used in patients with predominantly negative symptoms but is a suitable treatment for agitation and aggression in schizophrenia. These drugs have moderate sedative, antimuscarinic, and extrapyramidal effects.

Diphenylbutylpiperidines

The diphenylbutylpiperidines, of which the only drug is **pimozide**, is similar in action to the butyrophenones, being potent antipsychotics, but with extrapyramidal side effects. Pimozide can also cause cardiac side effects, notably prolonged QT interval (i.e. lengthening of the contraction phase of the cardiac cycle). This is the result of the drug blocking potassium channels, which prevents outward movement of potassium from the cardiac cells, and this delays repolarisation of the cell membrane (see Repolarisation, Chapter 3). This problem requires special precautions, including regular electrocardiograms (ECGs). It is not often used because of this risk to cardiac function.

Substituted benzamide

The only drug in this category is **sulpiride** (Figure 10.7c), which can control severe positive symptoms when given in high dosage or improve activity in those affected by dominant negative symptoms if given in lower dose. Sulpiride appears to have a greater affinity for the

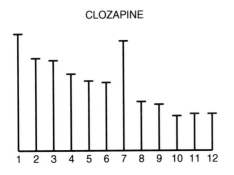

CLOZAPINE

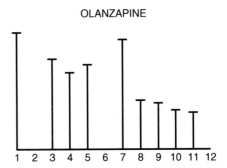

OLANZAPINE

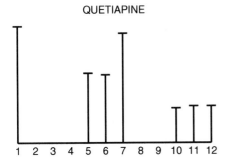

QUETIAPINE

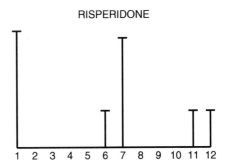

RISPERIDONE

Note: 1 = 5-HT2A; 2 = 5-HT1; 3 = 5-HT2C; 4 = 5-HT3; 5 = 5-HT6; 6 = 5-HT7; 7 = D2; 8 = D1, D3, D4;
9 = M1; 10 = H1; 11 = α1; 12 = α2

Figure 10.9 The receptor antagonistic properties of the major atypical antipsychotic drugs. (After Stahl 2003).

D_2 receptor than for any of the other dopamine receptors. It has fewer sedative effects and fewer extrapyramidal and antimuscarinic side effects than other drug groups.

The second-generation antipsychotics (atypicals)

The newer atypical antipsychotics include the drugs **clozapine** (Figure 10.8d), **risperidone, olanzapine, quetiapine, aripiprazole, amisulpride,** and **paliperidone**. Studies have suggested that these drugs appear to have three mechanisms of action that are distinct from the typical drugs, as follows:

1 As well as being dopamine antagonists, they also have significant other receptor antagonist properties, especially the 5-HT2A serotonin receptor (Figure 10.9, Table 10.5).
2 They produce fewer side effects generally, but especially fewer extrapyramidal side effects.
3 They appear to have a different 'hit and run' profile from that of the typical drugs.

Table 10.5 Receptor affinity for the major antipsychotic drugs (approximated from available data) (Labbate et al. 2010)

Antipsychotic	High receptor affinity	Intermediate receptor affinity	Low receptor affinity
Chlorpromazine	D2, α1, M, H1	D1	
Haloperidol	D2, D3, D4	5-HT2A, α1	D1, H1, 5-HT2C,
Olanzapine	5-HT2A, D2, 5-HT2C, 5-HT3, 5-HT6	D3, D4, D1 M1	H1, α1
Risperidone	5-HT2A, D2		5-HT7, α1, α2
Clozapine	D2, 5-HT2A, 5-HT1, 5-HT2C, 5-HT3, 5-HT7	D1, D3, D4, M1,	H1, α1, α2
Quetiapine	5-HT2A, D2	5-HT6, 5-HT7 α1, α2, H1	D1, D3, D4, 5-HT2C

The inclusion of the serotonin 5-HT2A receptor subtype within the antagonistic properties is a feature of all the atypical drugs but not the typical drugs. This is thought to be significant because serotonin has a regulatory role on dopamine release; i.e. serotonin limits dopamine release from the presynaptic bulb. By blocking the 5-HT2A receptor, the atypical drugs promote additional dopamine release. At first, this may sound counterproductive in a system where excess dopamine is thought to cause the symptoms of psychosis. The rationale suggested as to why this is helpful needs to be explained in the context of the four separate dopaminergic pathways.

- In the *mesolimbic pathway* (the main pathway involved in *positive* symptoms) the atypical drugs block the dopamine receptors and reduce the symptoms. Serotonin blockade in this pathway is restricted because there are lower numbers of 5-HT2A receptors in this pathway, so the increased dopamine produced is not enough to overcome the dopamine blockade (Figure 10.10).
- In the *mesocortical pathway* (the main pathway involved in *negative* symptoms) the dopamine blockade is reversed by the considerable amount of dopamine released by the blockade of 5-HT2A receptors, which are present in much higher numbers. The cerebral cortex is also served by the diffuse modulatory systems (see Depression, Chapter 11), which involves a serotonergic component, so the cortex is rich in serotonin receptors. Releasing dopamine in larger quantities provides significant improvement in the negative symptoms (Figure 10.10).
- In the *tuberoinfundibular pathway* (the pathway involved in the hormonal side effects), a reciprocal relationship exists between dopamine and serotonin receptor activity in the control of prolactin release from the pituitary. Blockade of the 5-HT2A serotonin receptors increases dopamine release, which then prevents the excessive prolactin release seen in treatment with the typical drugs.
- In the *nigrostriatal pathway* (the main pathway involved in extrapyramidal side effects), the blockade of 5-HT2A receptors causes increased dopamine release, which is enough to reverse the blockage of dopamine receptors and allows the dopamine to bind to these receptors. This prevents the onset of extrapyramidal side effects. This is very effective, as seen with the drug quetiapine, which has virtually no extrapyramidal side effects.

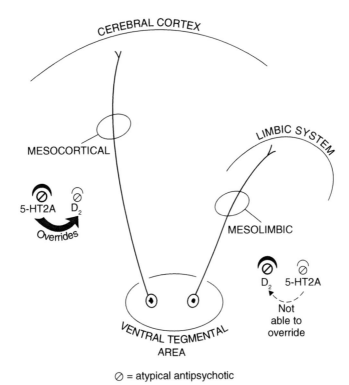

CEREBRAL CORTEX

MESOCORTICAL

LIMBIC SYSTEM

5-HT2A   D₂

Overrides

MESOLIMBIC

D₂   5-HT2A

Not
able to
override

VENTRAL TEGMENTAL
AREA

⊘ = atypical antipsychotic

Figure 10.10 The atypical antipsychotic effects on the mesocortical and mesolimbic systems. Low dopamine activity in the mesocortical system is thought to be the cause of the negative symptoms in schizophrenia, but high dopamine activity in the mesolimbic system is thought to cause the positive (psychotic) symptoms. In the mesocortical system there are more 5-HT2A serotonin receptors than D_2 dopamine receptors. The serotonin blockade by the atypical drugs reverses the blockade on dopamine receptors, thus causing increased dopamine activity, which improves the negative symptoms. In the mesolimbic system there are more D_2 receptors than serotonin receptors, so dopamine blockade dominates, relieving the positive symptoms.

In addition, the atypical drugs are said to have a different 'hit and run' profile from that of the typical drugs. This means that the mechanism of the atypical drug action on the dopamine receptors is different to that for the typical drugs (Figure 10.11). Typical drugs bind and block dopamine receptors (the 'hit') more tightly and for longer than atypical drugs. Atypical drugs release from the receptors and leave sooner (the 'run') than the typical drugs. This means the atypical drugs shorten the blockade time span and allow dopamine to return to the receptor quicker than with typical drugs, thus reducing the side effects caused by blockade.

Clozapine

Clozapine is an excellent atypical antipsychotic drug, probably the best currently available, with low side effects due to its low level of activity in basal ganglia. It is more active in

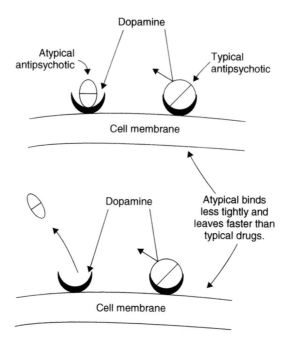

Figure 10.11 The 'hit and run' theory of atypical antipsychotic activity. Atypical drugs bind and block dopamine receptors (the 'hit') less tightly and for a shorter period than typical drugs. Atypical drugs release and leave quicker from the receptors (the 'run') than typical drugs. Atypical drugs therefore reduce side effects by shortening the blockade time span so that dopamine can return to the receptor quicker than with the typical drugs.

the mesolimbic pathway, the system implicated in psychosis. Some additional facts about clozapine are:

- Its affinity for D_2 receptor is only 10% that of chlorpromazine, and only 2% that of halo-peridol, yet it has a clinical potency twice that of chlorpromazine.
- It has a high affinity for the D_4 receptor.
- It is a CNS serotonergic 5-HT2 receptor antagonist, and the effects of this may include improvement of the negative symptoms of schizophrenia but also possibly weight gain (see Diabetes risk with antipsychotics on page 227).
- Its CNS histamine antagonistic action on the H1 receptor is 30 times greater than that of chlorpromazine, and this is probably the cause of the side effects of sedation, weight gain, and hypotension.
- Clozapine metabolites have been found to inhibit the growth of the **human immunodeficiency virus** (**HIV**, the known cause of **acquired immunodeficiency syndrome, AIDS**) and, while HIV is not known to be involved in schizophrenia, this discovery has added some weight to the theory that a virus may be involved in the cause (see Environmental factors on page 216).

Clozapine is used only for schizophrenic patients who do not respond to other drug treatments. This is because it can cause blood **dyscrasia** (a serious disturbance of the number of blood cells in circulation, sometimes causing dangerous falls in the leukocyte count). As a result, patients prescribed this drug must be treated by a specialist and registered on a special monitoring service.

Diabetes risk with antipsychotics

Schizophrenia is associated with an increased risk of developing diabetes. This risk is increased further with the use of antipsychotic drugs. The mechanism for this is not fully understood, but appears to involve two factors: (1) weight gain leading to obesity; and (2) insulin resistance. Obesity is linked to diabetes through insulin resistance at the insulin receptor. Part of the management of diabetes is weight loss, which helps to restore insulin receptor sensitivity.

Not all antipsychotics carry the same risk of weight gain. The biggest weight gain is linked to olanzapine and clozapine, moderate weight gain is linked to risperidone and quetiapine, and the least weight gain is linked to aripiprazole and amisulpride. The first generation of drugs carry a lower risk of promoting diabetes than the second generation. Of these, chlorpromazine and pericyazine carry the biggest risk; haloperidol and trifluoperazine have the lowest risk. Antipsychotics may also inhibit glucose transport into muscle, allowing it to remain in the blood and consequently promoting hyperglycaemia.

Patient compliance and suicide risk

Drug therapy has become the main mechanism in the management of patients' symptoms. However, one problem with drug therapy in schizophrenia is that of poor patient compliance, particularly within the community. Failure to take the drugs regularly results in the repeated return of some patients to hospital. To improve patient compliance, some drugs are available as **depot** injections, i.e. oil-based slow-releasing intramuscular medication that can be given by the nurse anything from weekly to 12-weekly.

Suicide risk in patients with schizophrenia can be affected by other drugs. Benzodiazepine administration to schizophrenic patients increases the risk of suicide by 91%, with most deaths occurring after 4 weeks of drug administration. However, those patients given antidepressants were found to carry a 43% lower risk of suicide.

High dosage of antipsychotic drugs

The dosage of antipsychotics used in acute psychotic patients is sometimes quite high. It is thought that as many as 25% of inpatients with schizophrenia are prescribed high doses by psychiatrists. High dose is defined as that which exceeds the maximum dose identified by the **British National Formulary (BNF)**. The problem has been highlighted because a number of patients on high dose antipsychotics have died suddenly, and electrocardiogram (ECG) changes (notably QT prolongation, see side effects on page 222) have been seen in patients on a high dose. The link between high-dose antipsychotics and sudden death is not accepted by everyone, but it would be a precautionary measure to maintain as many patients as possible on the normal dose ranges as identified in BNF. It should be kept in mind that use of high dosage in 'treatment-resistant' schizophrenia is unjustified. Careful assessment of every patient for risk of cardiac disorder before treatment begins is good practice, especially before high dosage is considered.

Rapid tranquillisation

When rapid tranquillisation is required with antipsychotic drugs, some general principles should be observed.

- Oral administration is preferred to parental route; and if parental route is used, patients should be moved onto oral as soon as possible.
- The best drugs to use are olanzapine or haloperidol, or the benzodiazipine lorazepam.
- Avoid a 'cocktail of drugs' if possible, but if several drugs are used then do not mix drugs in the same syringe, and do not mix anything with lorazepine (concurrent use of lorazepam and olanzapine is not recommended).
- Keep within the recommended dosage if possible.

Pharmacokinetics of the antipsychotics

Oral antipsychotics are well tolerated by mouth and absorbed quickly from the digestive tract. There is extensive first pass metabolism and this may be linked to the variable blood plasma concentration seen between patients on the same dosage of the same drug. The oral bioavailability is different between the various drugs (e.g. low for chlorpromazine at 10–33%, high for pimozide at up to 80%). The half-lives vary from some drugs with short half-lives (e.g. quetiapine = 6 hours, benperidol = 7 hours), to those with long half-lives (e.g. pimozide = 55 hours), and this will have an influence on the frequency that drugs are administered. As a general rule, drugs with short half-lives tend to be administered more frequently than those drugs with long half-lives. Depot injections are designed for slow release, so for this reason their half-lives are very long (even though the individual drug half-life may be quite short). Administration is therefore weekly or longer. Antipsychotics are metabolised in the liver and excreted from the kidneys.

Key points

- Schizophrenia is a polygenetic neurodevelopmental disorder.
- The symptoms of schizophrenia fall into two categories: positive (Type I) and negative (Type II).

Genetics

- The risk of developing schizophrenia is about 1% for the population as a whole.
- Multiple genes linked to schizophrenia have been found, and some environmental factors are implicated.

Brain pathology

- Some abnormalities have been reported in the brain. These include enlarged ventricles, a reduction in brain weight of about 5%, and a shortening of the length of the brain.
- The entorhinal cortex and the anterior hippocampus both show neuron losses of about 20%, and a change in the cytoarchitecture.
- Preschizophrenia, the pre-symptom childhood stages, causes the child to have a poor ability to mix and socialise with friends, and attention and language problems, causing them to underachieve at school.
- The mesolimbic system is thought to be the pathway most involved in positive symptoms.

Brain biochemistry

- Increased dopamine activity in the brain is thought to be the main cause of the positive symptoms of psychosis.

Environmental factors

- Two factors stand out as significant environmental contributors to the cause of schizophrenia: a history of birth trauma and maternal influenza during pregnancy.

The antipsychotic drugs

- The antipsychotic drugs fall into two main groups: the typical and atypical forms.
- These drugs are dopamine antagonists, i.e. they block dopamine receptors and reduce dopamine activity in the brain.
- The most important pathway in which to block dopamine for reducing the symptoms of psychosis is thought to be the *mesolimbic* tract, but antipsychotics also block dopamine receptors in other tracts, resulting in side effects.
- Extrapyramidal side effects are caused by blockade of dopamine receptors in the nigrostriatal pathway.
- Atypical drugs have a range of receptor blockade, but especially D_2 and 5-HT2A.
- This, and their different 'hit and run' profile results in fewer side effects.
- The problem of noncompliance in drug administration may be overcome by the use of depot injections.

References

Arnedo, J., Svrakic, D. M., del Val, C., Romero-Zaliz, R., Hernandez-Cuervo, H., Fanous, A. H., Pato, M. T., Pato, C. N., de Erausquin, G. A., Cloninger, C. R., and Zwir, I. (2014) Uncovering the hidden risk architecture of the schizophrenias: confirmation in three independent genome-wide association studies. *American Journal of Psychiatry*, **172** (2). Published online Sept. 15.

Blows, W. (2000) Neurotransmitters of the brain: serotonin, noradrenaline (norepinephrine), and dopamine. *Journal of Neuroscience Nursing*, **32** (4): 234–238.

Carlson, N. R. (2012) *Physiology of Behaviour* (11th edition). Pearson Education, Harlow, UK.

David, A. S. and Busatto, G. (1999) The hallucination: a disorder of brain and mind, *in* Ron, M. A. and David, A. S. (eds), *Disorders of Brain and Mind*. Cambridge University Press, Cambridge, UK.

Fletcher, P. (1998) The missing link: a failure of fronto-hippocampal integration in schizophrenia. *Nature Neuroscience*, **1** (4): 266–267.

Furlow, B. (2001) The making of a mind. *New Scientist*, **171** (2300): 38–41.

Greenhill, S. D., Juczewski, K., de Han, A. M., Seaton, G., Fox, K., and Hardingham, N. R. (2015) Adult cortical plasticity depends on an early postnatal critical period. *Science*, **349** (6246): 424. DOI: 10.1126/science.aaa8481.

Gyllenberg, D., Sourander, A., Niemela, S., Helenius, H., Sillanmaki, L., Ristkari, T., Piha, J., Kumpulainen, K., Tamminen, T., Moilanen, I., and Almqvist, F. (2010) Childhood predictors of later psychiatric hospital treatment: findings from the Finnish 1981 Birth Cohort Study. *European Child & Adolescent Psychiatry*, **19** (11): 823–833. DOI: 10.1007/s00787-010-0129-1.

Iyer, S. N., Boekestyn, L., Cassidy, C. M., King, S., Joober, R., and Malla, A. K. (2008) Signs and symptoms in the pre-psychotic phase: description and implications for diagnostic trajectories. *Psychological Medicine*, **38** (8): 1147–1156.

Labbate, A. L., Fava, M., Rosenbaum, J. F., and Arana, G. W. (2010) *Handbook of Psychiatric Drug Therapy* (6th edition). Wolters Kluwer, Lippincott Williams and Wilkins, Philadelphia, PA.

Maier, M. (1999) Magnetic resonance spectroscopy in neuropsychiatry, *in* Ron, M. A. and David, A. S. (eds), *Disorders of Brain and Mind*. Cambridge University Press, Cambridge, UK.

Nolen-Hoeksema, S. (2007) *Abnormal Psychology* (4th edition). McGraw-Hill, Boston, MA.

Ross, C. A. and Margolis, R. L. (2009) Schizophrenia: a point of disruption. *Nature*, **458**, 976–977.

Stahl, S. M. (2003) Describing an atypical antipsychotic: receptor binding and its role in pathophysiology. *Primary Care Companion Journal of Clinical Psychiatry*, **5** (suppl 3): 9–13.

SWGPGC (Schizophrenia Working Group of the Psychiatric Genomics Consortium) (2014) Biological insights from 108 schizophrenia-associated genetic loci. *Nature*, **511** (7510): 421–427. DOI: 10.1038/nature13595.

Thompson, P. M., Vidal, C., Giedd, J. N., Gochman, P., Blumenthal, J., Nicolson, R., Toga, A. W., and Rapoport, J. L. (2001) Mapping adolescent brain change reveals dynamic wave of accelerated gray matter loss in very early-onset schizophrenia. *Proceedings of the National Academy of Sciences of the USA*, **98** (20): 11650–11655.

11 Affective disorders

- Introduction
- Bipolar disorder
- Unipolar disorder
- Brain pathology
- Biochemistry
- Immunity
- Depression in young people
- Postpartum depression
- Seasonal affective disorder
- The antidepressant drugs
- Mood-stabilising drugs
- Key points

Introduction

It is normal sometimes to be unhappy as a result of certain life events, such as bereavement of a close family member, and this kind of reaction is expected. It is also expected that the sad state will resolve itself after a reasonable period of time, allowing the individual concerned to return to their usual state of mind and to function normally. Depressive illness (also called **affective disorder**; *affect* = 'mood') occurs either when the depressed state has no apparent cause or reason or when the period of depression is prolonged beyond what is considered normal, with no signs of recovery. The depth of depression is important also. A depressive illness dominates the person's life, committing them to an existence in misery with no end in sight. Suicide becomes an attractive way out of this despair, and many depressive patients succeed in killing themselves to end their suffering. Such patients need help to recover the purpose of living and, with treatment, many are returned successfully to a happier existence. Such an outcome is more likely now than it has ever been as a result of better understanding of what is happening in the brains of depressed patients and of the introduction of improved drug treatment. Depression has long been associated with other serious and long-term debilitating disorders, e.g. cancer, coronary artery disease, and chronic infections, and is often linked with the elderly (Hestad et al. 2009).

Depression is possibly the most common mental health disorder. The World Health Organization (WHO) estimate a worldwide incidence of depression at more than 350 million people of all ages, approximately 4% of the world's adult population. However, this may be an underestimate as a result of problems related to reporting and diagnosing cases in some regions of the world (Westly 2010).

Various attempts have been made to classify different depressed states and some of these classifications have been adopted and used more commonly than others (Table 11.1). The current view is that there are two main types of depressive illness, **unipolar depression** (having symptoms of depression only) and **bipolar depression** (having alternating periods of depression and mania, an acute borderline psychotic state involving symptoms of euphoria and disturbed behaviour; see Table 11.2). This classification is supported by growing evidence concerning the underlying biology of depression (Carlson 2012).

Table 11.1 Previous and current classifications of depression

Previous classifications	Explanation
1 Primary	Not associated with any other disorder
Secondary	As a result of some other disorder
2 Neurotic	Mild depression, associated with symptoms of a nervous nature, like anxiety
Psychotic	More severe depression, associated with psychotic symptoms akin to schizophrenia
3 Reactive	Caused by a sad or unfortunate life event, and continued from there
Endogenous	From within, i.e. no identifiable life event is recognised as the cause
Current classification	
Unipolar	Depressive symptoms only
Bipolar	Depressive symptoms plus bouts of mania

Table 11.2 The symptoms of depression

Symptom	Further explanation
Low level of mood (flattening of affect)	Misery that does not improve; looks very unhappy
Pessimistic thoughts	Feelings of hopelessness, unworthiness, no self-confidence
Low energy	
Psychomotor retardation	Slow body movements, delayed responses to stimuli
Sleep disturbance and tiredness	Early morning waking, difficulty in returning to sleep
Poor appetite and weight loss	
Slow speech and thought	Protracted conversations
Loss of libido	
Sometimes anxiety, agitation or restlessness	
Severe depression is sometimes associated with loss of reality and pessimistic delusions	These symptoms are akin to those of schizophrenia. Delusions are of doom and gloom
Sometimes mania (in bipolar depression)	Mania is the sudden outburst of overactivity, rapid speech and thinking, expanded optimistic ideas, increased appetite and libido, possibly aggression and psychotic symptoms such as hallucinations; manic events occur between depressive periods but are rare compared to the depressive phases. Bipolar I (BP I) indicates these manic states are severe. Bipolar II (BP II) indicates states of mild or very mild mania (hypomania), which may not impede everyday function

Depressed patients demonstrate the symptoms we now associate with disturbed receptor and neurotransmitter concentrations in the brain (Table 11.2). Gender differences in the symptoms are becoming better recognised. There are approximately twice as many women with depression than men (except in *bipolar I*, see below). Women's symptoms are typical of depression, i.e. various degrees of sadness, crying, and despair. Men, however, show symptoms of anger, irritation, and recklessness. These differences are thought to be due to social pressures on men not to succumb to what may be considered to be weak emotions (such as crying), rather than any biological differences (Westly 2010).

Another disorder, in which depressive symptoms appear to be chronic and directed *outwards* towards the world in the form of anger or irritability, is called **dysthymic disorder**.

Bipolar disorder

Bipolar disorder consists of mood swings from periods of depression to episodes of mania. It shares a lot of common ground with schizophrenia; the relationship between bipolar and schizophrenia is closer than the relationship between bipolar and unipolar depression. Bipolar depression has been considered by some to be a '*schizophrenia without the neurodevelopment error*'. It affects about 2 million people in the UK, and there has been a three-fold increase in numbers over the period 1995–2015.

Several types of bipolar disorder have been proposed as follows:

- **Bipolar I** (**manic-depressive disorder**) is characterised by periods of depression followed by episodes of mania. It occurs equally in both men and women.
- **Bipolar II** is a milder form with alternating periods of depression and **hypomania**, an elevated mood that does not reach the extent of full mania. Between the periods of mood change the patients live a normal life.
- **Cyclothymic disorder** shows episodes of hypomania followed by brief periods of mild depression.
- **Mixed bipolar** is where the patient suffers periods of mania and depression simultaneously. They can have flights of ideas (see Chapter 10) with grandiose delusions, while at the same time feel irritable, angry, and unhappy.
- **Rapid-cycling bipolar disorder** is defined as four or more episodes of mania and depression over a twelve-month period. Sufferers can switch from mania to depression or *vice versa* within one week, or even within one day. This type occurs more in women than in men, and increases the risk of suicide. In all the other types of bipolar disorder there appears to be no difference between the sexes.

The cause of bipolar disorder is becoming better understood. There may be an underlying disruption of the biological rhythms of the body, both **ultradian** (24-hour circadian rhythms; see Hormones, page 243) and **infradian** (rhythms longer than 24 hours, e.g. the female menstrual cycle) and this may contribute to the recurrent return of the symptoms. There also appears to be a tendency for it to develop more often in those persons born in the winter months (not unlike schizophrenia), leading to a suspicion of viral origin.

Intracellular signalling, a process involving pathways in which multiple chemicals interact, may be at the heart of bipolar disorder. The second messenger **cyclic adenosine monophosphate (cAMP)** (see Figure 4.2, Chapter 4), and **cyclic AMP-responsive element-binding protein (CREB)** (see Figure 8.5, Chapter 8) are both upregulated by antidepressant drugs.

In addition, the growth factor **brain-derived neurotrophic factor (BDNF)** (see Chapter 8, and the biology of stress, Chapter 9) is also upregulated by some classes of antidepressant drugs. The drugs achieve this over a period consistent with relief of symptoms, suggesting there may be a causal relationship. Raised concentrations of the **stimulatory G-protein (G_s)** and the enzyme **adenylyl cyclase (AC)** (see Figure 4.2, Chapter 4) are increased both in quantity (G_s) and activity (AC) in bipolar patients, although these changes are not thought to be due to gene abnormalities. There are also intracellular abnormalities found as the basis of the manic phases of this disorder (see Mania below).

Bipolar patients appear to be producing fewer than usual **oligodendrocytes** (see Chapter 3), and this reduces the myelin cover on neuronal axons, seriously affecting transmission of impulses along the axons.

Gene mutations have been implicated for many years because sometimes depression appears to be familial, particularly bipolar disorder. For the population as a whole, the risk of any one person developing bipolar depression is 1% (the same as for schizophrenia). The first-degree relatives (mother, father, brother, or sister) of a patient with bipolar depression have a concordance rate of 19%. The concordance rate for bipolar depression in monozygotic (identical) twins is about 65%, and in dizygotic (fraternal) twins the concordance rate is about 14%. Affected twins are most likely to have the same disorder, although occasional crossing over has been seen. The figures for family relationships are much greater than for the population as a whole (1%), suggesting a powerful genetic influence in the causation of this disorder.

A number of important genes are now known to be involved (**MAFD** = **major affective disorder**): *MAFD1* (18p); *MAFD2* (Xq28); *MAFD3* (21q22.3); *MAFD4* (16p12); *MAFD5* (2q22-24); *MAFD6* (6q23-24); *MAFD7* (22q12); *MAFD8* (10q21); *MAFD9* (12p13). Some additional gene mutations are also linked to bipolar disorder. For example:

- *P2X7* (or *P2RX7*) (12q24) is a gene that codes for an **adenosine triphosphate (ATP)** ionotropic cell-surface receptor component. The gene error is a point mutation (see Chapter 6) changing a glutamate amino acid to an arginine.
- *ANK3* (**ankyrin G**) codes for a protein that assembles **axonal sodium channels** (see Chapter 3), and the *CACNAC* gene codes for the **alpha 1C subunit** of one particular calcium channel. Both of these gene products are downregulated by the use of the drug **lithium**, which suggests they are involved in bipolar depression in humans.
- *GSK3β* gene codes for the enzyme **glycogen synthase kinase 3-β** which controls activity of **beta-catenin** (β-catenin), a protein acting on genes that promote cell survival, proliferation, and differentiation of the cell. The brain's ability to cope with stress and prevent depression may depend on the concentrations and activity of beta-catenin in the nucleus accumbens. Beta-catenin also acts on the gene *Dicer1*, which codes for proteins affecting expression of other genes, although how this affects depression is unknown. Mutations within this gene are known to be present in mood disorders, and drugs, including lithium, act through this pathway (see Lithium, page 259, and for a diagram showing GSK 3β and β-catenin see Figure 10.1, Chapter 10).

Mania

The biology of mania is now becoming clearer at the cellular level (Figure 11.1). **Protein kinase C (PKC)** is an enzyme involved in the activation and deactivation of many other

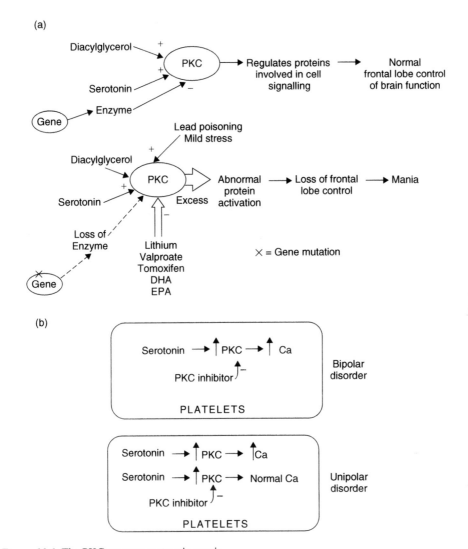

(a)

Diacylglycerol

PKC → Regulates proteins involved in cell signalling → Normal frontal lobe control of brain function

Serotonin

Enzyme

Gene

Lead poisoning
Mild stress

Diacylglycerol

PKC Excess → Abnormal protein activation → Loss of frontal lobe control → Mania

Serotonin

Loss of Enzyme

Lithium
Valproate
Tomoxifen
DHA
EPA

X = Gene mutation

Gene

(b)

Serotonin → ↑PKC → ↑Ca

PKC inhibitor ⌐−

PLATELETS

Bipolar disorder

Serotonin → ↑PKC → ↑Ca

Serotonin → ↑PKC → Normal Ca

PKC inhibitor ⌐−

PLATELETS

Unipolar disorder

Figure 11.1 The PKC enzyme system in mania.

proteins, some of which are part of the cell signalling mechanism (one method by which cells signal to each other) in many tissue types. Overactivity of the PKC cell signalling system, especially within the glutamate systems of the prefrontal cortex, is now strongly implicated in causing the symptoms of mania. PKC is itself activated by the second messenger **diacylglycerol** (see Chapter 4) and serotonin in brain cells. PKC activation is reduced by an enzyme that, if coded by a mutant gene, would fail to regulate PKC. Excessive PKC activity causes reduced prefrontal lobe function and ultimately loss of some prefrontal cells. This loss of prefrontal cortex function appears to be a key factor in the production of manic symptoms. Regulation of the PKC system is achieved by the drugs lithium, valproate, and tomoxifen given in therapeutic doses. Tomoxifen is used in breast cancer treatment as an anti-oestrogen, but it may be used in the future in bipolar disorder therapy. In addition, the omega-3 unsaturated fatty acids **docosahexaenoic acid (DHA)** and **eicosapentaenoic acid (EPA)** have an inhibitory effect on PKC, whereas mild stress and lead poisoning increase PKC activity (Figure 11.1a).

PKC activity in platelets is also increased in bipolar disorder, causing an increase in intracellular calcium. PKC inhibitors applied to platelets from depressed patients causes a reduction of calcium in unipolar depression but not in bipolar disorder, supporting the notion that these are distinct disorders with different pathologies (Figure 11.1b).

Unipolar disorder

Unipolar disorder is marked by periods of depression without episodes of mania. The incidence in females is double that seen in males, and the disorder carries a genetic risk to the general population of about 6% (i.e. 6 in 100 people will develop the disorder). Mild forms of depression carry a general population risk of approximately 10%. The concordance rate for first-degree relatives is also 10%.

Some genes have been linked to depression (**MDD** = **major depressive disorder**):

- *MDD1* (12q22-23.2) gene is linked to unipolar depression.
- *MTHFR* (1p36) gene codes for an enzyme involved in folate (folic acid) metabolism.
- *CREB1* (2q34) gene is linked to unipolar major affective disorder (MAFD).
- *FKBP5* (6p21) gene is involved in regulation of the hypothalamo–pituitary–adrenal (HPA) axis (see Chapter 5) and linked to the response to antidepressants and recurrence of episodes of depression.
- *DYT1* (9q34) gene is linked to early age (before 30) recurrent major depression.
- *DRD4* (11p15) dopamine D_4 receptor gene is linked to unipolar depression.
- *TPH1* (11p15) is the **tryptophan hydroxylase** gene.
- *TPH2* (12q21) is another tryptophan hydroxylase gene, which may be involved in some cases of unipolar depression.
- *SLC6A4* (17q) is the **serotonin transporter** gene linked to unipolar depression.
- *BRC* (21q11) gene is linked to major depression.

Several suggested environmental factors are possibly involved in the cause of depression, including maternal deprivation, unstable parental relationships, and disturbance in the home life, all factors resulting in an unhappy childhood. These factors will have led to various *losses*, i.e. loss of a loved one, loss of a job or a home. Sudden loss events, such as a bereavement or parental separation, may trigger the first bouts of depression in a vulnerable individual.

Biological factors that contribute to causing depression are poorly known. Zinc deficiency has been linked with depression, with depressed patients having blood zinc concentrations 14% lower than normal. Even lower concentrations than this have been recorded in severely depressed patients. However, nonprescribed zinc supplements should not be relied upon to treat depression without first getting medical advice. This is because the depression may be due to other factors, and because zinc is a trace element, i.e. very small amounts are normal, and it can quickly reach toxic levels if too much is taken.

Environmental factors appear to play a much bigger role in the aetiology of unipolar depression, whereas genetic factors are more important in bipolar disorder.

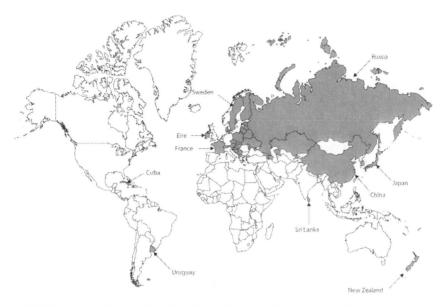

Figure 11.2 The areas of the world with a high suicide rate (shown as shaded countries).

Suicide

Suicide is a phenomenon that is often triggered by environmental factors such as poor social conditions or very difficult personal circumstances, all of which cause chronic stress. Somewhere in the world, one person dies from suicide every 40 seconds. The highest suicide rates in the world occur in northern and eastern European countries, Russia and Asian countries (notably China, Figure 11.2). The Indian rate of suicide may be five times higher than recorded because suicide there is a crime and families do not want this stigma recorded as the cause of death. Therefore many suicides are recorded as other causes of death. China has 22% of the world population but 40% of the world suicides. Here there are more women killing themselves than men (suicide in China accounts for one in four female deaths between the ages of 15 to 44 years), although everywhere else the male suicide rate is greater than the female rate (approximately four males die from suicide for every female suicide death). The high female rate in China may have something to do with the fact that Asian societies are male dominated and that women are given less value in society. Despite the high rate of suicide in these areas it is generally considered that mental illness, and in particular depression, probably accounts for only a low percentage of these deaths. In China, only about 50% of the suicidal deaths are caused by mental illness, the others are caused by their social conditions. The UK, when compared with these high rate countries, shows a significantly lower rate of suicide (Figure 11.2).

Genes linked to depression also increase the risk of suicide. Studies of monozygotic (identical) twins with depression where one twin killed themselves, between 13% and 19% of the second twins also committed suicide. This is very different to dizygotic (non-identical) twins where if one committed suicide, between 0% and 0.7% of the second twins killed themselves.

Connections between brain chemistry and suicide have been established: notably low concentrations of serotonin and its metabolite **5-hydroxyindolacetic acid (5HIAA)**, which confers a 10–20% increase in rate of suicide. There appears to be 30% more serotonin neurons in the brain stem, but they are smaller than normal and are defective in function. However, it does suggest that since they formed with the rest of the brain during fetal neuronal development, these people are born with the propensity to kill themselves. This does not mean they will commit suicide, but it does mean that they are more likely to kill themselves if they suffer depression. However, it is clear that there are other nonbiological factors involved, not least of all environmental factors and the social situation they find themselves in.

A number of **biomarkers**, i.e. factors that show up in the presence of disease, have been found to be strongly linked to suicide. High concentrations of certain biomarkers in the blood indicate a much higher risk of suicide. These biomarkers could form the basis of a blood test that could be used to predict the patient's risk of killing themselves with 92% accuracy. This would be a very valuable screening test to see who requires special precautions to prevent suicide. In addition, six metabolites in urine have been found to be important biomarkers that can help to distinguish between bipolar and unipolar disorder. These biomarkers will enable doctors or laboratories to perform a simple urine tests to help differentiate one diagnosis from the other.

One environmental factor linked to suicide is the parasitic infection toxoplasmosis (see Chapter 10), which causes 54% greater risk of women attempting suicide, with twice as many than usual succeeding, with or without a history of mental ill health. The suicide rate correlated well with the level of infection, i.e. the greater the infection the higher the suicide risk. The parasite ***Toxoplasma gondii*** affects the brain in a manner that alters behaviour so that sufferers become aggressive to themselves. Those women with the highest concentrations of antibodies against *Toxoplasma*, and therefore producing the highest concentrations of immune chemicals called **cytokines**, were 91% more likely to commit suicide than uninfected women.

Brain pathology

The evidence of physical changes identified in the brain during depression is limited. Changes are sometimes observed that are akin to those found in schizophrenia; for example, between 10 and 30% of depressed patients have some degree of ventricular enlargement, and some patients show a reduction in the size of the temporal lobe. The prefrontal cortex, ventral striatum, and hippocampus also suffer some cell losses (reduced grey matter volume), and therefore they shrink in size in depressed patients. This applies particularly to the frontal lobe, a pathology called **frontal lobe atrophy**, and to the hippocampus. Each episode of depression shrinks these brain areas further, notably the hippocampus, meaning that rapid symptom control can save a significant number of brain cells. Drug treatment, notably lithium, has been shown to stop this cell loss. Cell losses in depression also includes glial cells (see Chapter 3), and this adds to the problem in ways that are not yet fully understood. In bipolar disorder the medial prefrontal cortex is underactive, even when no symptoms are occurring. This underactivity is possibly the reason why bipolar patients find difficulty with multitasking. It would appear that bipolar patients are working harder with their emotional centres of the brain in compensation for the lack of medial prefrontal cortex activity. This may account for their inability to carry out complex tasks. Drug therapy can prevent cell losses and even correct some of the synaptic connections lost through episodes of depression.

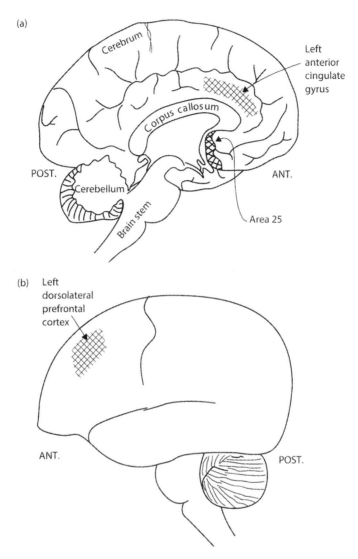

Figure 11.3 Areas of the brain involved in depression. Reduced blood flow is sometimes found in (a) the left anterior cingulate gyrus (seen here in midline section of the brain). Also shown is area 25, called the subgenual cingulate, which is overactive in depression. Blood flow is also often reduced in (b) the left dorsolateral prefrontal cortex (seen here in left lateral view).

Lesions are sometimes found in the periventricular white matter, i.e. the axons surrounding the ventricles. Studies of cerebral blood flow indicate various changes in the left anterior and right posterior areas of the cerebrum in a number of patients, including reduced blood flow to the left anterior cingulate gyrus and the left dorsolateral prefrontal cortex (Figure 11.3).

Part of the **cingulate region** of the brain, called the **subgenual cingulate** (Brodmann area 25), is a narrow band of frontal cortex folded beneath the corpus callosum (Figure 11.4).

Studies have demonstrated that this area is in a state of hyperactivity in major depression (Dobbs 2006). Normally area 25 has large amounts of **serotonin transporter (SERT)**, which moves serotonin from the synaptic cleft back into the presynaptic bulb, i.e. *reuptake* of serotonin. This has the effect of concentrating serotonin in the synapses of this area. Tiny variations in the length of the gene that codes for SERT (i.e. the *SLC6A4* gene at 17q.11.1-q12) were thought to affect this transporter in area 25 and contribute towards depression. Mixed results from the studies have failed to confirm this hypothesis one way or the other (see also Anxiety-related personality disorders, Chapter 9).

Overall, area 25 is thought to have a powerful influence over many brain areas involved in memory, the sleep–wake cycle, mood, thought, and self-esteem, and therefore is involved in feelings of guilt. Many of these functions are disrupted in depression, and guilt is thought to play an important role in the causation of depression. Overactivity of area 25 coupled with reduced frontal and limbic activity is found in most bipolar patients. Relief of depression using antidepressant therapy corrected these abnormal activity levels in area 25 and the frontal cortex. However, a number of patients that responded well to **cognitive behavioural therapy (CBT)** showed a significant reduction in area 25 activity to levels seen in nondepressed persons; plus they also had a *lowering* of frontal lobe activity. This is possibly because the group responding well to CBT had excessively high frontal activity, which settled down with therapy. It may be possible to distinguish between those patients who will recover best with drugs and those who will recover best on CBT on the basis of their frontal lobe activity levels. **Deep brain stimulation** is a surgical procedure in which electrodes are placed within the brain in white matter adjacent to area 25, and are connected to an electrical source that gives stimulation to the area. This appears to switch off area 25 activities and give good results in lifting depression.

Another brain region, the **lateral habenula**, has been shown to be the main part of the brain's disappointment circuit. The habenula is part of the limbic system, and is situated behind and slightly beneath the thalamus. Some neurons in this area are capable of secreting both **glutamate** (excitatory) and **gamma-aminobutyric acid (GABA**; inhibitory; see Chapter 4). This is very unusual, and in depression these neurons are underproducing GABA, so the disappointment circuit remains active all the time. Relief of depression using antidepressant therapy corrected these abnormal activity levels.

The left and right occipital lobes (at the back of the cerebrum) appear to be bent and wrapped around each other in about 35% of depressed patients. In fact, they have been found to be likely to have a three times greater chance of having wrap-around occipital lobes than nondepressed people, more so in females than in males. This is thought to be caused by brain growth inside the skull taking up more room than is available at that time, a problem solved by overlapping and bending the occipital lobes. It does cause some distortion to neighbouring structures such as parts of the ventricular system. The pathological significance and relevance to treatment of this anomaly is currently unknown.

Biochemistry

Serotonin

Serotonin (5-hydroxytryptamine, or 5-HT) is a major neurotransmitter in one of the two diffuse modulatory systems. The serotonergic system extends from the **raphe nuclei** of the brain stem to many other brain areas (Figure 11.4a) (Blows 2000a). Serotonin concentrations have been identified as a factor in depression. The neurotransmitter's metabolites (waste products

(a)

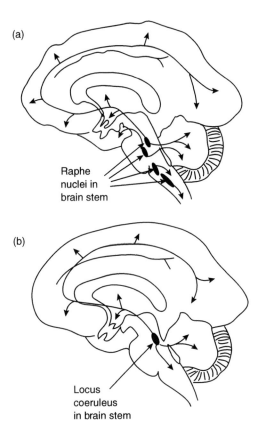

Raphe
nuclei in
brain stem

(b)

Locus
coeruleus
in brain stem

Figure 11.4 The diffuse modulatory systems. (a) The serotonin pathways from the raphe nuclei in the
brain stem extend to many areas of the brain. (b) A similar pattern of noradrenaline pathways
extends out from the locus coeruleus of the brain stem.

for excretion), derived from degraded serotonin and measured in the **cerebrospinal fluid**
(**CSF**), are significantly *reduced* in depression, indicating a lower than average turnover of
the transmitter at the synapses. Low concentrations of serotonin will also occur if the dietary
intake of the amino acid **tryptophan** is low, as it is required for the production of serotonin
(see Figure 4.8, Chapter 4). Male brains appear to suffer less than female brains from this
loss. Very low concentrations of serotonin have been linked to increased violent behaviour,
both against the self, as in suicide, or against others, as in violent crime including murder (see
Chapter 5). In addition, increases in the numbers of serotonin receptors have been identified
in some patients, and this greater receptor density is to be expected if the neurotransmitter is
low. The additional receptors are often of the subtype 2 (i.e. 5-HT2), and this is regarded as a
compensatory *upregulation* of the receptor to maximise the binding of what serotonin there is
present. The subtype 2 receptor is thought to be the most important of all the receptor subtypes
involved in mood regulation. There is some evidence indicating that the effects of low serotonin are further aggravated by a reduction in serotonin receptor activity (i.e. receptors function
less well even when the neurotransmitter binds) and by a loss in the number of neurons within
the serotonin pathways, leading to reduced serotonin synthesis.

Serotonin has some effect on the production of noradrenaline in the second diffuse modulatory system of the brain. As with the serotonergic system, this secondary system starts in the brain stem and passes out to many parts of the brain (see Noradrenaline below). Lower than normal serotonin concentrations reduce the noradrenergic neurons' ability to produce noradrenaline. Thus a low serotonin concentration has a *knock-on* effect in causing a lower noradrenaline concentration in the brain.

Serotonin is also taken up by **platelets (thrombocytes)**, which are blood cells important for the prevention of bleeding by the formation of a **thrombus** (a blood clot). Serotonin released from platelets has a local effect on blood vessels, which may have a bearing on migraine. The role of serotonin directly on platelets is to enhance their ability to become active as part of the thrombus formation process. In depression, the platelets show less ability to take up serotonin and thus are less able to be activated.

Noradrenaline

Noradrenaline pathways form the second of the two diffuse modulatory systems in the brain, noradrenaline being centred on the **locus coeruleus** in the brain stem, with pathways to many diverse parts of the cerebral cortex and limbic system (Figure 11.4b). Noradrenaline is the neurotransmitter of arousal, i.e. it causes increased levels of brain activity, and it is therefore most active during the day (Blows 2000a).

Some evidence indicates disturbance in the numbers and density of noradrenaline receptors in depression. Of the two major noradrenaline receptors that are known, **alpha-adrenergic** and **beta-adrenergic**, the increased density appears to be of the beta-adrenergic type. As already noted, some serotonin pathways from the raphe nucleus extend to areas that involve noradrenaline secretion, and it seems likely that noradrenaline concentrations are disturbed because there is a loss of serotonin regulation of noradrenaline secretion. This may cause a low concentration of noradrenaline in some synapses, and some antidepressant drugs act in raising these concentrations. In some cases of bipolar disorder, noradrenaline turnover in the cortex and thalamus is increased, reaching its highest point during a manic episode.

Glutamate

Coticosteroids are raised in **stress** (see Chapter 9, and Hormones in this chapter, on page 243), and high cortisol can stimulate the release of glutamate and increase the production of **NMDA glutamate receptors** in the CA3 region of the hippocampus in depression. This can lead to neurotoxicity, cell death, and atrophy of the hippocampus. Drugs that block the NMDA receptors appear to prevent this cell loss, and many of the antidepressant and mood-stabilising drugs do have indirect means of reducing this problem. Studies also show that decreased activity in the glutaminergic pathways linking the cortex with the limbic system is found in depression, whereas overactivity of these pathways occurs in mania.

Dopamine

Serotonin is not only a regulator of noradrenaline secretion, it also regulates the secretion of dopamine (the '*feel-good factor*'), so disturbance of the serotonin concentrations seen in depression is likely to have a knock-on effect on dopamine production. It is possible that severe bipolar depressive states that show psychotic symptoms such as hallucinations have some disturbance to the dopaminergic systems. Direct evidence of low dopamine in depression comes from low concentrations of **homovanillic acid (HVA)** in cerebrospinal fluid. HVA is the metabolite of dopamine (see Chapter 4). There is reduced firing rate of dopamine neurons in the **ventral tegmental area (VTA)** of the brain stem (see Chapter 8) resulting in less dopamine release in the limbic area. Also, dopamine agonist drugs have been shown to lift depression, although this is not currently standard treatment.

Hormones

Hormonal abnormalities are also well recognised in depression. Depressed patients often show reduced concentrations of secretion of several pituitary hormones, especially **growth hormone** and **thyroid hormone**. Depression is frequently associated with hypothyroidism, and thyroid hormone is given to a number of depressed patients along with their antidepressant medication (see Chapter 5). This combination is considered by many to improve the results from the antidepressants. Chronic stress, or prolonged corticosteroid therapy, in which persistently high concentrations of cortisol, and in particular prolonged elevated levels of **corticotrophin-releasing factor (CRF)**, can also lead to depression. This is accompanied by atrophy and death of CA3 cells in the hippocampus (see Chapter 10), resulting in reduced hippocampal volume. In chronic stress the HPA axis (Figure 11.5) goes into prolonged hyperactivity, resulting in enlargement of both the adrenal and pituitary glands. This hyperactivity is probably due to malfunction of the CRF-producing neurons in the hypothalamus and can happen either as a result of external chronic stress or as a result of a direct problem with the neurons. CRF produced in elevated quantities does more than just cause the release of **adrenocorticotropic hormone (ACTH**, Figure 11.5), it also suppresses sleep (causing insomnia), reduces appetite (causing anorexia), inhibits reproductive behaviour, and causes withdrawal in unfamiliar environments – all symptoms that are seen in depression. Some of these are disturbances of the body 'clocks', often called **circadian rhythms** because some, such as the sleep–wake cycle, take about a day to cycle (*circadian* = 'about a day'). Circadian rhythm disturbance is involved in causing many of the symptoms of depression, especially in children (see Childhood depression, on page 248). CRF concentrations are found to be high in the CSF of depressed patients but return to normal with treatment. The increased activity of the HPA axis results in persistently high concentrations of circulating cortisol, the protective hormone released in stress. Normally, a high concentration of cortisol in the blood is short-lived, as a result of the hormone binding to receptors in the brain; the brain responds to this by signalling the reduction of cortisol production and release through the HPA axis (Figures 11.5 and 11.6). In depression, these cortisol receptors are not functioning adequately; the brain's ability to suppress cortisol production is reduced and cortisol concentrations remain high.

In **dysthymic disorder**, there is less evidence for the involvement of the HPA, but there are indications of dysfunction of the **hypothalamus–pituitary–thyroid (HPT) axis** (Figure 11.5) causing thyroid hormones abnormalities in many cases.

Postmenopausal depression may be due to the low **oestrogen** that occurs, and a new form of **hormonal replacement therapy (HRT)**, an oestrogen called **10β, 17β-dihydroxyestra-1,4-dien-3-one (DHED)**, may help this situation. It is a prodrug (see Chapter 7) that is converted to oestrogen (**17β-oestradiol**) only in the brain, and this will reduce the side effects on the body sometimes caused by standard HRT.

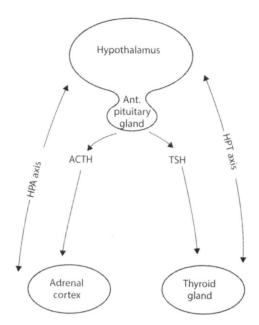

Figure 11.5 The hypothalamo–pituitary–adrenal (HPA) axis and the hypothalamo–pituitary–thyroid (HPT) axis. The HPA involves adrenocorticotropic hormone (ACTH), and the HPT axis involves thyroid-stimulating hormone (TSH). Depression often involves a prolonged hyperactivity of the HPA, whereas dysthymic disorder involves a dysfunction of the HPT.

Immunity

The relatively new science of **psychoimmunology** is pointing the way toward a better understanding of how the mind (or the brain) affects the immune system and *vice versa*. Stress and depression are said to be the major players in this field, with significant changes occurring in the immune system in both these disorders (Hestad et al. 2009). However, the problem of '*cause or effect*' comes into play, and much detail has to be worked out to determine whether the changes seen cause depression or whether they are the result of depression. Different researchers have reported a wide range of immune changes in depression (Brown 2001), but the main changes are as listed in Table 11.3.

Monocytes are phagocytic white cells; that is, they engulf **antigens** (foreign particles) as part of the fight against infection. **NK (natural killer)** cells are white blood cells that are normally active against virally infected and some malignant cells. **Lymphocytes** are white cells that provide the main defence against invading antigens. There are two types of lymphocyte: **B-cells**, which produce proteins called **antibodies** that attack antigens (B-cell defence is called **humoral immunity**), and **T-cells**, which attack and destroy specific antigens (T-cell defence is called **cell-mediated immunity**). Lymphocyte studies in depression appear conflicting, with overall numbers down but T-cells concentrations raised. This is possibly because different subgroups of depressive patients show different lymphocyte results, with overall disturbance affecting cell-mediated immunity more than humoral immunity. Humoral antibody production sometimes involves anti-serotonin antibodies, the presence of which is associated with a poor response to treatment. Understanding these variations

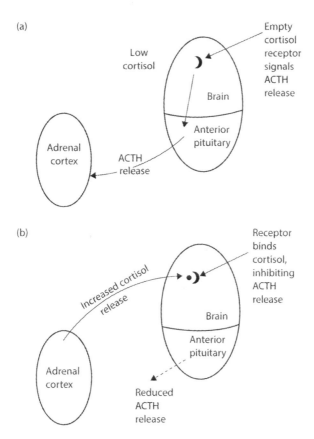

Figure 11.6 The effect of blood cortisol concentration on adrenocorticotropic hormone (ACTH). Low concentrations of cortisol in the blood cause a release of ACTH, which stimulates cortisol release from the adrenal cortex (a). This is because cortisol receptors in the brain remain empty and signal the anterior pituitary, where ACTH is produced. Increased concentrations of cortisol in the blood (b) bind with the brain receptors, and this deactivates the signal to the anterior pituitary, which reduces ACTH release. In depression, the receptors are possibly malfunctioning, and ACTH release is not turned off even when cortisol concentrations are high.

is a goal for further research. Regarding some terminology in Table 11.3, **gangliosides** are **glycolipids** (i.e. lipids with sugars attached) found in the brain and nervous system, and **high-density lipoproteins (HDLs)** are blood lipid particles containing **cholesterol**.

Cytokines are chemicals involved in *cell signalling* during an immune response. Those raised in depression are reported as **interleukin-1beta (IL-1β), interleukin-6 (IL-6), tumour necrosing factor-α, gamma-interferon (γ-IF; IFNγ)** and **prostaglandin E$_2$ (PGE$_2$)**. Cytokines are naturally produced during infections by activated immune cells, i.e. leukocytes such as monocytes and lymphocytes, but they are also given as drugs for various conditions, such as cancer therapy. Observations of people with active immune systems during infections, or during cancer treatment with cytokine therapy, show them often to be sad, not eating or sleeping well, with poor concentration and constant tiredness with

Table 11.3 The psychoimmunological changes reported in depression

Psychoimmunological change	Possible effects on the patient
Lower circulating active monocytes	?Affects immune response to infection
Lower circulating active NK cells	?May disturb sleep and cause psychomotor retardation
Lower lymphocyte proliferation	?Affects immune response to infection
Increased circulating cytokines, especially PGE_2, TNF-α and IF-γ.	?May be involved in the cause of depression (see text)
Raised acute-phase proteins (APP)	?Part of an acute immune response
Raised anti-serotonin antibodies	?Antibodies lower serotonin in blood + CNS
Raised anti-ganglioside antibodies	?Antibodies lower gangliosides (part of serotonin receptors) in CNS
Raised circulating T-cells	Unknown if any
Disturbed blood lipid concentrations, especially high-density lipoprotein (HDL)	Unknown if any
Lower circulating beta-endorphin	Associated with lower concentrations of NK cells
Raised leukocytes, e.g. neutrophils	Unknown if any

fatigue, and complaining of multiple aches and pains. These are symptoms akin to those of depression, and this is sometimes called 'sickness behaviour' or 'sickness syndrome'. It may be that antidepressants could have an anti-inflammatory effect and therefore have a role to play in treating people with sickness syndrome, and there is growing evidence that some antidepressant drugs could act as a *prophylaxis*, i.e. have a preventive effect, if given before or during cytokine therapy.

In depression, **PGE₂** and **Il-6** appear to enhance each other in a loop, which is suppressed by antidepressants. IL-1β and Il-6 appear to be involved in the disturbance of the HPA axis and in the disorder of serotonin metabolism. Brown (2001) reported that patients taking either one of two drugs to boost their immune systems to fight infection or cancer were becoming depressed, and even suicidal. These drugs are **alpha-interferon (α-IF)** and **interleukin-2 (IL-2)**, and it is this kind of observation that provides further weight in support of the *immune theory* of depression. The mechanism is still not fully identified, but it would appear that cytokines reduce the concentration of tryptophan, the precursor of serotonin, possibly leading to a serotonin shortage. Tryptophan is degraded by the enzyme **idoleamine 2,3-dioxygenase (IDO)**, which converts tryptophan into a metabolite in the brain. In depression, raised concentrations of **tumour necrosing factor-α** and **γ-interferon** cause raised concentrations of IDO. This creates more tryptophan metabolite than expected, and it is this increased metabolite concentration that appears to induce the depressive symptoms seen in sickness syndrome. Drugs that block the formation or action of IDO may become a valuable mechanism of treatment for the future.

The large circulatory cytokine molecules, such as **interleukin**, are not generally able to cross the blood–brain barrier, so their role is copied by smaller molecules such as **prostaglandins** and **nitric oxide** *inside* the brain. These smaller molecules stimulate glial cells in the brain to produce further inflammatory cytokines, which then bind to receptors on neurons of the cerebellum, the hippocampus, and the hypothalamus – areas where mood and behaviour are moderated.

As noted, cortisol concentrations are high in depression, and this has implications for the immune system. Apart from the glial cells of the brain, the immune cells in the blood also have cortisol receptors and can therefore bind cortisol. As well as the HPA axis,

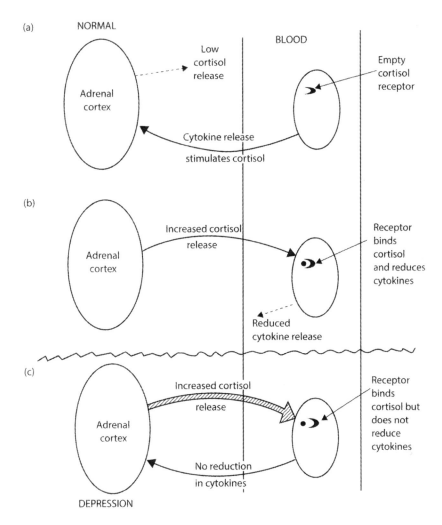

Figure 11.7 The relationship between cortisol concentrations and cytokine production. (a) Immune cells in the blood produce cytokines, which stimulate cortisol production when this is low. (b) As cortisol concentrations rise, cortisol binds to cortisol receptors in the immune cells, and this reduces cytokine production. (c) In depression, the receptors do not function so well, resulting in continued cytokine production when cortisol concentration is high.

inflammatory cytokines also trigger cortisol release, but the rise in cortisol concentration causes the inflammatory cells to reduce cytokine production in a *double feedback mechanism* (Figure 11.7). If brain cortisol receptors are not working well, inflammatory cell receptors may not be functioning properly either, and the high cortisol concentrations fail to reduce the cytokine concentrations. A vicious circle is created in which the cytokines continue to stimulate further cortisol release, which is then unable to turn the cytokines off.

Some of these findings may also be useful as **markers** of depression, as their blood measurement is fairly consistent and they could be used as part of the diagnostic procedure to identify depression. The markers include raised leukocyte (white cell) numbers, especially the **neutrophils** (phagocytic cells, of the **granulocyte** white cell group), raised cortisol concentrations, and the **HDL** findings.

Depression in young people

Compared with adult depression, the incidence of depression in children is less: about 2.5% of children, 8.3% of adolescents, and 16% of adults suffer the disorder. The symptoms in childhood may not involve sadness but irritability, boredom, or simply finding no enjoyment in life. Depressed children are likely to have relationship difficulties and problems at school. Each depressive episode lasts, on average, about 8 months, and about 20% are at risk of developing bipolar disorder, especially if they come from a family with a member suffering from bipolar disorder.

As identified above, there is growing evidence that bipolar depression is linked to disturbance of the body's biological rhythms (i.e. circadian rhythms), such as the sleep–wake cycle (e.g. insomnia), eating habits (e.g. anorexia), body temperature, and hormonal imbalance. The cycles from depression to manic states and back to depression again occur quicker in children than in adults. The changes in the circadian rhythms are in some way linked to these rapid mood swings, but the molecular mechanism remains unclear. Disturbances of the circadian rhythms are dominant among the symptoms of this disorder in children. However, in adolescence, manic states include not just euphoria and circadian disturbances, but also extreme optimism that defies normal judgement, excessive sexual desires, and outspokenness. These symptoms are contrary to the individual's normal state of behaviour when well.

It now appears that in children with bipolar disorder the disturbance to these biological rhythms may be due to as many as four mutations of the **RAR-related orphan receptor B** (**RORB**) gene at 9q22. The full function of the protein coded by this gene is unknown, but it possibly has some importance in the expression of other genes. It is involved in the regulation of the circadian cycles, which go wrong in depression. One example is sleep loss, which is a major symptom often seen early in childhood bipolar depression.

The long-term detrimental effects (i.e. the *'psychological scars'*) of a period of depression in childhood (to a greater extent) and in adolescence (to a lesser extent) are as follows:

- Impairment of social skills, in particular interpersonal skills: the childhood dependence on adults comes under considerable strain during depression, and the effects of this strain can be long-lasting.
- Developmental skills, especially the learning skills developed at school, are likely to suffer as a result of a depressive phase, with gaps in knowledge occurring that are difficult to make up at a later date.
- The development of the concept of 'self' is a feature of childhood (mostly) and adolescence. Depression at an early age may distort the perception of 'self' for years after.
- Extended periods of negative thinking may be reinforced by a depressive episode during childhood, causing low self-esteem, fatigue, poor social skills, difficulty with concentration and learning.

From about 13 years of age onward, depressive states become more common among girls rather than boys. The reasons are not entirely clear but may be partly due to hormonal changes that result in different ways boys and girls view the physical effects created by the hormones.

Social pressures to conform to certain stereotypes, often led by celebrities or advertising, have a greater impact on girls than on boys (Nolen-Hoeksema 2007).

Suicide is attempted in about 5 to 8% of adolescents, and it is a leading cause of death in this age group.

Postpartum depression

Depression can occur during pregnancy, with a peak of incidence between weeks 18 to 32 of gestation, but most cases of depression linked to pregnancy and childbirth happen soon after delivery of the baby. Suicide claims the lives of up to 20% of all postpartum deaths. A significant number of women have the comorbidities of anxiety with depression. Babies born to mothers who were depressed during the pregnancy are at higher risk of depression as adults.

Some women may show signs *before* the birth that suggest that a depressive illness could follow labour; such signs include lack of preparation for the baby, denying the pregnancy, or expressing future plans that clearly do not involve the baby. The range of severity is wide, from a mild form (often called 'baby blues') to an intense suicidal psychotic depression.

- **Postpartum blues** (baby blues): a mild depression that lasts 1 to 14 days after the birth, often peaking on the fifth day, in which the new mother feels low and cries easily. She may show hostility toward the baby or even the father. It affects between 20% and 75% of mothers; the figure varies between different studies.
- **Postpartum depression**: a more severe syndrome occurring at any time up to 6 months after the birth that lasts for most of the first year. These mothers show loss of emotion, anxiety, reduced appetite, sleep disturbance, and guilty feelings. Most of the women have no intentions of harming themselves or the baby. It affects between 10% and 15% of mothers.
- **Postpartum psychosis**: the most severe form, in which the mother loses contact with reality and shows signs of psychosis (hallucinations, delusions, and disorientation). The depression takes the form of unipolar or bipolar depression, with harmful tendencies towards the baby (who may be seen as the cause of the problem) or themselves. It affects about 0.2% of mothers.

The cause of these conditions is unclear, but a hormonal or immune imbalance, stress, or a genetic predisposition to mood disorders have all been suggested as contributing factors. **Oestrogen** and **progesterone** concentrations in the blood drop by about 90% within the first 48 hours after birth. Oestrogen has profound effects on the brain, notably affecting dopamine turnover, with similar effects on the serotonin and GABA systems. The *SERT* gene has been implicated in postpartum psychosis; the gene codes for the serotonin transporter that causes reuptake of serotonin at the synapse. In addition, other suspect genes are those that code for the serotonin receptors 5-HT2A and 5-HT2C. Protein deficiency has also been suggested as a potential cause, or a contributing factor to postpartum depression, given that the mother's protein intake over the period of gestation was required to accommodate for both the growing child and her own protein needs. This is easily corrected by providing an increase in the protein content of the mother's diet, and it may be a safe and valuable method of reducing the risk of postpartum depression in women who could be vulnerable.

During pregnancy, the uterine contents, notably the fotus, is *immunologically privileged* in the sense that the fotus is foreign, or alien tissue (i.e. it is potentially an **antigen**) that has to be tolerated by the mother's immune system. Very soon after birth, the mother's immune system changes significantly. There is an increase in those factors that promote inflammation, i.e. activation of **type 1 T-helper cells (Th1 cells)**, increased concentrations of **interferon gamma (INFγ)** and **tumour necrosing factor alpha (TNFα)**, and these factors are associated with postpartum depression. About one-third of all sufferers have a previous history of a psychiatric disorder and about one-quarter will have more than one episode.

Seasonal affective disorder

Seasonal affective disorder (SAD) is a depressive state that occurs during the winter months when shorter days are accompanied by less sun, i.e. when light levels are lower. Exposure to natural daylight is therefore at a minimum. Daylight is an important external cue for several biological rhythms that the brain goes through, each rhythm taking about a day (approximately 24 hours) to complete. As we have already seen, these rhythms are known as circadian rhythms and an example is the **sleep–wake cycle** (see Chapter 16). However, sunlight is also involved in mood regulation.

Serotonin is used by the **pineal gland** (located immediately behind the hypothalamus: Figure 11.8) to make a hormone called **melatonin**. **Pinealocytes** (cells of the pineal gland) concentrate serotonin, which is then converted first to *N*-acetylserotonin, then to melatonin. Melatonin can cross membranes better than serotonin and it binds to receptors to form complexes that interact with cellular activity. Melatonin receptors are of three types:

1   **MT1**, found in the **suprachiasmic nucleus (SCN)**, cerebellum, cerebral cortex, thalamus, and hippocampus and associated with the rod cells of the retina;
2   **MT2**, found in the retina, hippocampus, SCN, and cerebellum;
3   **MT3**, not yet found in humans.

The SCN is a pair of small cell clusters within the anterior ventral hypothalamus, just above the optic chiasma (where the optic nerves partially cross-over). The SCN controls behavioural, metabolic, and physiologic rhythms of the body. The pineal gland produces melatonin in response to light levels falling on the retina, i.e. part of the retinal output to the brain goes to the SCN in the hypothalamus (via the **retinohypothalamic tract**), and the SNC controls melatonin production by the pineal gland in response to these light levels. During the dark, the pineal gland produces melatonin from serotonin, and the melatonin concentration then rises. The concentration of melatonin feeds back from the pineal gland to the SNC, which then moderates production according to light levels on the retina. Melatonin may be the true trigger of sleep, as it is involved in the normal sleep–wake cycle (see Chapter 16). Melatonin concentrations are very low during the day. The winter months of long nights and lower daytime light levels can maintain a higher than expected melatonin concentration during the day, and this may trigger a persistent depressive mood throughout the winter. In addition, people suffering from SAD produce higher than expected levels of the **SERT** protein, which as we have seen normally moves serotonin back into the presynaptic bulb (reuptake), where it is stored and becomes inactive. They then lack serotonin in the synaptic cleft, a feature seen in unipolar and bipolar depression.

SAD can sometimes be treated with artificial light (called **phototherapy**) (Birtwistle and Martin 1999).

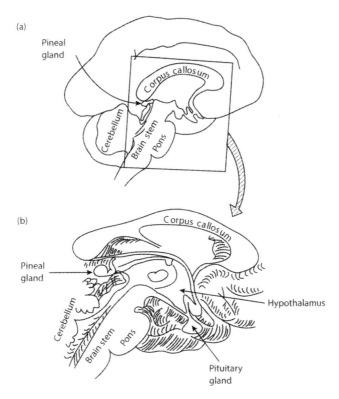

Figure 11.8 Location of the pineal gland. (a) Midline section through the brain, view from the right. (b) Close-up of the upper brain stem, hypothalamus, and corpus callosum, showing the pineal gland.

The antidepressant drugs

The main neurotransmitters involved in depression are the *monoamines* serotonin and noradrenaline (Blows 2000a, b). The **monoamine hypothesis** of depression came from two important observations made in the 1950s:

- Some patients treated for hypertension with a drug called **reserpine** were becoming depressed.
- Some patients were treated for tuberculosis with a drug that is no longer in use for this purpose, called **para-amino salicylic acid (PAS)**. Some of these patients were becoming happier.

Reserpine was later found to deplete the synapses of both their serotonin and noradrenaline, thus inducing a depressive state. PAS, however, was noted to block the enzyme that breaks down the neurotransmitter, thus allowing the neurotransmitter to increase in the synapse and therefore relieving depression. The enzyme concerned is monoamine oxidase, which is found in association with the mitochondria of the presynaptic bulb. After use in the synaptic cleft, many neurotransmitters are returned to the presynaptic bulb (*reuptake*; see Chapter 3) for

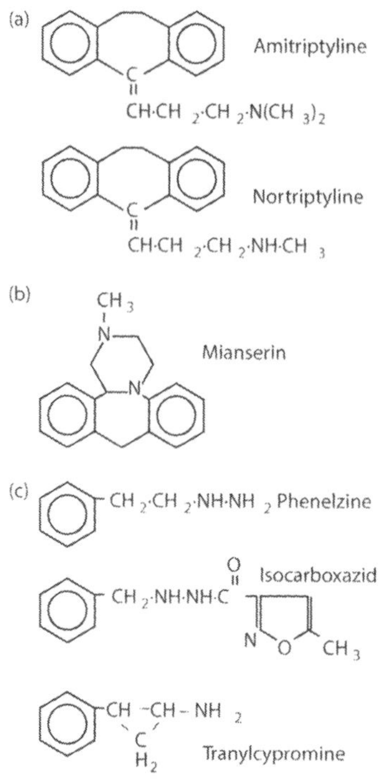

Figure 11.9 Structure of some important antidepressants: (a) tricyclic drugs; (b) tricyclic-related (tetracyclic) drug; (c) monoamine oxidase inhibitor (MAOI) drugs.

conversion to a metabolite before removal from the brain. This creates two possible mechanisms for increasing the amounts of neurotransmitter in the synaptic cleft:

* Blocking the reuptake so that the chemical stays in the cleft. This is the principal mode of action of the **tricyclic antidepressants** and *some* **atypical antidepressants**.
* Blocking the breakdown by inhibiting the enzyme so that the chemical builds up in the synapse. This is the principal mode of action of the **monoamine oxidase inhibitors (MAOIs)**.

Tricyclic antidepressants

These drugs are named after the three-ringed (*tri-cyclic*) nature of their chemistry, known as the **dibenzazepine** structure (Figure 11.9a). They work by blocking the reuptake of the neurotransmitters serotonin and noradrenaline into the presynaptic bulb, with the result that these transmitters accumulate in the synaptic cleft. Two of the drugs in early use were **imipramine** (the first antidepressant, which came into clinical practice in the late 1950s), which is more selective in blocking noradrenaline, and **amitriptyline** (Figure 11.9a), which has approximately equal activity in blocking both neurotransmitters. Other tricyclic antidepressant drugs are **doxepin, clomipramine, dosulepin, lofepramine, nortriptyline**, and **trimipramine**.

This drug group had the problem that symptoms of depression were not relieved until up to 6 weeks into treatment (known as a **therapeutic delay** or **latency period**). This was difficult to understand; after all, the very first dose of the drug given was active in raising the neurotransmitter concentrations at the synapse, so why was mood taking so long to return to normal? It is now thought that the delay is due to the time it takes to downregulate receptors or to improve receptor sensitivity. This therapeutic delay can increase the risk of suicide because during this time the patient acquires more energy and severely depressed patients with more energy are a greater suicide risk. There had to be another way round this delay. One step forward was the development of drugs that were more selective for blocking the reuptake of either serotonin (the **selective serotonin reuptake inhibitors**, or **SSRIs**) or noradrenaline (Table 11.4). These drugs are said to have a shorter therapeutic delay than the tricyclic drugs.

The side effects of the tricyclic antidepressants are drowsiness, dry mouth, blurred vision, urinary retention, and constipation, all of which are **antimuscarinic** effects. Muscarinic receptors (see Chapter 4) normally bind the neurotransmitter acetylcholine. As muscarinic antagonists, the tricyclic antidepressants prevent acetylcholine from binding to muscarinic receptors, and in this way cause the side effects. Some of these side effects may become less troublesome as tolerance develops. Other side effects include weight gain, **hyponatremia** (low blood sodium levels) in the elderly, and occasionally **cardiac arrhythmias** (abnormal rhythms of heart activity) such as **heart block** (failure of electrical conduction through the heart) and changes on the **electrocardiogram** (**ECG**). These cardiovascular changes are a potential problem in overdose. Central nervous system side effects include anxiety, dizziness, drowsiness, agitation, confusion (aggravated by hyponatremia), and sleep disturbance, and these may occur more often in the elderly. Serious side effects, such as hallucinations, convulsions, and **extrapyramidal side effects** (**EPS**; see Chapter 10) are rare, occurring in about 5% of patients on these drugs.

The most likely tricyclic drug interactions are with the MAOI drug group. The switching of treatment from tricyclic to MAOI, or from MAOI to tricyclic medication, should only be done after a time gap of 2 weeks or more.

Tricyclic-related (tetracyclic) antidepressants

Mianserin and **trazodone** are tetracyclic drugs, i.e. they are not based on a three-ring structure (tricyclic) but a four-ring structure. They work in a similar manner to the tricyclic drugs, i.e. they block the reuptake of neurotransmitters into the presynaptic bulb at the synapse. They also have similar side effects. Mianserin can cause blood **dyscrasia**, a serious reduction in the blood cell count, and patients require a full blood count every 4 weeks for the first 3 months of treatment. Trazodone is useful for treating anxiety as well as depression, and is therefore suitable for treating depressed patients who show additional symptoms of anxiety.

Selective serotonin reuptake inhibitors (SSRIs)

SSRIs selectively inhibit the reuptake of serotonin, therefore increasing the serotonin concentrations in the cleft. They do this by binding to **SERT**, which normally locks onto serotonin and moves it back into the presynaptic bulb. SSRIs prevent this protein from moving the serotonin, which then accumulates in the synaptic cleft. **Fluoxetine** was one of the first SSRIs to be introduced into clinical practice in the late 1980s. It is perhaps still the best known and most often prescribed antidepressant. Other SSRI drugs include **citalopram**,

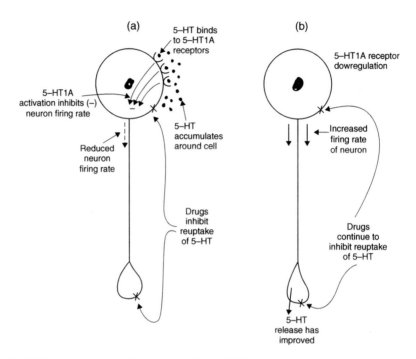

Figure 11.10 The short-term and long-term effects of SSRI drugs on the serotonin neurons. (a) In the short-term, the blockage of reuptake at the synapse and cell body causes serotonin to accumulate around the neuron. This raised serotonin concentration actively stimulates the 5-HT1A autoreceptor on the cell body, which in turn decreases neuronal firing. (b) In the longer term, this causes the cell to downregulate the 5-HT1A autoreceptor so the neuron can restore the impulse firing rate. This increases serotonin release at the synapse; reuptake is prevented, and therefore serotonin accumulates.

escitalopram, paroxetine, sertraline, and **fluvoxamine**. These drugs are thought to have a short-term and a long-term effect in raising serotonin levels in the cleft, both of which are explained in Figure 11.10.

SSRIs apparently do not work well for mild depression, and are therefore used more effectively in severe depression. There appears now to be other mechanisms through which these drugs lift depression, and these mechanisms work on a longer time scale. Fluoxetine has been found to increase neurogenesis in the brain. The drug causes a 50% increase in the activation of **progenitor** cells, i.e. those cells from which new neurons are produced. Antidepressants may partly prevent atrophy of the hippocampus by improving synaptic plasticity and stimulating neurogenesis.

SSRIs are said to have fewer side effects and are safer than tricyclic drugs if taken as an overdose because they have fewer cardiac effects. They are less sedating and have fewer antimuscarinic and cardiovascular effects than the tricyclics, but they do sometimes cause varying degrees of nausea and vomiting, constipation, rashes, dizziness, fatigue, and headache. Some of these unwanted effects become less troublesome as patients begin to tolerate the drug.

Table 11.4 Selective serotonin and noradrenaline inhibitors

Serotonin-selective reuptake inhibitors	Noradrenaline-selective inhibitors
Fluoxetine, Sertraline, Paroxetine, Citalopram, Fluvoxamine Escitalopram	Nortryptiline Reboxetine

Table 11.5 Some atypical antidepressants

Antidepressant	Notes
Mirtazapine	Blocks presynaptic α_2-adrenoceptors, which causes an increase in noradrenaline release
Agomelatine	A melatonin receptor agonist and selective serotonin receptor antagonist
Flupentixol	An antipsychotic that can be used as an antidepressant in low dose

Serotonin and noradrenaline reuptake inhibitors (SNRIs)

Venlafaxine and **Duloxetine** are SNRI drugs that, in a similar way to the tricyclic drugs, block the reuptake of both serotonin and noradrenaline – but as with the SSRIs they have much fewer side effects and shorter therapeutic delay than the tricyclic drugs. Venlafaxine has variable effects at different dosages. At low dose it inhibits the reuptake of serotonin, at intermediate dose the inhibition of reuptake of noradrenaline becomes important, and at higher dose it inhibits the reuptake of serotonin, noradrenaline, and dopamine.

Selective noradrenaline reuptake inhibitors (NRIs)

Reboxetine inhibits the reuptake of noradrenaline only, and the resulting increase in noradrenaline is thought to enhance the neurotransmission of the serotonergic pathways. Reboxetine has fewer side effects than the tricyclic drugs, including fewer cardiac effects.

Other antidepressants

These drugs (**mirtazapine, agomelatine**, and **flupentixol**) are newer than the other groups and have different means of antidepressant activity (Table 11.5, Figure 11.9b). The fact that some relieve depression without interfering with the reuptake of neurotransmitter adds weight to the notion that blocking reuptake may not be the primary mechanism for relieving depression. These drugs modify the function of serotonin or noradrenaline receptor sites (Table 11.5). Drugs of this group appear to relieve symptoms faster than the tricyclic drugs and are known to be active in the limbic areas of the brain. Because some do not block transmitter reuptake, they tend to cause fewer side effects than the tricyclic group.

Monoamine oxidase inhibitors

MAOI drugs, as we have seen, block the action of the MAO enzyme, which breaks down the monoamine neurotransmitters after reuptake (see Chapter 4). MAO is located on the outer membrane of mitochondria in the presynaptic bulb, particularly in the dopaminergic, adrenergic, and serotonergic pathways. When the enzyme is blocked with the inhibitor drug, the neurotransmitter cannot be reduced to its metabolites for excretion and remains in the synapse. The transmitter levels then rise in the bulb and cleft. This action is more pronounced in noradrenergic and serotonergic synapses than in dopaminergic synapses.

Two forms of MAO exist – **MAO-A** and **MAO-B** – but the human brain has mostly MAO-B. Both forms of the enzyme degrade all three neurotransmitters (dopamine, noradrenaline, and serotonin) when these transmitters are in high concentration, but when they are in lower concentration the enzymes become more specific. Both forms of the enzyme also exist in many tissues outside the brain, in particular the gut wall and the liver. The purpose of having the enzyme in these digestion-related sites is to facilitate the degradation of monoamines found in the diet, mostly **tyromine**. If tyromine enters the blood unmodified by MAO, it can cause a **hypertensive crisis**. A throbbing headache is an early sign of this potentially dangerous condition, but other symptoms include neck stiffness, palpitations, chest pain, sweating, and cold, clammy skin. This is what happened to some patients given MAOI drugs for depression before it was realised that dietary monoamines were the cause of their crisis. To allow continuation of the treatment with the MAOI drugs it became necessary to remove monoamines from the diet. Patients were then issued with a list of foods to avoid, particularly those that contain the monoamine tyromine: foods such as cheese, broad bean pods, pickled herring, salami, pepperoni, overripe bananas, sauerkraut, tofu and soya sauce, red wine, and yeast or meat extracts, to name a few. On the surface, it does seem paradoxical to issue potentially suicidal patients with tablets and a list of foods that may, in combination with the drugs, kill them! In reality, of course, it was more selective and controlled than this picture would suggest, with potentially suicidal patients admitted for observation. However, occasional fatalities did occur, and it became apparent that this was not the ideal way to cope with the problem.

All the original MAOI drugs worked by the *irreversible* blocking of the enzyme MAO, which meant that the enzyme had to be degraded, removed, and replaced by a new enzyme. The problem of potentially dangerous hypertensive crisis led to the development of the newer *reversible* **MAOI (RIMA)** drugs. These work by locking onto and inhibiting the enzyme when the monoamine concentrations are low, thus allowing the concentrations to accumulate and rise (as in the brain in depression). Should there be a sudden rise in mono-amines – in the digestive tract and the liver following the eating of a cheese sandwich, for example – the drug unlocks from the enzyme, which then becomes free to act on the monoamines in the diet. Meanwhile, the same drug remains active in the brain, where the monoamine concentrations are low, thus exerting its antidepressant qualities. The action of the drug is therefore dependent on the amine levels in the area where it is found. As a result, the presence of monoamines in the diet has become a less important issue, although patients should still avoid consuming large amounts of these foods. The only RIMA drug currently available in clinical practice in the UK is listed in Table 11.6, but others are available outside the UK.

MAOI drugs can cause side effects such as **postural hypotension** (low blood pressure on standing up from a sitting or lying position, a particular problem for elderly patients on these drugs) and dizziness. Other noted side effects include dry mouth, drowsiness, insomnia, headache, fatigue, gastrointestinal disturbances, difficulty with **micturition** (passing urine), and many more, some potentially serious. For all these reasons, MAOI drugs are usually a second-line choice of treatment, used when the SSRI or atypical drugs have failed.

Table 11.6 MAOI antidepressants

Irreversible MAOI drugs	Reversible MAOI drug (RIMA)
Phenelzine	Moclobemide (MAO-A specific)
Isocarboxazid	
Tranylcypromine	

The relief of depression is not entirely dependent on the increase in neurotransmitter concentrations in the brain, so how else do antidepressants work? All the antidepressant drugs appear to relieve depression through a number of possible mechanisms, including:

- readjustment of the sensitivity of the receptors for serotonin and noradrenaline;
- modification of the transport of these neurotransmitters across the presynaptic membrane;
- correction of abnormal activity levels in area 25 and the frontal cortex;
- blocking the NMDA receptors, which prevents cell loss in the front lobe and hippocampus.

It seems likely that depression is the combination of defective neurotransmitter transporter, poor receptor activity, and low neurotransmitter concentrations at the synapse and other errors involving GABA and glutamate receptors. The antidepressants correct these defects, and in so doing readjust the HPA axis to normal. They may also go some way in correcting the immune system abnormalities.

Pharmacokinetics and pharmacotherapeutics of the antidepressants

All these drugs are well absorbed from the gut, so oral administration is not normally a problem. The tricyclic drugs have variable first pass metabolism, and this means the dose does not always correlate with the therapeutic response. They are highly protein bound in circulation and tend to have long half-lives. The SSRI drugs half-lives run into several days, and they have good bioavailability following first pass metabolism. The SNRI venlafaxine has limited first pass metabolism, resulting in a high bioavailability (more than 90%). The half-life of 5 hours for this drug is extended by the fact that the major metabolite is the primary active agent, with a half-life of 11 hours. Reboxetine (the NRI drug) has 100% bioavailability, i.e. no first pass metabolism, and a 15-hour half-life. MAOI drugs tend to have short half-lives (typically 1 to 3 hours) and so may need to be given more frequently.

Because antidepressants are not addictive in the classical sense of the word, withdrawal of antidepressants should not be a problem provided it is done slowly. Sudden withdrawal after long-term use may induce unwanted effects, such as stomach upset, flu-like symptoms, sweating, insomnia, anxiety, dizziness, tremor, confusion, vivid nightmares, sexual dysfunction, and sensations similar to small electric shocks (described as 'brain zaps', 'brains shocks', or 'head shocks'). These unwanted effects are often referred to as '**SSRI discontinuation syndrome**' (sometimes called '**SSRI withdrawal syndrome**' or '**SSRI cessation syndrome**').

There is no clinical justification for administering two different antidepressants for the same patient at the same time. This is likely to cause dangerous drug interactions. The MAOI drugs must never be administered *immediately* before or after the tricyclic drugs. At least a 2-week gap should be allowed before commencing one of these groups after stopping the other. The potential for causing a hazardous interaction between these drug groups is very high. RIMA drugs are particularly dangerous if prescribed with other antidepressants owing to the prospect of hazardous drug interactions.

Serotonin syndrome

Serotonin syndrome (sometimes called 'serotonin toxicity', 'serotonin storm', or 'hypersero-tonemia') is a potentially life-threatening adverse drug reaction in which excessive serotonin is produced in the brain and leaks into the blood. The result is overactivity of serotonergic receptors in both the brain and the body. The cause may be very high antidepressant dosage, or sometimes even normal dosage of one antidepressant drug, or a reaction between two anti-depressant drugs (which should never happen; see above), or the use of some illicit drugs. The symptoms occur rapidly, and they include confusion, mania, agitation, hallucinations, headache, shivering, sweating, low blood pressure, nausea, muscle twitching and tremor, raised body temperature, fast pulse rate, diarrhoea, and dilated pupils. These symptoms can range from quite mild to very severe – even fatal. Discontinuation of any antidepressant drugs must be the first line of treatment, followed in severe cases with the administration of a serotonin antagonist. Benzodiazepine sedation may also be useful.

Antidepressants versus placebo and alternative therapies

There is a debate concerning how effective antidepressants are when compared with placebo. Current studies suggest that placebos are about 75% as effective in relieving depression as antidepressants, with about 50–60% of patients improving on antidepressants compared to 25–30% of patients improving on placebos. Some argue that because placebos cause no side effects at all, they are the better option. However, many patients will get better anyway with no treatment at all after an average period of 8 months of illness, providing they do not com-mit suicide. Another small percentage of patients do not respond at all to antidepressants. As it stands, the evidence points to the fact that antidepressants have a very important role in treating depression and should be used. How much they benefit the patient is variable, from no benefit at all to full restoration of normal health, and every patient should be given that chance to restore their health.

The use of alternative therapies, e.g. psychotherapy, has been compared with antidepressant use, and the general consensus is that although alternative therapies are effective, antidepres-sants work faster. Some people would say that the combination of drugs with alternative therapies is the best approach.

Withdrawal from antidepressants

Although antidepressants do not actually cause addiction, about one-third of all patients who stop taking them have withdrawal symptoms. These include dizziness, flu-like symptoms, anxiety, stomach upsets and bizarre dreams. They are usually mild but can be severe in a small number of people. Gradual withdrawal by slowly lowering the dose over a period of weeks or months is the best way to prevent this problem. Antidepressants should, in any case, be continued for a minimum of 6 months after the patient feels better to prevent relapse back to depression.

Use of antidepressants in other disorders

Antidepressants are gaining acceptance for use in a wider range of disorders even though they are not all licensed for that disorder. These include **obsessive compulsive disorder**

(**OCD**; see Chapter 15), **panic attacks**, **bulimia nervosa**, and **post-traumatic stress disorder** (all in Chapter 9), impulsive behaviour, **premenstrual tension**, and even chronic pain.

Ketamine and related drugs that may be used in depression

Ketamine (see Chapter 9) is an anaesthetic often used by teenagers as a recreational drug, but now it is gaining ground as a potential treatment for depression. It works very fast, relieving depression within 2–24 hours, unlike the usual antidepressant drugs, which take days or weeks to improve symptoms. It is thought to work by blocking the NMDA glutamate receptor, although how this relieves depression is not fully understood. Katamine has also been shown to quickly activate the **mammalian target of rapamycin (mTOR)** cell signalling pathway. This acts as a regulator of cell growth, proliferation, and metabolism. Activation of this pathway by ketamine results in increased numbers of synapses, i.e. synaptogenesis (see Chapter 2), and improved function of synapses. There are some problems that prevent its current widespread use in depression therapy. The side effects may be troublesome at therapeutic dosages, e.g. **out of body experiences (dissociative effect)** that last about an hour. At higher dosage it can also cause a psychotic state, the so-called '**K-hole**' effect, where those taking the drug experience a severe disorientation with acute, vivid hallucinations. Also, the problems of long-term use are not known. Ketamine, and variants like ketamine, are effective in lifting depression in those persons who do not respond to conventional antidepressants.

New variations of ketamine are under development in an attempt to reduce these side effects. A ketamine-like drug called **GLYX-13** shows promise in lifting depression without the ketamine side effects. It is also an antagonist of the glutaminergic NMDA receptor and relieves depression within 24 hours, the effects lasting about a week. Another drug called **decoglurant** is still in clinical trials.

Mood-stabilising drugs

The drugs described in this section are those used to prevent the swings in mood associated with bipolar depression, in which long periods of deep depression are interrupted by occasional bouts of mania. **Lithium carbonate** is very effective in this role by controlling the manic state when used in a prophylactic manner, i.e. over a long time period. It has no role to play in the management of unipolar depression or in restoring to normal an acute manic state.

Lithium is given orally and is rapidly absorbed from the gut, peak levels being reached in the blood within 24 hours of commencement. The drug shows several biochemical effects occurring together, and, until recently, which of these resulted in the desired effect was difficult to determine.

Lithium is a **cation** (a positively charged particle) and can act as a substitute for other cations such as sodium (Na^+), potassium (K^+), magnesium (Mg^{2+}), or calcium (Ca^{2+}). Lithium can penetrate the neuronal cell body membrane and accumulate within the cytoplasm. This increases the intracellular cation population, repelling some K^+, which is forced out of the cell. This results in a partial *depolarisation* of that neuron, and in turn slows the *repolarisation* phase, thus reducing the excitation of the neuron (see Chapter 3). However, the main action of lithium in prevention of mania appears to be its role in inhibiting the PKC enzyme, which becomes excessively active and does not shut down normally in mania. Lithium indirectly inhibits this enzyme, thus preventing the PKC cause of mania (look back at Figure 11.1).

Lithium has several other effects (Figure 11.11):

- It inhibits **ATPase** (the enzyme that produces **ATP**, the cell's high-energy molecule), causing a reduction in the concentration of ATP in the cell.
- It inhibits **glycogen synthase kinase-3 (GSK-3)**, and as such it helps to regulate the functions of the GSK-3 pathway, notably synaptic plasticity and cell survival (Figure 11.1). This is important in reversing the atrophy seen in the frontal lobe and hippocampus. GSK-3 also influences the circadian rhythms of the body, and lithium therefore has an important role in regulating these rhythms.
- In the long-term it causes an increase in **N-acetylaspartate (NAA)**, a derivative of aspartate and an important neuronal marker, and as such suggests both improved neuronal viability and an increase in the total amount of grey matter in the brain, and helps to reverse frontal lobe atrophy.
- Long-term lithium also increases activity in the **mitogen-activated protein (MAP)** kinase pathway, which is involved in a wide range of cellular functions through gene transcription.
- It has an inhibitory effect on **cAMP** and **inositol**.
- It slows down the uptake of choline into the neurons that synthesise acetylcholine, and this neurotransmitter is therefore reduced.
- It causes reduced release of serotonin and reduced serotonin receptor density in the hippocampus.
- It prevents dopamine receptors in the corpus striatum from becoming supersensitive to dopamine, a possibility that can occur after long-term use of the **neuroleptic** drugs. This particular action of lithium is probably quite an important mechanism leading to the desired anti-manic effect.
- It has significant antiviral effects, especially against the **herpes virus**.
- It has modulatory effects on cell-mediated and humoral immunity. This suggests a possible role for viral infections in depression.

Toxic concentrations of lithium are achieved rapidly if the dose is not carefully controlled. Blood concentrations of the drug are monitored. The toxic effects of lithium, which may be worsened by a low blood sodium concentration, include tremor, **ataxia** (unsteady walking), nausea, dizziness, convulsions, and coma. Lithium can also cause a wide range of other side effects, such as endocrine disturbance – notably **thyroid disorders**, by inhibiting iodine uptake into the thyroid gland and reducing thyroid hormone production. Alterations of the thyroid receptor concentration in the hypothalamus as a result of lithium treatment may have some bearing on its mood-stabilising role given the importance of the thyroid for brain activity. Lithium can also cause **polyurea** (a large urine output) with **polydipsia** (excessive thirst), weight gain, oedema, and gastrointestinal disturbances. Changes in the electrical rhythm of the heart may be noticed on the **electrocardiogram (ECG)**. Clearly, the decision to use lithium is not taken lightly, and usually involves specialist advice.

Carbamazepine is also available for the prophylaxis of mania, especially in those patients who are unresponsive to lithium. It is particularly useful in patients who have a rapid cycle of manic and depressive episodes (i.e. four or more such episodes per year). This drug is a sodium channel blocker and as such it is important antiepileptic, as discussed in Chapter 12. Like lithium, **valproate**, another antiepileptic drug, inhibits **GSK-3** but by a different (and as

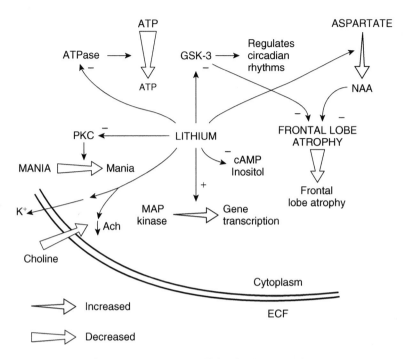

Figure 11.11 The action of lithium. ECF = extracellular fluid; see text for other abbreviations.

yet uncertain) mechanism to lithium. **Tamoxifen** (an anti-oestrogen) is also known to inhibit **PKC** and at sufficient dosage may reduce mania. Work is proceeding to determine the possible clinical use of tamoxifen as an anti-manic drug.

Key points

Depressive illness

- Depressive illness occurs when the depressed state has no apparent cause or when the period of depression is prolonged beyond what is considered normal.
- Two main types of illnesses occur: unipolar depression (depression only) and bipolar depression (symptoms of depression with periods of mania).

Risk

- For the population as a whole, the risk of developing unipolar depression is 6%, and for bipolar depression the risk is 1%.
- First-degree relatives of a bipolar depressed patient have a concordance rate of 19%, while for unipolar depression the concordance rate is 10%.
- The concordance rate for bipolar depression in monozygotic twins is about 65%; in dizygotic twins the concordance rate is about 14%. This indicates that bipolar depression is a genetically based disease.

Cause

- A number of important genes are implicated in the causation of major affective disorder.

Brain pathology

- There are some limited physical changes in the brains of depressed patients; some have ventricular enlargement and a reduction in the size of the temporal lobe and hippocampus.
- Brodmann area 25, the subgenual cingulate, appears to be hyperactive in depression, and deep brain stimulation can treat depression by reducing this activity.
- Oligodendrocyte numbers are lower in bipolar disorder, causing demyelination.
- The lateral habenula is the brain's disappointment area, and in depression it appears to be undersecreting GABA, thus remaining active all the time.

Biochemistry and immunity

- Serotonin and noradrenaline are reduced in depression, and a low turnover of these transmitters occurs at the synapse of the diffuse modulatory systems.
- Very low levels of serotonin have been linked to increased violent behaviour, such as suicide.
- The serotonin subtype-2 receptor (5-HT2) is thought to be the most important receptor involved in mood regulation.
- A prolonged hyperactivity of the hypothalomo–pituitary–adrenal (HPA) axis occurs, causing chronic corticotropin-releasing factor (CRF) and cortisol release.
- Raised cortisol can cause raised glutamate and increased NMDA receptors in the hippocampus in depression, leading to atrophy of the hippocampus.
- There are significant immune system changes in depression.

Postpartum depression

- Postpartum depression, in which women become depressed after birth, is an umbrella term for three conditions: postpartum blues (a mild depression), postpartum depression (a more severe syndrome), and postpartum psychosis (the most severe form).

SAD

- Seasonal affective disorder (SAD) is a depressive state occurring during the winter months when there are shorter days and low light levels.
- It can be treated with phototherapy.

Tricyclic antidepressants

- Tricyclic antidepressants work by blocking the reuptake of serotonin and noradrenaline into the presynaptic bulb, so these transmitters accumulate in the synaptic cleft.
- Some tricyclic antidepressants are more selective for noradrenaline.

SSRI antidepressants

- Selective serotonin reuptake inhibitor (SSRI) drugs are more selective for blocking the reuptake of serotonin.
- These antidepressants reduce the side effects seen in other drugs and shorten the therapeutic delay.

MAOI antidepressants

- Monoamine oxidase inhibitors (MAOI) block the enzyme monoamine oxidase, which normally breaks down neurotransmitters.
- Antidepressant drugs relieve depression mainly by increasing neurotransmitter concentrations, by readjusting the sensitivity of the receptors for serotonin and noradrenaline and by modifying the transport of these neurotransmitters across the presynaptic membrane.
- MAOI drugs require restriction of oral intake of the monoamine tyromine to prevent hypertensive crisis.
- Different antidepressant drugs should not be prescribed without at least a 2-week gap between them to prevent drug interactions.

Lithium

- Lithium is a prophylactic mood-stabilising drug used to control the manic phases of bipolar depression on a long-term basis.
- Lithium works mainly by inhibiting both the PKC enzyme system and the GSK 3β pathway within the neuron, and this prevents cell death and atrophy.
- Lithium can reach toxic concentrations quickly and must be carefully monitored.

References

Birtwistle, J. and Martin, N. (1999) Seasonal affective disorder: its recognition and treatment. *British Journal of Nursing*, **8** (15): 1004–1009.

Blows, W. T. (2000a) Neurotransmitters of the brain: serotonin, noradrenaline (norepinephrine), and dopamine. *Journal of Neuroscience Nursing*, **32** (4): 234–238.

Blows, W. T. (2000b) The neurobiology of antidepressants. *Journal of Neuroscience Nursing*, **32** (3): 177–180.

Brown, P. (2001) A mind under siege. *New Scientist*, **170** (2295; 16 June): 34–37.

Carlson, N. R. (2012) *Physiology of Behaviour* (11th edition). Pearson Education, Harlow, UK.

Dobbs, D. (2006) Turning off depression. *Scientific American Mind*, **17** (4): 26–31.

Hestad, K., Aukrust, P., Tønseth, S., and Reitan, S. (2009) Depression has a strong relationship to alterations in the immune, endocrine and neural system. *Current Psychiatry Reviews*, **5**: 287–297.

Nolen-Hoeksema, S. (2007) *Abnormal Psychology*. McGraw-Hill, Boston, MA.

Westly, E. (2010) Different shades of blue. *Scientific American Mind*, **21** (2): 30–37.

12 Epilepsy

- Seizures: types and causes
- The electroencephalogram in epilepsy
- Factors involved in the cause of epilepsy
- The epileptogenic focus
- Tonic–clonic (grand mal) seizures
- The hippocampal involvement in seizures
- Temporal lobe seizures (psychomotor epilepsy)
- Jacksonian seizures
- Infantile spasms and febrile convulsions
- Childhood epilepsies
- The anticonvulsant drugs
- Key points

Seizures: types and causes

Epilepsy is a term used to cover a very wide range of complex disorders, all character-ised by the presence of seizures and sometimes convulsions. **Seizures**, or **fits**, are brief periods of high-frequency, high-voltage electrical discharges from the brain. They are associated with an **altered state of consciousness** and accompanied by changes in sen-sory and motor function, causing momentarily abnormal behavioural patterns. The altered state of consciousness may mean a short period of either total or partial loss of conscious-ness, or simply a state of unawareness. **Convulsions** are powerful, often violent, rhythmic muscular contractions of the trunk and limbs occurring during a seizure. The word *ictal* is used to indicate a fit, with *interictal* meaning the period between two successive fits. Seizures occur in a variety of major or minor types, and are basically the result of **cerebral irritation**, meaning anything that directly disturbs the function of neurons in the brain. The majority of these *one-off* fits are caused by temporary, self-correcting, or curable problems.

    Idiopathic, or **primary**, epilepsy (indicated as **1°**) is of unknown cause; that is, the existing pathology cannot be explained, and may be due to a developmental malformation of the brain structure. **Symptomatic**, or **secondary**, epilepsy (indicated as **2°**) is caused by distinct and explainable brain pathology, either in structure or function. There are also various syndromes involving fits and special forms of epilepsy.

Between 1% and 2% of the world's population suffer from epilepsy. It is estimated that the total number of people in the UK who have ever had a fit is about 5% (including febrile convulsions). The occurrence of one fit does not mean the sufferer has epilepsy, and of this 5% only about 0.5% will go on to develop true epilepsy after their first fit.

A standard classification of seizures is as follows:

A   **Generalised seizures**

    1   Absences
    2   Generalised tonic–clonic
    3   Myoclonic
    4   Atonic

B   **Partial** (or **focal**) **seizures**

    1   Simple
    2   Complex

Generalised seizures

Generalised seizures are characterised by changes in consciousness due to spread of an electrical discharge to many areas of the brain, and they are often associated with convulsions. They account for about 30% of all epilepsies. *Generalised epilepsies* can be classified into four types: **absences**, **generalised tonic–clonic**, **myoclonic**, and **atonic**. Of these four types, the first two are the most common.

Absence (formally the **petit mal** or **minor fit**) describes a transient loss of awareness during which the person will stop what they are doing, stare vacantly into space for about 30 seconds or so, perhaps fumble with objects around them, then return to normal. There is no perceptive or cognitive function for the duration of the fit and afterwards there is no memory of the event. The person does not fall to the ground because normal **muscle tone** is maintained. Occasionally **automatism** (mechanical-like automatic movement) is seen, particularly if the duration of the fit is longer than 30 seconds. Petit mal usually starts at around the age of 5–7 years and stops at puberty, but can go on into adulthood. **Atypical absences** show a similar clinical picture, but the person may also show muscle twitching or some other abnormal movement.

Generalised tonic–clonic fits (the **grand mal** or **major fit**), are those in which the person loses consciousness, falls to the ground, and convulses. They are discussed in Tonic–clonic (grand mal) seizures on page 273. This form of epilepsy is the type most people think of as a fit in the full sense of the word. Such fits occur in three ways: as **primary generalised epilepsy**, where there is no other neurological abnormality; as a **partial seizure**, which becomes generalised; and as a symptom associated with **diffuse brain dysfunction**.

Myoclonic fits (*myo* = 'muscle', *clonus* = 'rapid alternating contractions and relaxations of skeletal muscle') are those in which muscle jerks occur in the arms or legs for a short period of about 1–5 seconds.

Atonic (*a* = 'without', *tonic* = 'tone') are also called **drop attacks**. They are fits in which there is a sudden loss of muscle tone, resulting in collapse of the person. They last only a few seconds.

Partial (or focal) seizures

Focal seizures are centred in one particular part of the brain with some spread of the impulses, but spread is more limited than in generalised seizures. These are the most common types of seizure. The neurons involved fire rapid bursts of action potentials, which are then synchronised in other neuron groups as the wave of impulses spreads.

Consciousness is often preserved (**simple partial**), but sometimes lost (**complex partial**) depending on the cause of the seizure, the location of the initial site, and the spread of the electrical impulse. Behavioural changes are often a feature. The areas of the brain usually involved are:

- **Frontal lobe:** seizures originating here cause predominantly motor symptoms, especially of the legs and the head. These seizures last for just a few seconds and occur several times a day.
- **Parietal lobe:** seizures originating here can cause sensory and motor symptoms, as in **Jacksonian epilepsy**.
- **Temporal lobe:** seizures originating here cause personality symptoms, as typified in **temporal lobe epilepsy**.
- **Occipital lobe:** seizures originating here cause disturbance of the visual cortex, resulting in the patient seeing visual phenomena such as flashing lights or sparks.

A proportion of partial seizures are localised to start with but then evolve into full generalised seizures.

There is some evidence to suggest that at least one form of partial seizure, called **Rasmussen's encephalitis (RE)**, may be **autoimmune** in origin (Acharya 2002). *Autoimmune* means that the immune system reacts to a normal part of the body as though it was a harmful agent introduced from the environment. Research in this area is currently limited, but changes in the body's immune response are part of the pathology of this disease.

The electroencephalogram in epilepsy

The electroencephalogram (EEG) is a very useful tool in the investigation of epileptic syndromes but cannot be used alone to diagnose epilepsy. It does have a value in helping to distinguish between the different categories of epilepsy. Basically, the EEG is a recording of the overall pattern of electrical signals generated by millions of active neurons across the brain surface. A characteristic epileptic feature on the EEG is the *spike*, a pointed feature in the wave pattern not seen on the normal tracing, as shown in Figure 12.1. During seizures the wave patterns and spikes show increased frequencies and abnormal irregularities as the seizure spreads. The following patterns are usually seen.

- Absences show a 3 Hz (three-per-second) 'spike and wave' activity (Figure 12.2). This wave pattern appears to generate from a **thalamocortical loop** (i.e. neurological loop connections between the thalamus and the cortex). Rhythmic oscillations of this loop are seen in sleep (i.e. sleep spindles; see Chapter 16), and they also appear to be responsible for the full manifestation of absences.
- Simple partial seizures show localised slow but sharp wave activity (Figure 12.3).
- Complex partial seizures show a medium-voltage spike activity centred on one brain area, increasing in intensity as it spreads (Figure 12.4).
- Generalised tonic–clonic seizures show rhythmic high-voltage activity leading to the clinical appearance of convulsions, with bilateral multispiked wave patterns during convulsions (Figure 12.5).

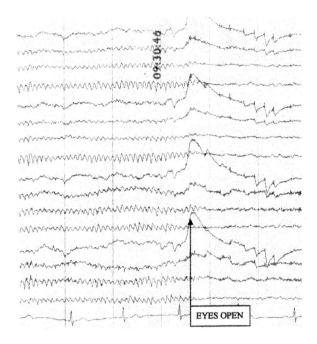

Figure 12.1 The normal electroencephalogram (EEG) tracing. There is no 'spike' feature often seen in epilepsy.

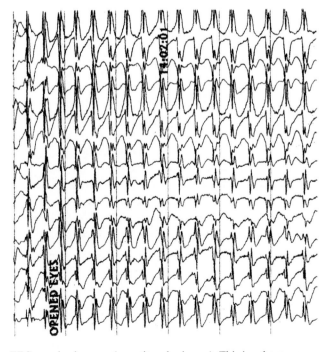

Figure 12.2 The EEG seen in absences (or petit mal seizures). This is a three-per-second wave pattern.

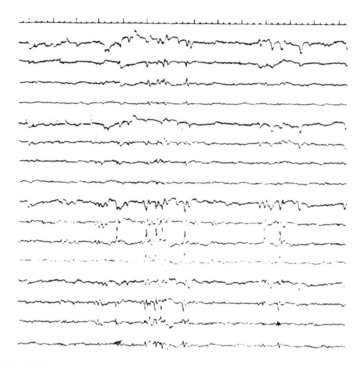

Figure 12.3 The EEG seen in simple partial seizures.

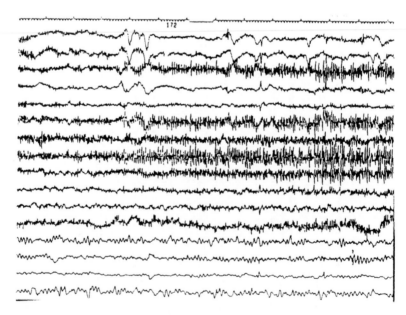

Figure 12.4 The EEG seen in complex partial seizures.

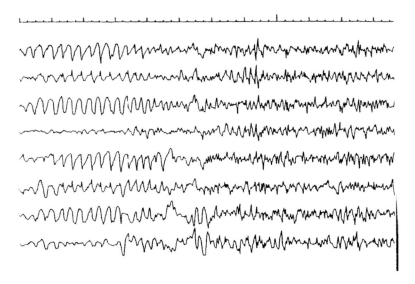

Figure 12.5 The EEG seen in general tonic–clonic (or grand mal) seizures.

Table 12.1 The known causes of seizures

Cause of seizures	Notes
Congenital defects	Caused by disruption to neuronal function
Genetics	Causing a genetic syndrome of which epilepsy is one symptom
Head injury (accidental or birth)	Caused by brain damage or raised intracranial pressure (RICP)
Brain tumours and central nervous system disorders	Caused by pressure and disruption to neuronal function
Intracranial infections	Caused by irritation of the brain surface
Febrile convulsions	Caused by high temperature in children under 7 years of age
Drugs and alcohol withdrawal	Caused by removal of depressive effect on neuronal function
Metabolic	Caused by toxic disturbance of neuronal biochemistry
Bright or flashing lights	Caused by excessive activation of some brain pathways
Psychological	Invented by the patient for a specific purpose

Factors involved in the cause of epilepsy

Fits are either of known or unknown aetiology. The designation *unknown* probably means that the underlying pathology remains undetected. Examples of those caused by known pathology are listed in Table 12.1.

Other factors include:

- **Age:** the incidence of fits increases with age; 12 per 100,000 people between 40 and 59 years of age are affected, and this figure rises to 80 per 100,000 in the population over 60 years. One-quarter of the epileptic population is over 60 years old. Age also accounts for different types of epileptic syndromes (see Childhood epilepsies, page 277).

Table 12.2 Some genetic epileptic disorders

Genetic epilepsy	Notes
West syndrome (generalised); at Xp22	About 17% of West syndrome is caused by genetic factors. Involves infant developmental delay, muscle spasms and long-term intellectual handicap.
Lennox-Gastaut syndrome (generalised); at 4q21.3	Multiple tonic or atonic seizures per day, sometimes absences, drop attacks, or myoclonus. Slow mental development or even intellectual regression with learning difficulties.
Myoclonic epilepsy and ragged red fibres (MERRF) Mitochondrial gene	Seizures with myopathy (muscle deterioration) (see text).
Lafora disease (or **Lafora progressive myoclonic epilepsy**) 2 genes at 6q & 6p22	Neurons and other tissue cells have Lafora bodies (intracellular inclusions). Starts in adolescence with myoclonus, seizures, and drop attacks associated with gradual dementia. Usually fatal around mid-twenties.
Progressive epilepsy with mental retardation; at 8q	Generalised tonic–clonic seizures begin at 5 to 10 years of age, increasing until puberty, and then declining in frequency to 35 years, when the person remains seizure-free. Intellectual deterioration begins about 5 years after seizures begin and requires nursing care.
Benign familial neonatal convulsions (BFNC); at 20q	Seizures from 2nd or 3rd day after birth cease at about 6 months of age. Development after that is normal.

- **Genetics**: epilepsy can be familial, but the picture is often complicated by the effects of several genes involved acting together (polygenic), or by varying amounts of genetic penetrance (see Chapter 6). There are over 250 genetic causes of epilepsy, and many are disorders that carry an increased risk of epilepsy as a common feature. Some are **autosomal recessive** whereas others are **autosomal dominant**, **X-linked**, or even **mitochondrial DNA** (see Table 12.2).

Not all the genes responsible for epilepsy are found in the karyotype. DNA, the molecular basis of genes, is also found in **mitochondria**, the cellular organelles charged with the task of energy production. Mitochondria need their own genes to code for the proteins involved in the energy cycle. One mitochondrial gene mutation that can cause seizures is **myoclonic epilepsy and ragged red fibres (*MERRF*)** (Figure 12.6, Table 12.2). The 'ragged red fibres' are the accumulations of mitochondria seen on biopsy below the cell membrane of skeletal muscle. A change from the DNA base adenine to guanine in the normal gene causes a mutation that reduces mRNA production and thus protein synthesis. Skeletal muscle then deteriorates and the person becomes deaf and demented before the seizures, myoclonus, and ataxia begin (Mancuso et al. 2004).

The epileptogenic focus

A number of epileptic fits are caused by an **epileptogenic focus** (Hickey 2013; McCance et al. 2014). This is a lesion at any specific site in the brain where, as a result of damage or changes in their biochemistry, the neurons are in continuous state of partial depolarisation and are therefore hyperexcitable. The surrounding gamma-aminobutyric acid (GABA) neurons inhibit the excessive activity of the focus, but on occasions the focal activity exceeds

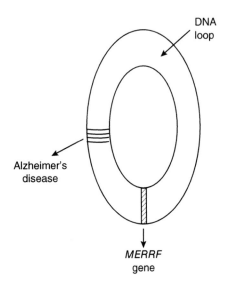

Figure 12.6 The mitochondrial DNA loop. Two genes on this loop are important for mental health, one associated with Alzheimer's disease, and the myoclonic epilepsy and ragged red fibres (*MERRF*) gene, which causes a syndrome that includes epilepsy.

the inhibitory neurons, sometimes due to low GABA concentrations, and a seizure results. The abnormal discharges spread to other parts of the brain, e.g. the cerebral cortex (affecting consciousness) and subcortical parts, and this spread causes a generalised fit. It is useful to think of a fit as an electric *storm* in the brain spreading from one particular point. Where the epileptogenic focus is known and has been studied, several interesting characteristics have been found (Figure 12.7):

- The neurons of the focus may suffer some degree of **deafferentation**, i.e. a loss of the branches from dendrites (**dendritic spines**), the afferent component of the neuron (see Chapter 3). This means there is a reduction in synaptic density because dendritic spines are the location of many synaptic connections. The reason for this loss is not fully understood, but it causes a chronic state of depolarisation and excitability in the neurons.
- The normal passage of an action potential is from the cell to the synapse, and this is described as an **orthodromic** impulse. There is some evidence to suggest that the epileptogenic focus can sometimes generate **antidromic** impulses, which return abnormally from the synapse back up the axon. This is possibly one reason for a rapid depolarisation in the axon of the focal neurons. The antidromic impulses may also generate other orthodromic impulses, creating a cycle.
- There are neurotransmitter differences at the focus. Focal neurons have reduced GABA activity; i.e. less inhibition from the GABA neurons that occur in the vicinity of the focus. This creates an imbalance between excitation and inhibition, with excitation overwhelming the inhibitory activity. The process is made worse by increased excitatory activity at the NMDA and AMPA glutamate receptors (Chapter 4). The focus is also more sensitive to acetylcholine (ACh), which binds to ACh receptors for longer than it does on normal neurons.

- The cells of the focus and other neurons have increased permeability to ions. This is due to an increase in the numbers of ion channels within the cell membrane, a process called **upregulation**. Chief among the ion channels involved in epilepsy are calcium and potassium channels. Calcium (Ca^{2+}) is normally in greater concentrations outside the neuronal cell body, with potassium (K^+) inside. There are several types of calcium channel in the cell membrane, and the channels involved in epilepsy are known as **T-type channels**. Changes in the genetic expression of these channels results in an increase in T-type channels in the membrane. A gene disorder that affects ion channels is sometimes called a **channelopathy**. T-type calcium and potassium channelopathies are the best studied in relation to epilepsy. During a seizure, focal neurons leak calcium *into* the cell through the T-type channels, and this displaces potassium *out of* the cell. These ionic changes cause increased depolarisation of the membrane and further hyper-excitability of the neuron (McCance et al. 2014). Some drugs that block T-type calcium channels to reduce cellular hyperexcitability and therefore help to prevent fits are now in clinical use.

- Occasionally, a **primary (1°)** epileptogenic focus (the real focus) can induce changes in normal brain cells nearby so that they act as a **secondary (2°)** focus (false focus) during a seizure. This induction process is known as **kindling**. In some cases, the primary focus is present in one hemisphere of the brain (either cortical or subcortical), while a secondary focus (also called a **mirror focus**) can be traced in the opposite hemisphere (Figure 12.8) (Hickey 2013). The primary focus communicates with the false secondary focus through the corpus callosum. The secondary focus is essentially normal brain tissue acting along with the true focus to cause the seizure. However, given enough time, the secondary focus will be converted to epileptogenic tissue, which can function independently. This means that early surgical removal of the primary focus is important, as is possible in some patients, before this permanent conversion of the secondary focus occurs. This surgery, if done early enough, can often result in the restoration of normal structure and function of the secondary focus (Acharya 2002).

The net effect of all these changes at the epileptogenic focus is to produce a small area of neurons that are hyperactive with a low threshold for firing impulses. They are likely to discharge action potentials easily and rapidly, up to 1000 impulses per second during a fit, sparking off a wave of high-voltage abnormal electrical activity across the brain.

During a fit the brain increases its use of adenosine triphosphate (ATP) as an energy source by 250%. This huge energy requirement must be met by an increase in the blood supply, which also increases by 250%. The oxygen consumption of the neurons increases by 60%, but still this massive supply becomes depleted. The brain moves into anaerobic metabolism, with the result that lactic acid production, acidosis, and cellular exhaustion occur (McCance et al. 2014). Fits rarely last for more than one or two minutes. What causes the fit to stop has been controversial. Previously it was considered to be due to either the neurotransmitters becoming depleted or because of the rapid accumulation of waste products that cannot be removed fast enough from the cell body. A more modern view suggests that since the fit was the result of excessive excitatory activity, the cessation of the fit may be due to restoration of inhibitory activity to restore the balance (see Tonic–clonic (grand mal) seizures, below). In either case, any further abnormal neuronal activity would be prevented.

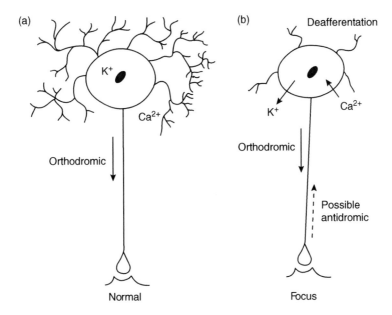

Figure 12.7 Changes at the epileptogenic focus neuron. Deafferentation, calcium entry, and possible antidromic impulses are some of the features that cause greater electrical activity at the focus.

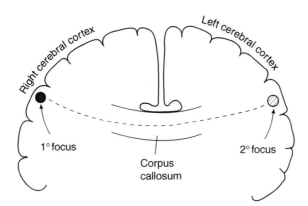

Figure 12.8 The primary (1°) focus sometimes causes a secondary (2°) focus to form at the mirror image position on the other side of the brain. They link through the corpus callosum. Removal of the primary focus causes the secondary focus to disappear.

Tonic–clonic (grand mal) seizures

Generalised tonic–clonic fits may be due to an epileptogenic focus or caused by a more widespread irritation of brain cells. Some factors that lead to this form of grand mal seizure are listed in Table 12.1, and this list illustrates why those having an epileptic-type fit for the first time must undergo extensive investigations to identify the presence or absence of a focus and, if the latter, the cause.

The fit occurs in four stages, as shown in Table 12.3. The **tonic stage** involves muscle rigidity due to a strong increase in muscle tone. This is caused by the spread of abnormal impulses to the subcortical regions, notably the thalamus, brain stem, and spinal cord. The **clonic stage** is the convulsive stage, and this involves inhibitory responses from the thalamus, basal ganglia, and cortex that interrupt the tonic phase to allow brief moments of muscle relaxation followed by restoration of rigidity. These bursts of inhibitory impulses become more dominant and gradually gain control of the fit, causing the fit to stop.

Table 12.4 indicates the immediate first aid care required at each stage of the fit.

Two important myths associated with the management of fits are discussed further here:

- **Do not put anything in the mouth**. The placing of a hard object between the teeth to stop the person from biting their tongue is usually done *too late* and therefore becomes a dangerous procedure. By the start of the tonic phase the jaw will already be clenched tightly shut, and to open the jaw would require a considerable force, causing injury to the patient's mouth. Bleeding into the mouth and dental damage would cause a further risk of

Table 12.3 Stages of a tonic–clonic fit

Stage of the fit	Notes
1 **Aura**, or warning	Occurs in the form of confusion, aggression, or hallucinations such as flashing lights or strange smells. Many patients do not have an aura, and some who have an aura do not recognise it as such.
2 **Tonic**	Fall to the ground followed by increased muscle tone, which causes stiffness and arching of the body on the ground. Lasts about 15–30 seconds, during which breathing stops and the patient becomes somewhat cyanosed.
3 **Clonic**	The convulsive stage. The patient thrashes about with rapid, powerful muscle contractions. They may be incontinent. Breathing is spasmodic and excessive salivation causes frothing at the mouth. Lasts for about 30–60 seconds.
4 **Recovery**	Starts when the patient stops moving. Breathing gradually settles down. Patient goes from unconsciousness into sleep, and then wakens. They may be a little confused or disorientated, but should recover from this quickly. There is no memory of the event. Lasts about 5–10 minutes or so.

Table 12.4 Immediate first aid required at each stage of the fit

Stage of the fit	Action at each stage
1 **Aura**	Assist the patient to the ground in a clear area to avoid injury when falling or convulsing. Loosen tight clothing at the neck, chest, and waist. Note the time.
2 **Tonic**	Work from the head end away from the body. Do not restrain the patient. Keep other people away from the patient's body. Keep the airway as clear as possible. Do not try to put anything between the teeth, as this will cause oral damage and bleeding into the mouth. Clear the area around the patient.
3 **Clonic**	Continue to work from the head end away from the body. Do not restrain the patient. Observe and facilitate breathing by clearing the airway of any obstruction. Check the pulse (carotid is best) and skin colour for cyanosis.
4 **Recovery**	Turn into the recovery position when convulsion stops. Stay at head end to maintain clear airway and check breathing, pulse, and skin colour. On the patient's awakening, get them into a resting position gradually. Note the time again.

airway obstruction and distress when the patient wakes up. If the person is going to bite their tongue, this will have happened by the start of the tonic phase. Any such damage to the tongue is not common and can be treated. The aura, therefore, is the only stage at which it is possible to take preventative action. Since an aura does not always occur, and if it does it is over very quickly, it is best to relegate this procedure to the history books.

- **Do not restrain the patient**. The restraining of the body during the convulsion is another very dangerous practice. Anyone attempting this is putting themselves and the patient at considerable risk of injury, and it is unnecessary. The patient's limb movements are powerful, and they may kick, punch, or throw off anyone holding them. In addition, it has been shown that restraint causes more limb injuries to the patient than allowing them to be free. Emptying the space around the patient's body to give them room is a useful thing to do, to prevent them hitting against hard objects. Everyone should keep clear of the patient's body, while the carer stays at the head end.

The patient should be placed in the *recovery position* as soon as the clonic phase ends, i.e. the **recovery stage**. The carer should remain with the patient at all times, unless there is no choice but to leave to get help. If going to get help is the only choice, leave the patient in the *recovery position* or wait until they are awake. The patient may go into a second fit, so someone should, whenever possible, remain to assist in case this happens. Staying at the head end, the carer should *maintain a clear airway* and *observe for breathing, carotid pulse, and cyanosis* (*cyanosis* = 'blue colour of the skin, indicating a lack of oxygen'). Check the patient's *level of consciousness* every few minutes by talking to them (Blows 2012). On return to consciousness, allow the patient time to rest, reassure them, and help them orient themselves to time, place, and what happened. The patient can sit up *slowly*, when ready to do so. The carer should make a note of the time at each stage of the fit, but especially the time taken for recovery. A prolonged time of the recovery phase, i.e. longer than 30 minutes, may be a sign of complications. Be aware of the possibilities of complications and seek help if required. Some of the possible complications are:

- The patient may go into another fit. If this happens then they must receive urgent medical care to prevent further fitting. **Status epilepticus** means the occurrence of multiple fits lasting 30 minutes or more without regaining consciousness between fits, and this is a very serious complication. **Impending status epilepticus** (multiple fits lasting 5 minutes or more without regaining consciousness between fits) often precedes status epilepticus and acts as a warning that the patient may be deteriorating. Status epilepticus is dangerous because patients can die from exhaustion or heart failure and prolonged convulsions create a shortage of oxygen to the brain, causing brain damage.
- **Postepileptic (interictal) twilight state** is a prolonged period of confusion and disorientation following a fit. Restless wandering and abnormal behaviour can accompany a twilight state. Patients do not know what they are doing and may unknowingly carry out bizarre, dangerous, and even criminal acts. Again, urgent medical help is needed to safeguard the patient and others around him or her.

The hippocampal involvement in seizures

Some seizures are triggered by abnormal activity from the hippocampus. The hippocampus is described in Chapter 1, and also in Chapter 10 in relation to schizophrenia. The cells most prone to epilepsy within the hippocampus are those of the **CA3** cell collection because they have strong excitatory connections. The least prone to epilepsy are the **granulate cells** of the dentate gyrus, because they have strong inhibitory connections. Normally, granulate cells provide inhibitory impulses that resist any onset of epileptogenesis within the hippocampus. Variation in the synaptic circuitry may change granulate cells to epileptogenic status, which may then initiate a fit. The exact changes that cause granulate cells to trigger a fit are still under examination, but they centre on the formation of abnormal synaptic connections and the local reduction of inhibition (Acharya 2002).

Astrocytes also get involved in hippocampal-related epilepsy. One of the many functions of astrocytes is to absorb glucose from the blood, transform it to **lactic acid**, and pass this to the neurons for energy. Loss of the **GluT astrocytes** (see Chapter 3) in **hippocampal sclerosis** (i.e. a hardening of the tissues, see Temporal lobe seizures, below) reduces the energy available to the hippocampal neurons. GluT astrocytes are normally joined in networks that remove waste molecules and ions from the neuronal environment. A lack of GluT cells allows such molecular material to increase, overstimulating the neurons and possibly triggering a seizure. **GluR astrocytes** (Chapter 3) in the sclerotic hippocampus have below normal numbers of potassium channels, and slow-acting glutamate receptors, causing neurons to fire impulses easily and quickly, which may trigger fits.

Temporal lobe seizures (psychomotor epilepsy)

Epilepsy caused by temporal lobe lesions has a specific set of characteristics. The main occurrence is an abrupt change in personality and restless automatic behaviour patterns, with or without a concluding loss of consciousness. Hallucinations of an **olfactory** (smell) or **gustatory** (taste) nature sometimes occur and the patient may experience **déjà vu**, i.e. the sense of events repeating themselves, or **jamais vu**, the sense of being a stranger in familiar company or environments. Psychotic symptoms can present with aggressive overtones and emotional or mood swings. This sudden change in the behaviour and personality can be very frightening to the witness, who is often a member of the patient's family. The sudden onset of the symptoms and the quick return to normal are strong indications that the cause is a seizure, even in the absence of convulsions.

The temporal lobe lesion responsible is often **medial temporal sclerosis**, a hardening of the temporal brain tissue, which occurs often in the hippocampus (also called **hippocampal sclerosis**), notably that part called **Ammon's horn** (see the anatomy of the hippocampus, Chapter 10, Figure 10.5). This lesion is associated with cerebral anoxia, especially as a fetus, or can result from febrile convulsions early in childhood, particularly if they were complicated or prolonged. The child grows up free from seizures for many years, but then develops temporal lobe epilepsy in early adulthood.

One part of the temporal lobe is the *limbic portion* (i.e. the area that connects and works with the limbic system), and epilepsy caused by a lesion here is referred to as **medial temporal epilepsy syndrome** (or simply **limbic epilepsy**). Again, the characteristics of this syndrome involve behavioural difficulties and psychotic, schizophrenia-like symptoms. There is also an **interictal syndrome** (i.e. symptoms occurring between fits), identified by reduced sexual behaviour, increased religious convictions (e.g. compulsive church attendance), and **hypergraphia** (excessive compulsive writing). The presence of psychosis as part of an epileptic illness is confusing, as without the fits these patients may well be diagnosed as schizophrenic. Often this raises the question: *Does the epilepsy cause this psychosis, or* *is this a schizophrenic illness with the patient having fits as well?* One suggested distinction between the 'psychosis of epilepsy' and the 'psychosis of schizophrenia' is that the former is a milder psychosis with fewer negative symptoms, no thought disorder, full preservation of affect, and a distinct increase in religious delusions.

Jacksonian seizures

Jacksonian fits begin with a unilateral twitching of muscles in one part of the body – for example, the small finger of the *left* hand – and from there the convulsion spreads to all other parts of the same side of the body, and then onto the other side. The patient becomes unconscious and has a full convulsion. The muscles involved at the start indicate which part of the cerebral primary motor cortex was generating the fit, i.e. the focus of the lesion. In the example given here, the lesion would be in the *right* motor cortex (Brodmann 4), the area that controls the little finger. Notice that the *right* motor cortex controls the *left* side because the motor fibres cross to the other side, mostly within the brain stem. The lesion in the motor cortex could be a tumour, inflammation, or scar tissue. The disease manifestations are extremely varied, and other symptoms include sudden head and eye movements, tingling, numbness and smacking of the lips. Keen observation by those present can pinpoint the muscles involved at the start of the twitching and thereby assist the doctor in the diagnosis and location of the lesion.

Infantile spasms and febrile convulsions

Infantile spasms are attacks of head nodding and flexing of the body that begin in the early months of life. They cause a type of EEG trace known as **hypsarrhythmia**, which is a very disorganised and chaotic brain wave recording with no recognisable patterns. Gross abnormalities of the brain are one cause of this form of epilepsy, and in this case it can lead to progressive intellectual disability. However, another cause is a deficiency of **vitamin B$_6$ (pyridoxine)** in the diet, and treatment simply involves replacing the vitamin.

Infantile (or febrile) convulsions are not true epilepsy and very few cases go on to develop epilepsy later in life. The cause is a high temperature in children below the age of 7 years when the temperature control centre in the hypothalamus is still immature. Prevention of the convulsion can sometimes be achieved by the administration of **paracetamol** in syrup form when the child is conscious and able to swallow, during the early stages of a raised temperature. Paracetamol is thought to help reduce body temperature, although scientific evidence for this is lacking. Measures are aimed at body temperature reduction, and include reducing the clothing, cooling the *room* (not the child directly) with a fan, or tepid sponging. If consciousness is lost and convulsions commence, do not attempt to give anything further by mouth. Maintain a clear airway, continue cooling the child, and seek medical assistance as quickly as possible (Blows 2012). Drug treatment, usually with **diazepam** administered by injection or rectally by a doctor, may be required to stop the fitting, as prolonged fits can cause brain damage.

Childhood epilepsies

Epilepsies appearing in childhood increase the risk of developmental delays, affecting the normal expected milestones. Some childhood epilepsies are benign. The term *benign* here means infrequent mild seizures that are not linked to cognitive or psychosocial disturbance. The opposite of benign are severe frequent seizures with an impact on cognitive or psychosocial development, high risk of injuries from falls, and a poor response to treatment.

- **Rolandic epilepsy (RE)**, or **benign rolandic epilepsy (BRE)**, occurs in 1 in 500 children between 3 and 12 years of age, 60% being boys, 40% girls. The disorder stops during the teenage years in nearly all cases, and the number that become epileptic in adulthood is no higher than seen in the general population. The seizures are of the simple partial type, starting with sounds in the larynx followed by sensory and motor symptoms affecting the mouth, tongue, face, and speech. They occur mostly during sleep just prior to waking. A characteristic that is diagnostic of RE is the presence of **centrotemporal sharp waves (CTS)**, which are seen on the EEG during a seizure. The disorder is due to a gene mutation within the **elongator protein complex 4 (*ELP4*)** gene on chromosome 11. This gene normally produces a protein that is involved in **transfer RNA (tRNA)** modification and gene transcription during central nervous system (CNS) neuronal migration and development (see Chapter 2). RE probably stops during the teenage years because the brain reaches full developmental maturity, and the gene becomes less active.
- **Benign occipital epilepsy** causes seizures of any type with chains of spike waves on EEG originating from the occipital lobe. A subset of children have 'Panayiotopoulos syndrome' starting from 4 to 8 years of age. These children have night seizures, vomiting, and eye deviation.
- **Childhood absence epilepsy (CAE)** has an onset age range between 4 and 10 years of age. Absence attacks are frequent and last 5 to 15 seconds each. This type of epilepsy is often associated with learning difficulties, which continue after the seizures disappear, and may go on for life. Cognitive problems are a serious outcome and may have detrimental effects on mental and social development.
- **Generalised epilepsy with febrile seizures plus (GEFS+)** is a syndrome in which febrile convulsions extend beyond the age of 7, often into the teens. As teenagers, these fits take the form of tonic–clonic seizures. Two gene mutations are involved: **sodium channel voltage-gated type I alpha subunit (*SCN1A*)** on chromosome 2q24, and *SCN1B* on chromosome 19q13. These genes are involved in sodium channel subunits, and mutations cause defects in the sodium channels (a **channelopathy**) along the neuronal axon.
- **Autosomal dominant nocturnal frontal lobe epilepsy (ADNFLE)** is another channelopathy that begins in childhood with short, nocturnal seizures with motor system involvement. The two mutations identified in this syndrome are on gene *CHRNA4* on chromosome 20q13.2, and a second gene at 15q24. Both genes code for subunits of nicotinic receptors, which normally bind acetylcholine (see Chapter 4).

The anticonvulsant drugs

There are several classes of drugs used in the treatment of epilepsy (Table 12.5). They act in two main ways:

1 on the epileptogenic focus and other cells to prevent the abnormal electrical discharge from happening;
2 on the brain as a whole to prevent spread of the discharge.

Table 12.5 The classification of the antiepileptic drugs

Group	Drugs	Function
Aldehydes	Paraldehyde (in children)	Not fully established; it may reduce activity within the reticular formation of the brain stem
Barbiturates	Phenobarbital	GABA receptor enhancer
Benzodiazepines	Clobazam, clonazepam, diazepam, midazolam, lorazepam	GABA receptor enhancers
Carboxamides	Carbamazepine, oxcarbazepine, eslicarbazepine	Sodium channel blockers
Fatty acids	Sodium valproate, vigabatrin, tiagabine	Increases amount of GABA
Fructose derivatives	Topiramate	Sodium channel blocker and GABA receptor enhancer
GABA analogs	Pregabalin, gabapentin	Reduces calcium influx
Hydantoins	Phenytoin, fosphenytoin	Sodium channel blockers
Pyrimidinediones	Primidone	Metabolites reduce glutamate activity and enhance GABA receptor
Pyrrolidines	Levetiracetam	Reduces neurotransmitter release
Succinimides	Ethosuximide	Calcium channel blocker
Sulfonamides	Zonisamide	Sodium channel blocker, reduces calcium entry
Triazines	Lamotrigine	Sodium channel blocker
Others	Rufinamide, lacosamide	Prolongs the inactive state of sodium channels

Rufinamide is used in Lennox-Gastaut syndrome (Table 12.2).

Lacosamide acts on sodium channels at sites that have long-term depolarisation, such as the epileptogenic focus, and is used for partial onset seizures.

Vigabatrin and progabide are also analogs of GABA.

There are a number of different mechanisms of drug action (several drugs have multiple activities) (Figure 12.9):

1   Those acting on sodium channels along the axon:

 - *Sodium channel blockers* act by blocking the channels through which sodium influxes through the axonal membrane during an action potential. This prevents the action potential from traveling any further down the axon, and the discharge is blocked from spreading. In this way these drugs stabilise the axonal membrane. The drugs in this group are **phenytoin, fosphenytoin, carbamazepine, oxcarbazepine, eslicarbazepine, lamotrigine, sodium valproate,** and **topiramate** (these last two drugs have a wide spectrum of anticonvulsive activities). **Zonisamide** has a similar action, i.e. it blocks repetitive firing of sodium channels (and another action, see Calcium channels, below).
 - Promoting the slow inactivation of sodium channels, which decreases the number of sodium channels available for depolarisation. The result is a more stable axonal membrane, which cannot accommodate the rapid firing required during seizures. The drug

here is **lacosamide**. Although the mechanisms of activity of **rufinamide** are largely unknown, one of its main functions appears to be the prolongation of the inactive state in sodium channels, thus making them less responsive to action potentials.

2   Those acting on GABA:

- Promoting GABA activity by binding to the GABA$_A$ receptor complex (Figure 4.13 in Chapter 4, and Figure 12.9). This enhances the action of GABA, which opens the chloride channels and causes inhibition of any further action potentials, preventing spread of the discharges across the brain. The drugs in this group are the **benzodiazepines (diazepam, clonazepam, clobazam, midazolam,** and **lorazepam),** which are used in several types of epilepsy (Table 12.6) and the **barbiturates (phenobarbital** is the drug of this group used in epilepsy) and the drugs **tiagabine** and **topiramate**.
- Increasing the amount of GABA available in the brain is another way of improving inhibition of action potentials. There are three ways this can be achieved:
  - o   by preventing the breakdown of GABA, i.e. inhibiting the enzyme GABA transaminase (GABA-T) which metabolises GABA (the drugs are **vigabatrin** and **sodium valproate**);
  - o   by promoting the production of GABA through enhancing the GABA-producing enzyme GABA decarboxylase (GAD), and it is thought the drug **sodium valproate** achieves this;
  - o   by preventing the reuptake of GABA from the synapse (the drugs are **sodium valproate** and **tiagabine**).
- These actions cause GABA to build up in quantity at the synapse.

3   Those acting on glutamate:

- **Phenobarbital** suppresses glutamate activity, glutamate being the excitatory neurotransmitter of the cerebrum. Suppressing the excitatory action of glutamate, particularly on the NMDA receptors, will reduce the ability of the abnormal discharge to spread across the cerebrum. This drug is especially useful in having a dual role in combating the spread of seizures (see also the GABA$_A$ receptor).
- Metabolites of the drug **primidone** are **phenobarbitol** and **phenylethylmalonamide,** both of which will suppress glutamate activity and promote GABA-A inhibitory receptor activity.
- Inhibition of the AMPA glutamate receptor by **topiramate** and **perampanel** (AMPA antagonists) is another way to reduce the excitatory effect of glutamate activity.

4   Those acting on calcium channels:

- *Calcium channel blockers* have been tried as anticonvulsant therapy, with some success in clinical trials. They prevent the influx of calcium into the neuron cell body, and this reduces the ability of the epileptogenic focus to discharge action potentials. The drug **ethosuximide**, currently regarded as the best treatment for infantile absences, has long been considered to be a T-type calcium channel blocker. **Zonisamide** also reduces calcium flow through T-type calcium channels.
- Binding to the alpha2-delta calcium channel subunit, which then reduces calcium influx. The drugs **gabapentin** and **pregabalin** do this.

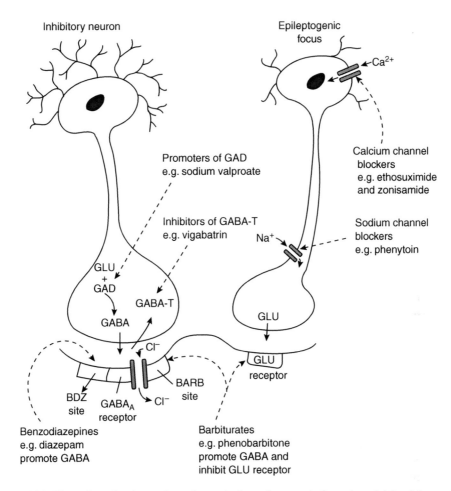

Inhibitory neuron

Epileptogenic focus

←Ca²⁺

Promoters of GAD
e.g. sodium valproate

Calcium channel blockers
e.g. ethosuximide and zonisamide

Inhibitors of GABA-T
e.g. vigabatrin

Na⁺

Sodium channel blockers
e.g. phenytoin

GLU
+
GAD

GABA-T

GABA

GLU

Cl⁻

GLU

GLU
receptor

BDZ
site

GABA_A
receptor

Cl⁻

BARB
site

Benzodiazepines
e.g. diazepam
promote GABA

Barbiturates
e.g. phenobarbitone
promote GABA and
inhibit GLU receptor

Figure 12.9 The action of anticonvulsant drugs. At the epileptogenic focus (top right) calcium enters abnormally and excites the cell. Calcium channel blockers may be useful to prevent cell excitation. The abnormal action potentials (impulses) from the focus pass down the axon where sodium influxes. Blocking the sodium channels would halt the progress of the impulses. At the synapse, glutamate is released. Blocking the glutamate receptor will halt the impulses at that point. The inhibitory neuron (top left) produces gamma-aminobutyric acid (GABA), which blocks impulses. Promoting glutamic acid decarboxylase (GAD) or inhibiting GABA-transaminase (GABA-T) will increase the level of GABA at the synapse. Drugs that increase GABA activity at the GABA_A receptor will help to inhibit abnormal impulses.

5   Those modifying the release of excitatory neurotransmitter:

   •   **Levetiracetam** is a drug that binds to the presynaptic vesicle protein 2A and reduces the release of these vesicles, thus less neurotransmitter into the synaptic cleft, during an action potential. The effect is greatest during rapid firing of action potentials, which is exactly what happens during a seizure.

Table 12.6 Drugs used in specific epileptic categories

Epileptic category	Drugs used in the treatment
Partial seizures	
Simple	Carbamazepine, lamotrigine, sodium valproate, oxcarbazepine
Complex	Carbamazepine, lamotrigine, sodium valproate, oxcarbazepine
Generalised seizures	
Absences	Ethosuximide, sodium valproate,
Tonic–clonic	Carbamazepine, lamotrigine, sodium valproate
Myoclonic	1st: sodium valproate, 2nd: clonazepam, levetiracetam
Status epilepticus	Diazepam, clonazepam, lorazepam, paraldehyde, phenytoin, phenobarbital (preventive)
Infantile spasms	Clonazepam, also effectively treated with ACTH
Infantile (febrile) convulsions	Diazepam

6   Those acting on potassium (K) channels:

- **Retigabine** is unique in being the first drug to act on K channels along the axon. By opening these channels for longer, more potassium leaves the axon, thus rapidly promoting the repolarisation and resting membrane potential phases of the action potential. This calms the neuron and reduces rapid firing.

Particular drugs are used to treat specific epileptic categories, as indicated in Table 12.6.

The pharmacokinetics of the antiepileptic drugs

Most antiepileptic drugs are well tolerated by mouth, making oral administration easy. Carbamazipine absorption is slow and incomplete. Oral administration involves **first pass metabolism** (see Chapter 7). Binding to protein (mostly albumin) in plasma varies between 80 and 90% (phenytoin) to 50% (phenobarbital). Induction of liver enzymes occurs, particularly with phenobarbital and phenytoin, and this may cause drug interactions if given with other medication. Some drugs have short half-lives (e.g. oxcarbazepine at 1–2.5 hours) whereas others have intermediate half-lives (e.g. phenytoin at 7–60 hours, valproate at 7–15 hours) or much longer half-lives (e.g. phenobarbital at 50–150 hours). Drugs with long half-lives may be administered less often or in lower dosage than those with shorter half-lives. Most drugs are metabolised in the liver and excreted through the kidneys.

The side effects of the anticonvulsant drugs

The side effects of anticonvulsant drugs are quite extensive and relate to the specific drugs listed in Table 12.5. Sedation is a problem with some drugs, notably the benzodiazepines and phenobarbital, and this may cause difficulties with some activities. The side effects of phenytoin are numerous, including dizziness, nausea, skin rashes, insomnia, gastrointestinal disturbance, **nystagmus** (rapid, involuntary flicking of the eyes), **ataxia** (unsteady walking), and **diplopia** (double vision). However, it still has a valuable contribution to make to anticonvulsive therapy. Carbamazepine and ethosuximide both have similar lists of extensive side effects, including headache, dizziness, drowsiness, ataxia, and gastrointestinal problems. More serious side effects, such as **agranulocytosis** (reduced white blood cell counts), **aplastic anaemia** (low red blood cell counts due to reduced bone marrow activity), and even mental depression, are less often reported. Sodium valproate can cause nausea, ataxia, gastric irritation, tremor, increased appetite and weight gain, transient hair loss, and occasional blood disorders. This drug can also be toxic to the liver and can disturb the blood clotting mechanism, so careful patient selection and persistent monitoring of blood clotting and liver function are important.

Anticonvulsant drug interactions and withdrawal

Drug interactions are also a problem with the anticonvulsants, and this is a good reason for patients to be given **monotherapy**, i.e. treatment with one drug only. The patient is unlikely to benefit from several drugs at once and toxic effects can occur quickly, with an unpredictable outcome. Care must be taken to ensure that the anticonvulsant drug prescribed is compatible with any other form of medication the patient may be taking. It is important to check with the drug interaction information in the prescription information text and British National Formulary (BNF). Withdrawal of any anticonvulsant drug must be done slowly, with staged reductions in dosage. This particularly applies to the benzodiazepines and barbiturates. Abrupt withdrawal of the drug, or sudden change of one drug to another, may cause *rebound seizures* to occur.

Key points

Types of seizures

- Generalised fits are characterised by unconsciousness; partial (or focal) seizures, are centred on one particular part of the brain with limited spread.
- Generalised fits include absences, and generalised tonic–clonic, myotonic, and atonic seizures.
- Partial fits may be simple (no loss of consciousness) or complex (loss of consciousness), and may become generalised.
- The generalised tonic–clonic (the grand mal, or major fit) causes the patient to loose consciousness, fall to the ground, and convulse.

Electroencephalogram

- EEGs have value in helping to distinguish between the different categories of epilepsy.

Factors involved in the cause of epilepsy

- The incidence of fits increases with age.
- Some epilepsies are genetic and run in families.

The epileptogenic focus

- Many epileptic fits are caused by an epileptogenic focus, a lesion at a specific site in the brain that can trigger a fit.
- The neurons of the focus appear to suffer some degree of deafferentation, abnormal glucose and protein metabolism, changes in ion permeability, reduced GABA activity, and possibly the production of an orthodromic–antidromic loop.
- The primary focus is sometimes linked to a secondary focus.

Tonic–clonic (grand mal) seizures

- The four phases of a grand mal fit are aura (if present), tonic, clonic, and recovery.
- Do not force anything between the patient's teeth during a fit.
- Do not restrain a convulsing patient.
- Work from the head end during a fit to clear the airway and maintain observations.
- Place the patient in the recovery position when the recovery stage begins.
- Get help if complications arise, such as in status epilepticus or postepileptic twilight state.

The hippocampal involvement in seizures

- The **CA3** cells are most prone to epilepsy within the hippocampus.
- Reduced GABA inhibition and abnormal synaptic connections may be responsible for hippocampal induced seizures.

Temporal lobe seizures (psychomotor epilepsy)

- Temporal lobe epilepsy (or psychomotor epilepsy) is characterised by an abrupt change in personality and restless automatic behaviour patterns, with or without a concluding loss of consciousness.
- The lesion is medial temporal sclerosis, a hardening of the temporal lobe brain tissue, often in the hippocampus.
- Interictal syndrome (symptoms occurring between fits), involves reduced sexual behaviour, increased religious convictions, and hypergraphia.

Jacksonian seizures

- Jacksonian fits begin with a unilateral twitching of muscles in one part of the body, and it spreads from there to all other parts of the body.

Infantile spasms and febrile convulsions

- Infantile spasms involve head nodding and flexing of the body, which begin early in life.
- Infantile (or febrile) convulsions are not true epilepsy.
- The cause is a high temperature in children below the age of 7 years, due to the hypothalamic temperature control centre being immature.

Anticonvulsant drugs

- Benzodiazepine and phenobarbital act by binding to the $GABA_A$ receptor and promote the opening of the GABA-mediated chloride channels to inhibit any action potentials.
- Some drugs, e.g. phenytoin, sodium valproate, and carbamazepine, are sodium channel blockers, blocking the entry of sodium into the axon during an action potential.
- Monotherapy is preferred to prevent drug interactions and toxicity.
- Withdrawal of anticonvulsants should be gradual.

References

Acharya, J. N. (2002) Recent advances in epileptogenesis. *Current Science*, **82** (6): 679–688.

Blows, W. T. (2012) *The Biological Basis of Clinical Observations*. Routledge, Abingdon, Oxon.

Hickey, J. V. (2013) *The Clinical Practice of Neurological and Neurosurgical Nursing* (7th edition). Lippincott, Williams and Wilkins, Philadelphia, PA.

Mancuso, M., Filosto, M., Mootha, V. K., Rocchi, A., Pistolesi, S., Murri, L., DiMauro, S., and Siciliano, G. (2004) A novel mitochondrial tRNAPhe mutation causes MERRF syndrome. *Neurology*, **62** (11): 2119–2121.

McCance, K. L., Huether, S. E., Brashers, V. L., and Rote, N. S. (2014) *Pathophysiology, the Biological Basis of Disease in Adults and Children* (7th edition). Elsevier-Mosby, London, UK.

13 Subcortical degenerative diseases of the brain

- Introduction: the basal ganglia
- Parkinson's disease
- The anti-Parkinson drugs
- Huntington's disease
- Wilson's disease and Harvey's disease
- Key points

Introduction: the basal ganglia

The subcortical degenerative diseases, often called the **subcortical dementias**, are caused by degeneration of the basal ganglia, i.e. those parts of the brain below the conscious cortex, which have a powerful influence over body movements and muscle tone (Aird 2000). The basal ganglia (see Chapter 1) form part of a loop that regulates motor function (Figure 1.8). This loop starts with the **frontal cortex**, which projects fibres to the **corpus striatum**. The striatum has connections with both the **globus pallidus** and the **substantia nigra pars reticulata**, which then connect to various nuclei of the **thalamus**. Finally, the thalamus connects back to the frontal lobe, completing the loop (Figures 1.8, 13.1). Degeneration of any part of this loop can cause both motor symptoms (basal ganglia) and psychotic symptoms (frontal lobe). Central to the production of symptoms in these disorders is the disturbance to dopamine metabolism. Dopamine depletion in the basal ganglia causes motor deficits, while dopamine problems in the frontal lobes generate cognitive and psychotic symptoms.

The basal ganglia are five separate nuclei of neuronal cell bodies (see Chapter 1, Figure 1.7). The main pathways between the nuclei and their connections with other brain areas are shown in Figure 13.2. The **caudate nucleus** and the **putamen** (together called the **corpus striatum**) have an input from the cerebral cortex (the *higher centres* of the brain) that involves the neurotransmitter **glutamate**. Two outputs from the caudate nucleus to the **globus pallidus** use GABA as the neurotransmitter; one is an inhibitory pathway to the **medial globus pallidus (GPm)**, the other is an inhibitory pathway to the **lateral globus pallidus (GPl)**. The putamen has an output to part of the **substantia nigra** called the **pars reticulata** (abbreviated to **SNr**). The other part of the substantia nigra, the **pars compacta (SNc)**, has dopaminergic feedback loops to both components of the corpus striatum, i.e. an excitatory loop back to the putamen, an excitatory loop back to the GPm caudate nucleus output, and

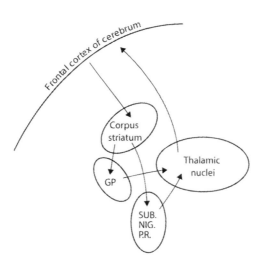

Figure 13.1 The motor loop, from frontal cortex to the corpus striatum, then to both the globus pallidus and the substantia nigra pars reticulata (SUB. NIG. P.R). From here the connection is with the thalamus then back to the cortex.

an inhibitory loop back to the GPI caudate nucleus output. The output from GPI to the **sub-thalamic nucleus (ST)** utilises GABA, while the outputs from the ST to both the SNr and the GPm are facilitated via glutamate. Both the SNr and the GPm have GABA-mediated outputs to the **thalamus**. All these pathways can be visualised using Figure 13.2. In Chapter 1 we saw that the substantia nigra is responsible for lowering muscle tone, and it does this through its dopaminergic pathways to the corpus striatum. This statement is fundamental to our understanding of Parkinson's disease.

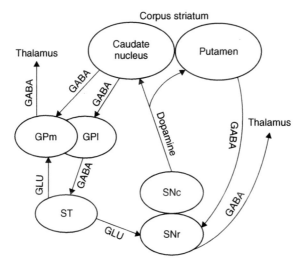

Figure 13.2 Normal basal ganglia pathways. Compare with Figure 13.3. GLU = glutamate, GABA = gamma-aminobutyric acid, SN = substantia nigra, ST = subthalamus.

Parkinson's disease

James Parkinson (1755–1824) was an apothecary surgeon working in Hoxton, an area of Shoreditch, East London. During his regular walks through East London he noticed six people who had a stiffness to their gait and shaking limbs. In 1817 he wrote a description of these people, and this was published as *An Essay on the Shaking Palsy* (a disease he called *paralysis agitans*, which means 'agitated paralysis'). It became known as Parkinson's disease (PD) some 60 years later.

PD affects about 2 people per 1000 in the UK population. Muscle stiffness (or **rigidity**) and shaking of the limbs (or **tremor**) have become the classic signs of the disease. The major features of Parkinson's disease are therefore as follows.

- Progressive muscle rigidity due to increasing muscle tone: the body and limbs become stiff and movement is very limited (i.e. an **akinesia** = a muscular paralysis, or a **bradykinesia** or **hypokinesis** = slow voluntary movements) (Borrell 2000) causing difficulty in initiating movement, which is sometimes known as **freezing**. These are often relieved during sleep.
- Shaking of the limbs, both *coarse* tremors of the whole limb and *fine* tremors of the hand and fingers: these are reduced during intentional movement of the limb, but become very marked at rest. Fine tremors of the hand are sometimes called *pill rolling*, because they resemble the hand movements used to roll hand-made pills before the days of quality control.
- People with PD adopt a forward stance, i.e. leaning slightly forwards, and walk with a shuffling gait. When walking, the top half of the body tends to move forwards faster than the feet, and there is a risk of falling forwards onto the face. In one study, 59% of people with PD had falls, and of these falls 49% resulted in injuries (Gray and Hildebrand 2000). Factors that increase the risk of falling were identified as the severity of the symptoms of the disease, the effectiveness of the medication, the activities and the location of the person at the time of the fall and the degree of fatigue they were suffering at the time (Gray and Hildebrand 2000).
- The arms are held in a bent fashion, in a position similar to that seen in the insect called a praying mantis.
- The facial muscles are paralysed by the excessive muscle tone and this results in the inability to adopt a facial expression, known as the **Parkinsonian mask**.
- Speech becomes difficult over time and is reduced to a low, mumbled, and hurried voice that is almost impossible to understand.
- The mouth tends to hang open and produce excessive saliva (called **sialorrhoea**). This results in patients dribbling saliva down their front. Having one's mouth open all the time is embarrassing, so patients often try to solve both these problems by putting a handkerchief in their mouth. The handkerchief soaks up the excess saliva and blocks the open mouth.
- Swallowing becomes difficult as the disease progresses and towards the latter stages other methods of feeding are required, e.g. nasogastric tube feeding.
- The patient's handwriting becomes impossible to read and communication with the patient becomes very difficult.
- **Oculogyric crisis** is a phenomenon that occurs perhaps several times a day. The eyes rotate upwards so that the iris is hidden under the upper lid and they are held there for a minute or so before returning to normal. This muscular spasm of the eye muscles is involuntary and unpredictable and is said to be very painful.

- Other associated symptoms include constipation, sexual dysfunction, **orthostatic** or **postural hypotension** (low blood pressure on standing), and bladder dysfunction, all due to disturbance of the **autonomic nervous system** (i.e. the component of the nervous system that maintains automatic organ functions) (Herndon et al. 2000).
- Sleep disturbances occur often (Crabb 2001).
- Psychiatric symptoms, such as **depression** (up to 16.5% of PD patients) and **hallucinations** (up to 37% of PD patients) require specific management.
- **Dementia** has been identified in as many as 25% of patients with PD (Herndon et al. 2000), further complicating both the clinical appearance of the disease and its management.

What is happening in this disorder is that, for reasons that remain unclear, the substantia nigra is gradually degenerating, i.e. neurons of this nucleus are dying and are not being replaced. Since the function of the substantia nigra is to lower muscle tone (and the function of the cerebellum is to increase muscle tone), there is normally a balance between the two. The gradual loss of the substantia nigra upsets that balance in favour of the cerebellum (which remains normal). Muscle tone therefore increases unopposed, but the symptoms only become apparent quite late in the disorder because the deterioration of the substantia nigra is very slow and because the neurons are able to compensate to some extent for the losses. Symptoms do not usually appear until the substantia nigra has lost 60% of its cells, so patients diagnosed with PD have had the disorder for many years without symptoms. This is one reason why the disease usually affects those over 60 years of age, although occasionally it is seen in some patients earlier in life. The substantia nigra ('black substance') is so called because its neurons contain a large quantity of **neuromelanin**, a pigment that gives the cells a dark colour. As these cells die in PD, the neuromelanin is released, and antibodies in the blood that are specific to neuromelanin are increased. This increase *may* prove to be useful as a test in the early detection of the disease long before symptoms arise (Nowak 2000).

Prior to the cell losses, affected cells also develop **Lewy bodies**. These are intracellular collections of neurofilamentous material (i.e. made of neurofilaments) surrounding a central core of a protein called **α-synuclein** (see below). These Lewy bodies occur prior to neuronal degeneration and death. In PD, the substantia nigra is the main site of Lewy body formation, although Lewy bodies can sometimes be identified in other parts of the brain, for example in the cortex when dementia or psychoses also occur.

As part of their role, the neurons of the substantia nigra pars compacta (SNc) produce dopamine, but the loss of cells in PD means that the SNc becomes unable to produce dopamine. Within the pathway that extends from the substantia nigra to the corpus striatum, i.e. the **nigrostriatal pathway**, dopamine levels drop very low. The symptoms of the disease are related to this effect (Figure 13.3), but there is a threshold of 60% loss of dopamine in this pathway before symptoms occur. Clearly a loss of 60% dopamine takes a long time to achieve.

The gradual loss of the doperminergic nigrostriatal pathway has a knock-on effect on the remaining basal ganglia (follow these steps by comparing Figure 13.2 with Figure 13.3):

- Low dopamine excitation from the SNc to the putamen results in lower GABA activity from the putamen to the SNr. This reduced GABA inhibition of SNr allows an increased GABA inhibition of the thalamus.
- Low dopamine inhibition from the SNc to the caudate nucleus allows an increase in the GABA inhibitory effect from the caudate nucleus on GPI. GPI inhibition is increased, causing low GABA inhibition of the subthalamus (ST).

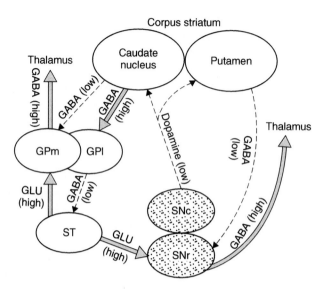

Figure 13.3 Parkinson's disease. The lack of dopaminergic pathways from the dying substantia nigra (shaded) to the corpus striatum causes increased GABA activity in the other pathways shown. The result is excess motor disturbance to the thalamus. (Abbreviations as in Figure 13.2.)

- The loss of the inhibitory effects of GABA from the GPI on the ST allows the ST to increase the excitatory glutamate pathways to both the GPm and the SNr, and thus cause increased GABA inhibition of the thalamus.
- Low dopamine excitation from the SNc of the caudate nucleus reduces the caudate nucleus GABA activity to GPm. This results in a low caudate nucleus GABA inhibition of the GPm. The GPm is now free to increase its own GABA inhibition of the thalamus.
- The thalamus is now receiving increased GABA inhibition from both the GPm and the SNr, causing inhibition of the thalamus in its vital motor loop role.

The cause of PD is unknown, although a number of factors are emerging as candidates.

Genetics

Mutations in the **LRRK2, PARK2, PARK7, PINK1**, and **SNCA** genes are known to cause PD (Table 13.1). In addition, mutations of the **GBA, SNCAIP**, and **UCHL1** genes increase the risk of developing PD. A smaller number of patients are found in family groups and in those presenting with symptoms under 50 years of age, and these are likely to be the result of inherited genetic factors. However, most cases are sporadic (no family history), and these appear to be the result of interactions between genes and environmental factors.

The genetic component of the majority of sporadic cases of PD is now better understood. Mutations of the **α-synuclein (SNCA)** gene (Table 13.1), which is found in some PD families, codes for **α-synuclein** protein. This protein is found accumulating within Lewy bodies, mostly in dopamine neurons, prior to the neuron's death. There are various

Table 13.1 The genetic involvement in Parkinson's disease

Gene	Locus	Notes
LRRK2	12q12	Codes for the poorly understood kinase enzyme called **dardarin**, or **leucine-rich repeat kinase 2**. Mutations are a cause of PD.
PARK2	6q25.2-q27	Codes for the protein **parkin**, which has a part in destruction of unwanted or damaged proteins. Mutations are a cause of PD.
PARK7	1p36	Codes for the protein **DJ-7**, which appears to have multiple but poorly understood functions in the cell. Mutations are a cause of PD.
PINK1	1p36	Codes for **PTEN-induced putative kinase 1**, a poorly understood enzyme related to mitochondrial function. Mutations are a cause of PD.
SNCA	4q21	Codes for the protein **α-synuclein**, which has a poorly understood role in synaptic function (see text). Mutations are a cause of PD.
GBA	1q21	Codes for the lysosomal enzyme **beta-glucocerebrosidase**, which breaks down unwanted cellular products. Mutations increase the risk of PD.
SNCAIP	5q23	Codes for two proteins: **synphilin-1** and **synphilin-1A**, which have poorly understood roles in synaptic function. Mutations increase the risk of PD.
UCHL1	4p14	Codes for the protein **ubiquitin carboxyl-terminal hydrolase L1**, which is involved in the degradation of unwanted proteins. Mutations increase the risk of PD.

It is interesting that a single gene locus, 1p36, contains two gene mutations capable of causing PD.

forms of α-synuclein, and it is a gene variant that produces an elongated variety of the protein that causes most of the sporadic cases of PD. This gene variant is more common than previously known, so many people who are not from families with a history of PD are still at risk. The α-synuclein protein is folded prior to use, and errors in folding (called **misfolding**; see also Chapter 14), caused when the protein folds too slowly, precedes the accumulation in Lewy bodies. A similar process involving misfolded synuclein occurs in **Shy-Drager syndrome (SDS**, also known as **multiple system atrophy, MSA)**, a disorder similar to PD. In PD, toxins in the environment appear to promote the formation of the elongated form of the protein, and may even cause the folding error; therefore exposure to these toxins puts the individual at higher risk of developing PD than expected (see Environment, below). The elongated version of the α-synuclein protein, and the slow folding error, may become future targets for drug therapy, in order to inhibit its production and accumulation. Also, the elongated form of the protein has been found in the blood of PD patients, and this may one day serve as the basis of a blood test to see who is at high risk of the disease.

Deletions of some mitochondrial DNA, i.e. the genes that code for enzymes of the energy chain within the mitochondria, have been found in some PD patients. Loss of these genes would result in the failure of energy production within the neuron, leading to cell death (Figure 13.4). Mitochondrial DNA mutations are known to be a factor in the cause of **Alzheimer's disease** (see Chapter 14), and **Leigh syndrome**, a progressive loss of movement and speech due to basal ganglia degeneration in children.

Environment

A neurotoxin has been identified that induces PD in animals and also in those humans who have accidentally made contact with it. The neurotoxin is called ***N*-methyl-4-phenyl-1,2,3, 6-tetrahydropyridine (MPTP)**. Some drug addicts in the USA injected this substance into themselves by mistake, as it is a by-product of 'home-made' cocaine, and they soon developed advanced, irreversible PD. MPTP probably works by being changed first to **1-methyl-4-phenylpyridinium (MPP⁺)** by the action of the enzyme MAO-B. By interfering with the energy cycle within the mitochondrion, and by inducing the formation of damaging chemical agents called **superoxide radicals**, MPP⁺ is more neurotoxic than its precursor MPTP. As such, the presence of MPP⁺ results in depleted energy levels, neural damage, and cellular losses (Figure 13.4). The discovery of MPTP has opened the way to new research that may lead to a better understanding of this disease. Some other possible neurotoxins are also suspected to cause sporadic PD, mostly pesticides used in the agricultural industry. Increasing evidence is pointing to an association between organophosphate pesticides used in farming or agricultural work and PD. They probably cause the disease by increasing the level of elongated α-synuclein protein produced in the brain, or slow down the folding process (see Genetics, above). There is a seven-fold greater risk of developing PD in people exposed to these pesticides.

Biochemical

There is evidence that a metabolite of dopamine, called 3,4-dihydroxyphenylacetaldehyde (**DOPAL**) is toxic to neurons, and contributes to neuronal losses in PD. DOPAL is 1000 times more toxic to neurons than dopamine itself. This appears to be because of DOPAL's ability to generate intracellular **free radicals**, chemicals that react and damage cellular

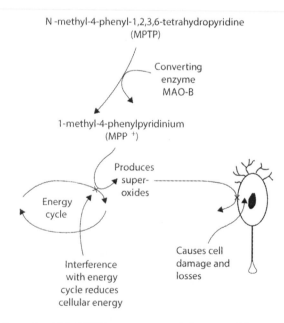

Figure 13.4 The pathway in which MPTP causes neuronal damage and losses.

components. Free radicals appear to cause α-synuclein to aggregate, with resulting loss of function. DOPAL may also be a target for future anti-Parkinson's therapy.

The anti-Parkinson drugs

It might sound reasonable to treat Parkinson's disease by simply replacing the missing neurotransmitter, dopamine, with dopamine in drug form, thus restoring the muscle tone balance between the substantia nigra and the cerebellum. There are two main problems with this scenario:

- Dopamine does not cross the blood–brain barrier, and, moreover, raised dopamine outside the brain (in general circulation) causes unpleasant side effects, and is particularly harmful to cardiac function.
- Simply replacing dopamine does not stop the relentless deterioration of the substantia nigra, the main cause of the symptoms.

Nevertheless, this notion of replacing dopamine in order to improve the quality of life has become the mainstay of treatment. Since dopamine could not be given directly by mouth or by injection (see above), the precursor called **levodopa (L-DOPA)**, which does cross the blood–brain barrier, was used. Conversion from levodopa to dopamine is carried out in the neurons of the basal ganglia. Remember, however, that the dopaminergic neurons of the substantia nigra are slowly dying, so their ability to convert levodopa to dopamine is in gradual decline. In the 1960s, the use of levodopa was shown to have dramatic effects in relieving symptoms. Some decades on, it has become clear that levodopa has some serious long-term problems:

- The amount of conversion of levodopa to dopamine in the brain is somewhat unpredictable. While the dose of levodopa administered can be controlled, what happens after that cannot be controlled. The same levodopa dose can have different results on different days. A way around this problem is to give the minimum dose in combination with other drugs.
- The amount of conversion of levodopa to dopamine declines with time. After 5 years of treatment with levodopa, the patient needs higher dosages to achieve a reasonable result. Higher dosages mean more side effects. One cause of this is that dopamine receptors lose their sensitivity and more neurotransmitter is needed to stimulate them. A way around this is to give the patient a drug holiday. This means removing them from all their medication (except antibiotics if they happen to be on them) for about 2–4 days. During this drug-free time the patient suffers the full symptoms, but the dopamine receptors are resensitised and on reinstatement of levodopa the patient will have reduced symptoms on a lower levodopa dosage. However, this problem is minimised in modern treatment by using low-dose levodopa in combination with other drugs.
- The enzyme that converts levodopa to dopamine, called **dopa decarboxylase**, is found also in other tissues outside the brain, so part of the levodopa dose is converted to dopamine in the body. Of course, once converted to dopamine it cannot cross the blood–brain barrier. So the dopamine levels in circulation build up, causing side effects, especially involving the heart. To prevent this, another drug, called a **dopa-decarboxylase inhibitor**, is given to block the enzyme *outside* the brain (but *not inside*

the brain, as the inhibitor drug cannot cross the blood–brain barrier) so that more of the levodopa enters the brain and is converted there. These inhibitor drugs are **benserazide** and **carbidopa**. In modern Parkinson's disease therapy, the inhibitor drug is given built into the levodopa; for example, benserazide with levodopa is called **co-beneldopa**, and carbidopa with levodopa is called **co-careldopa**.

- Some patients suffer the **on–off phenomenon**, which means the sudden switching from a near symptom-free state to severe symptoms, and back again, several times throughout the day. This gets worse as the length of the treatment period increases. The sudden nature and severity of this switching is distressing, but it can be reduced by splitting the dose from once per day to several times throughout the day, or by giving **modified-release** (i.e. slow-release levodopa) medication. This gives a better regulation of blood levels of levodopa, and improves the control of symptoms.
- **End of dose deterioration** means that the period of symptom-free benefit after each dose becomes progressively shorter. Again, a change to modified-release preparations can help to overcome this problem. The drug **selegiline**, a **monoamine oxidase B** inhibitor, can help to reduce this problem when used with levodopa. Monoamine oxidase B is an enzyme that breaks down neurotransmitters, including dopamine, and inhibiting this enzyme allows dopamine to increase in the brain.

The side effects of levodopa are anorexia, nausea, dizziness, **tachycardia** (fast pulse rate), **arrhythmias** (abnormal changes in heart rhythm), insomnia, and **postural hypotension** (low blood pressure when standing upright).

Other drugs

Antimuscarinic drugs are antagonists (or blockers) of acetylcholine muscarinic (M) receptors. These drugs work by reducing the effects of acetylcholine on the receptors. Acetylecholine is a neurotransmitter of the parasympathetic nervous system and activates muscarinic receptors. Excessive acetylcholine, and therefore excess parasympathetic activity, has occurred as a result of low dopamine in PD, and these drugs help to restore the normal balance between the two systems. The drugs are **trihexyphenidyl, orphenadrine, and procyclidine**. They are less effective than levodopa in controlling symptoms, but may be useful in reducing some symptoms, notably the sialorrhoea (excess of saliva). They also facilitate some decrease in rigidity and tremor. However, their use is limited to the early stages of the disease, as they become less effective as the symptoms worsen, and the dopamine agonists are more effective. They are also associated with cognitive impairment.

Dopamine agonists are drugs that act like dopamine in the brain and stimulate dopamine receptors. However, since they are not dopamine they have no problems crossing the blood–brain barrier and require no enzyme conversion. The first-line drugs in this group are **pramipexole, ropinirole**, and **rotigotine**. Less often used are **bromocriptine, carbergoline**, and **pergolide** because they have been linked to fibrotic reactions. These drugs are being used to augment the role of levodopa, and they can also help to prevent the *on–off phenomenon*. They can cause some side effects, such as nausea, vomiting, headaches, dizziness, hypotension, drowsiness, and confusion. **Ropinirole** and **bromocriptine** are D_2 receptor agonists and **pramipexole** is an agonist for both the D_2 and D_3 receptors. **Apomorphine** is a potent D_1 and D_2 receptor agonist, which is useful in the management of the *on–off phenomenon*, but it is an **emetogenic**, i.e. it causes vomiting, which may contribute to poor patient compliance. It should be prescribed and initiated by a clinical specialist.

Monoamine oxidase B inhibitors (rasagiline and **selegiline)** are drugs that, at low dosage, selectively block the enzyme **monoamine oxidase (MAO) B**. MAO breaks down neurotransmitters after reuptake from the cleft has taken place. Two types of MAO occur in the brain: MAO-B is found in the corpus striatum, whereas MAO-A is widely found in the central nervous system and elsewhere. Selegiline prolongs the action of levodopa and is used with levodopa to relieve the end of dose deterioration. It also reduces the required dose of levodopa by about one-third, reducing levodopa side effects.

Amantadine is a weak dopamine agonist, but it is thought to improve dopamine release from the presynaptic bulb and block dopamine reuptake from the cleft. It has only a short-lived effect on PD, because the patient develops tolerance.

Catechol-*O*-methyl transferase (COMT) inhibitors (e.g. **entacapone** and **tolcapone)** are, as the name indicates, drugs that inhibit the COMT enzyme, which breaks down between 10% and 30% of levodopa outside the brain. When combined with a dopamine decarboxylase inhibitor, this drug doubles the half-life of levodopa and creates a 50% increase in motor activity per dose of levodopa. It is useful in the prevention of the end of dose deterioration problem. Tolcapone carries a risk of hepatotoxicity, so should only be used by a specialist when other drugs have failed to stabilise the patient's symptoms.

Modern treatment of PD is tailor-made to suit the patient, because so many factors are involved, such as the patient's age, stage of the disease, and drug reactions. Many patients are treated with a combination therapy of some levodopa together with an enzyme-inhibiting drug, and perhaps another additional drug given as an adjunct therapy to overcome the problems of levodopa.

Other treatments

Surgery has been attempted to try and reduce the symptoms and allow the patient to be drug free. Most procedures centre on the introduction of dopamine-producing cells into the basal ganglia. Use of fetal cells has had mixed results, and the difficulties of supply and other ethical considerations makes this approach problematic. Now the use of stem cells is becoming a possibility. The animal trials were very successful, and human trials could begin by 2017.

Deep brain electrical stimulation (DBS) of the basal ganglia has proved to be disappointing in PD, but DBS of the **pedunculopontine nucleus (PPN)** has been very beneficial in helping to control two important and distressing symptoms of PD, i.e. freezing of gait **(akinesia)** and postural instability. These symptoms respond poorly to drug treatment and are responsible for the falls and injuries associated with PD. The PPN is situated in the brain stem, between the midbrain and the pons. Its function is part of the control of locomotion and posture, having direct connections with the basal ganglia and cerebellum.

Huntington's disease (HD)

George Huntington (1850–1916) was an American doctor in general practice. He was the son and grandson of doctors and all three of these men had noticed the strange symptom, known as **chorea**, that this disease produced in several American families. In 1872, at the age of just 22 years, George Huntington published a paper in which these patients were briefly described. The affected families, ultimately involving about 1000 patients occurring over 12 generations, were centred on the east end of Long Island, New York.

Huntington's disease (HD) is a neurodegenerative disorder of the GABA neurons within the basal ganglia, notably the caudate nucleus first, followed by the putamen (i.e. the corpus striatum), with concurrent enlargement of the lateral ventricles (Figure 13.5) (Carlson 2012). It is one of nine **polyglutamine** (or **polyQ**) disorders (Table 13.2). The disorder starts to produce symptoms most often between the ages of 30 and 45 years, in other words usually after the affected person has had their family and has passed the affected gene to the offspring. Up to 10 years prior to the onset of movement disorder, a number of patients show mild psychotic and behavioural symptoms, possibly due to the stress of living in a family with a genetic problem. A reduced cognitive ability, including learning and memory deficits in presymptomatic gene carriers, may be present compared with their non-carrier relatives.

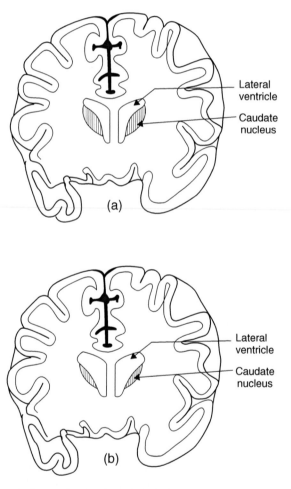

Figure 13.5 Huntington's disease. Section through the brain showing (a) the size of the normal ventricles and (b) the increased size of the ventricles in Huntington's disease due to destruction of the caudate nuclei (shown by the cross-hatched area).

Table 13.2 The polyglutamine (PolyQ) diseases

Disease	Gene	Locus	Protein	Symptoms	Normal repeat number	Disease number of repeats
HD (Huntington's disease)	HTT	4p16.3	Huntingtin	Psychiatric, motor and cognitive	6–35	36–250
DRPLA (Dentatorubropallidoluysian atrophy)	ATN1 (DRPLA)	12q	Atrophin-1	Epilepsy, ataxia and dementia	6–35	49–88
SBMA (Spinal and bulbar muscular atrophy)	AR	Xq11-12	Androgen receptor	Muscular atrophy	9–36	38–62
SCA1 (Spinocerebellar ataxia type 1)	ATXN1	6p22-23	Ataxin-1	Ataxia	6–35	49–88
SCA2 (Spinocerebellar ataxia type 2)	ATXN2	12q23-24	Ataxin-2	Ataxia	14–32	33–77
SCA3 (Spinocerebellar ataxia type 3) (Machado-Joseph disease)	ATXN3	14q24-31	Ataxin-3	Ataxia	12–40	55–86
SCA6 (Spinocerebellar ataxia type 6)	CACNA1A	19p3	CACNA1A	Ataxia	4–18	21–30
SCA7 (Spinocerebellar ataxia type 7)	ATXN7	3p12-21	Ataxin-7	Ataxia, retinal degeneration	7–17	38–120
SCA17 (Spinocerebellar ataxia type 17)	TBP	2q13	TATA-BP	Ataxia	25–42	47–63

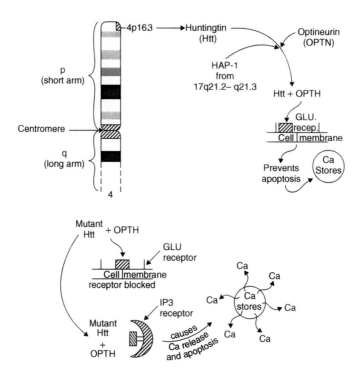

Figure 13.6 Chromosome 4 with the huntingtin gene at 4p16.3. Huntingtin binds with huntingtin-associated protein-1 (HAP-1) from chromosome 17.

HD is a progressive disorder for which there is no cure, so the survival rate is anything from 10 to 20 years from the onset of symptoms. The symptoms involve involuntary, uncontrollable, jerking movements of the limbs, head, and trunk. These jerky movements are called **chorea** (*chorea* = 'dance') and they disrupt the patient's normal daily existence and dominate their every purposeful movement. These patients also suffer an ataxia, an eventual loss of speech called **dysarthria** (*dysarthria* = 'imperfect articulation of speech'), and behavioural changes, including depression, apathy, and irritability (Hofmann 1999). There is often an intellectual decline associated with the disorder. Some patients develop a degree of dementia and others have schizophrenic-like psychoses, with excitable outbursts. The psychotic symptoms are suspected to be caused by the degeneration of the dorsal part of the caudate nucleus (Hofmann 1999).

The cause of this disorder is a genetic error on **chromosome 4**, specifically **4p16.3** (Figure 13.6). This is an **autosomal dominant gene**, and an affected parent has a 50% chance of passing the mutated gene to any of their offspring. The normal gene codes for a protein named **huntingtin (Htt**; see Table 13.2) and patients with HD usually produce both the normal and abnormal forms of the protein.

The gene mutation is called a **trinucleotide repeat**, where the repeated bases are **CAG** (**cytosine–adenine–guanine**), which normally codes for the amino acid **glutamine**. The normal gene has between 6 and 35 CAG repeats, but by duplicating this CAG trinucleotide base many times the number of repeats can reach abnormally high numbers, i.e. between

36 and 250 repeats (Table 13.2). Most people have fewer than 34 repeats, and do not develop the disorder, but the presence of more than 36 repeats causes symptoms of the disease. The number of repeats also affects age of onset of symptoms. Juvenile HD (early-age onset HD) is caused by more than 70 repeats (see also **anticipation**, Chapter 6). Early-age onset HD is characterised by slow speech, awkward gait, and difficulty in starting a movement coupled with slow movements (**bradykinesia**), abnormal eye movements, abnormal muscle spasms (**dystonia**), occasional fits, and muscle rigidity. It is the later-age onset HD (40 years old or more) that is usually characterised by chorea (uncontrollable jerky movements).

If the gene is passed to the offspring from the mother, the number of repeats tends to be copied faithfully: given a mother with, say, 43 repeats, the offspring will receive 43 repeats. But if the mutant gene is passed to the offspring from the father (which is more common), variation can occur in the number of repeats the offspring receives.

Multiple repeats of CAG result in a mutant form of Htt with a long glutamine 'tail' (called an **expanded polyglutamine tract**). Much research has cast light on how the mutant form of this protein can cause the disease.

Normal huntingtin. It is known that the normal huntingtin protein (Htt) is expressed widely in the brain and is essential for normal brain development, but importantly, it protects the cell against **apoptosis (programmed cell death)**. Htt binds to two other proteins; **huntingtin-associated protein-1 (HAP-1)** and **optineurin (OPTN)**. There is now evidence to suggest that normal huntingtin, after binding to optineurin, acts by further binding to specific glutamate receptors that have a cellular protective role, i.e. they prevent neuronal cell death (apoptosis). Apoptosis would be achieved by releasing the stored calcium in the cell. The presence of normal Htt, bound to specific glutamate receptors, would prevent the loss of neurons by blocking this natural destruction of cells (Figure 13.6). Normal Htt also controls the formation of **cilia**, i.e. extensions on the surface of cells, and these structures are abnormal in HD.

Mutant Htt. The mutant form of huntingtin (mutant Htt), is a misfolded version of the normal Htt protein. Proteins often fold up quite normally after production, but the folding process is poorly understood and can go wrong, causing errors. The proteins with the misfolding errors are capable of moving from cell to cell, causing normal cells to become involved in the disease. Mutant Htt, bound to OPTN, also binds to the specific glutamate receptors but has the effect of antagonising (blocking) these receptors. This stops the inhibitory function of the receptors, which then allow apoptosis to continue. At the same time, mutant Htt binds to excessive quantities of HAP-1. HAP-1 can then become an inhibitor of huntingtin, blocking its normal role. The two proteins, Htt and excessive amounts of HAP-1, then bind to **IP3** receptors (for IP3 see Chapter 4). In response to this, the IP3 receptors (in the presence of inhibited glutamate receptors) cause Ca^{2+} (calcium) to be released from cellular stores, triggering cell apoptosis (Figure 13.6).

Apopain is a proteolytic enzyme (an enzyme for breaking down proteins), and this enzyme splits the normal huntingtin protein, a process that is increased with the mutant abnormal huntingtin protein (Figure 13.7). The result is the accumulation of huntingtin fragments, some of which form clumps inside the nucleus. These clumps within the nucleus are called **neuronal intranuclear inclusions (NII)**. They contain mutant huntingtin fragments together with accumulated **mammalian target of rapamycin (mTOR;** see Chapter 11 under Ketamine) and another protein called **ubiquitin**. MTOR is a protein kinase in two forms: **TOR complex-1 (TORC1)**, which regulates cell growth and proliferation and mRNA translation, and **TOR complex-2 (TORC2)**, which promotes cytoskeletal formation, cell survival, and the cell cycle. The presence of mTOR proteins promotes the destruction of the mutant Htt, therefore

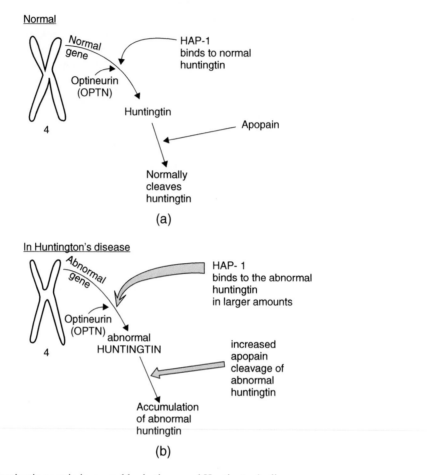

Figure 13.7 Huntingtin protein in normal brain tissue and Huntington's disease.

protecting the cell against the toxic effects of mutant Htt. Ubiquitin is a universal protein found throughout nature (the name comes from the word *ubiquitous*) and it appears to join with other proteins when those proteins are to be destroyed. It is one of the proteins found in the core of **Lewy bodies** (see Parkinson's disease, above). The presence of ubiquitin seems to slow down the process of cell damage and encourages the formation of NII as a means of tying up the harmful huntingtin fragments to help to prevent the damage (Quarrell 1999). However, these processes are probably only a delaying tactic, as the Htt continues to accumulate and these protective proteins fail to prevent the toxic effect of the mutant Htt. Promoting the functions of these protective proteins may be a mechanism for future therapy.

This means that there are several molecular processes that account for the possible effects we see in this disease (Figure 13.7):

- increased inhibition of huntingtin by HAP-1, allowing increased apoptosis;
- increased inhibition of specific glutamate receptors, which would normally help to block apoptosis;

- increased cleavage of huntingtin by apopain, resulting in damage to the nucleus;
- ultimate failure of the protective proteins to save the cell from damage and cell death.

Mitochondrial DNA damage is a feature found in ageing cells and contributes towards age-related neurodegeneration by reducing cellular energy levels. The ageing of mitochondrial DNA leading to damage is caused by **oxidative stress** within the cell (oxidative stress is discussed in relation to Alzheimer's disease, Chapter 14).

The formation of highly damaging oxidative species within the mitochondria is due to the nature of the mitochondrial role, i.e. energy production. Manufacturing **adenosine triphosphate (ATP)**, the high-energy molecule needed by all cells for energy purposes, generates oxygen-based radicals, which can damage DNA. Normally these radicals are neutralised by **antioxidants**. Raised concentrations of these oxygen-based radicals have been found in the cells of selective areas of the brain in HD, although the reason for this is not fully understood. Mutant Htt has also been shown to damage mitochondrial membranes, which causes disturbance to Ca^{2+} concentrations within the mitochondria, increasing the risk of cell death by calcium-induced **excitotoxicity**. This refers to neuronal cell death caused by activation of excitatory amino acid receptors, such as glutamate receptors. Mitochondrial DNA damage appears also to be implicated in the pathogenesis of not only Huntington's disease but also in Parkinson's disease and Alzheimer's disease (Yang et al. 2008).

Treatment of HD is not really an option at present. There is no cure and little in the way of drug treatment to improve the quality of life. **Tetrabenazine** can help to control the abnormal movements. This drug reduces dopamine synthesis in doperminergic neurons, but it has caused some patients to develop depression as a side effect. Possible new treatments are under development. The level of a particular lipid (or fat) called **monosialotetrahexosylganglioside (GM1**, a **ganglioside** found normally in the brain) is lower than normal in HD. GM1 is important for a number of cell functions, including myelination and myelin maintenance, cell to cell interactions, and calcium homeostasis within the cell. Low GM1 can contribute towards cell death. GM1 replacement has shown remarkable ability to restore normal movements during the early phases of research. Now clinical trials of GM1 are planned to see if the same excellent response occurs in people with HD.

Genetic testing has become available for families with HD, to see who in the family carries the gene and who does not. However, the implications of this are enormous, given the 100% penetrance of the gene (i.e. if present, the gene will definitely cause the disease). Any individual learning that they carry the gene will know that they will suffer and die from this disease. Worse still, they may have to live with the thought that they may have passed it on to their children. The only advantage would be for those who know they carry the gene and who are without children, as they would then have the ability to make a conscious decision whether or not to have children. It may be worth considering that sometimes not knowing is the better choice to take.

Wilson's disease and Harvey's disease

Wilson's disease

Dr S. A. Wilson (1878–1937) described a familial lenticular degeneration in 1912. Wilson's disease, as it was later called, is an autosomal recessive disorder of copper metabolism (Figure 13.8). The word *lenticular* refers to the **lentiform nucleus**, a combination of the

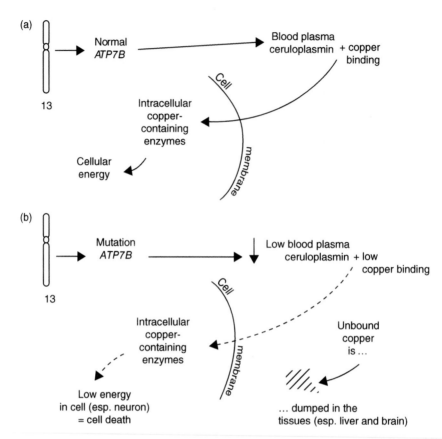

Figure 13.8 Wilson's disease. (a) Normal ceruloplasmin (coded by the *ATP7B* gene on chromosome 13) binds copper in the plasma and assists its movement into the cell. Here it is used by the enzymes that generate cellular energy. In Wilson's disease, (b) a gene error (mutation) causes low ceruloplasmin, and copper cannot enter the cell. The cell runs low on energy and the spare copper accumulates in the tissues, mostly the liver and the brain.

putamen and globus pallidus. The genetic problem is one of several possible mutations of the gene *ATP7B*, which is localised to 13q14.3–q21.1. The genetic error causes a reduction in the amount of a blood plasma component called **ceruloplasmin**. Ceruloplasmin is normally synthesised in the **Golgi apparatus** of cells, a structure within the cytoplasm that packages, modifies, and transports cellular products to a storage site within the cell or out of the cell altogether. Ceruloplasmin is involved in the transportation of copper into the cells, where it becomes integrated into copper-containing enzymes such as **cytochrome oxidase**. Cytochromes are proteins involved in the energy-producing chain found on the inner mitochondrial membrane. Ceruloplasmin is low in the majority of patients with this disorder. This prevents copper from entering the cell and being used to form enzymes, and that limits the cells' ability to generate energy. Cytochrome oxidase is usually found to be in a low state of activity in Wilson's disease. Copper that cannot enter the cells builds up in the body and is deposited in various tissues, notably the liver, the brain, and the eyes. The result is both neurological deficits and liver **cirrhosis** (i.e. hepatic **necrosis**, the death of liver cells).

The damage in the brain occurs mostly to the lenticular nuclei, and some degree of cerebral dementia can occur. Symptoms include severe involuntary movements at a young age (10–25 years), leading to progressive mental deterioration. Liver failure occurs later in the course of the disease. Unlike brain cells, liver cells are able to regenerate to a certain extent, so the effects of liver involvement are not felt until the disease is more advanced. **Hypercalciuria**, excessive calcium in the urine, is seen in many cases of Wilson's disease and is sometimes found early, before the neurological symptoms occur. It is due to **renal tubular acidosis**, a kidney problem in which the proximal tubule fails to control bicarbonate excretion. The excessive renal calcium can cause stones (or **renal calculi**) to form in the kidneys.

Treatment of Wilson's disease is based on the administration of a **chelating agent** called **penicillamine**. Chelating agents form soluble molecular compounds with a metal. Penicillamine forms a compound with the excess copper, and this promotes the elimination of copper from the body. If it is treated early enough, all further progress of the disease can be halted. However, the damage already done cannot be repaired. Patients intolerant of penicillamine can be treated with the drug **trientine**.

History: the strange case of Harvey's disease

During training as a psychiatric student nurse between 1965 and 1968 at Bexley Hospital, Kent (now closed, demolished, and redeveloped), the author was allocated to a ward called East Hospital. On arrival at this ward, the author was instructed to read a certain set of notes belonging to a patient who was on the ward at that time. The patient was suffering a form of genetically inherited subcortical dementia, which was only present in that one family. The disease had already killed everyone else in his family and our patient was the last family member to die. On his death, the disease would never be seen again as the gene was not passed on to any other generation, nor found in any other family. This was then a very rare example of a genetic disorder becoming extinct.

The symptoms were similar to those of Parkinson's disease or Wilson's disease, but the copper metabolism was normal. The patient had lost his speech; his mouth was held open and was filled with a handkerchief. He had a very unsteady stiff gait, walking almost on tiptoes, and falling over frequently due to the imbalance caused when the legs could not keep up with the top half of the body.

On the ward his condition was named after him with the family name of Harvey. However, the author has never been able to find any publication concerning this now extinct condition. Surely it must have occurred to a doctor at that time, given the uniqueness of the case, that publication of a paper describing the disease would be useful. Apparently not, and this very brief history, based as it is on the author's memory of the events, may be the only published record of this genetic disease that killed an entire family.

Key points

The basal ganglia

- The subcortical dementias, essentially degeneration of the basal ganglia, are often associated with depression and psychoses.
- The basal ganglia form part of a loop that regulates motor function. This loop consists of the frontal cortex, the corpus striatum, the globus pallidus, the substantia nigra pars reticulata, the thalamus, and back to the frontal lobe.

Parkinson's disease

- Muscle rigidity and tremor of the limbs are the classic signs of Parkinson's disease.
- The symptoms of Parkinson's disease are caused by a gradual loss of the substantia nigra cells. Muscle tone therefore increases unopposed.
- The nigrostriatal pathway develops very low dopamine concentrations, below a threshold of 60% loss of dopamine, before symptoms of the disease occur.
- The low dopamine level causes inhibition of the thalamic role in modifying control of movement by the frontal lobe.
- Both genetic and environmental factors are involved in the cause of this disease.
- Levodopa replaces dopamine in the nigrostriatal pathway and thus improves the quality of life. Long-term problems of levodopa have largely been overcome by multiple drug therapy.
- Carers must be aware of the constant risk of falls in PD patients due to their instability while walking, which is the result of a forward stance combined with a shuffling gait.

Huntington disease

- Huntington's disease is an autosomal dominant inherited disorder characterised by a deterioration of the corpus striatum caused by a mutation of a gene on chromosome 4.
- The main signs of Huntington's disease are involuntary jerky movements called chorea, speech loss, and intellectual decline.
- The gene mutation is a trinucleotide repeat of the bases CAG (cytosine–adenine–guanine), which causes a glutamine tail repeat sequence on the normal huntingtin protein.
- Accumulations of abnormal huntingtin protein fragments in the neuron nucleus and loss of normal huntingtin from the cytoplasm probably cause the cellular degeneration.

Wilson's disease

- Wilson's disease is a familial lenticular degeneration caused by an autosomal recessive gene that results in disorder of copper metabolism.
- Mutations of the gene *ATP7B* cause a reduction in the amount of ceruloplasmin in blood, which disturbs copper transport into neurons.
- Energy-producing enzymes that use copper fail to function.
- The result is both neurological deficits, caused by damage to the lenticular nuclei, and liver cirrhosis.
- Treatment of Wilson's disease is with the drug penicillamine, which promotes the elimination of copper from the body.

Harvey's disease

- Harvey's disease may have been a very rare example of a familial genetic basal ganglia degenerative disorder that became extinct in the 1960s when the last affected member of the family died.

References

Aird, T. (2000) Functional anatomy of the basal ganglia. *Journal of Neuroscience Nursing,* **32** (5): 250–253.

Borrell, E. (2000) Hypokinetic movement disorders. *Journal of Neuroscience Nursing,* **32** (5): 254–255.

Carlson, N. (2012) *Physiology of Behaviour* (11th edition). Pearson Education, Harlow, UK.

Crabb, L. (2001) Sleep disorders in Parkinson's disease: the nursing role. *British Journal of Nursing*, **10** (1): 42–47.

Gray, P. and Hildebrand, K. (2000) Fall risk factors in Parkinson's disease. *Journal of Neuroscience Nursing*, **32** (4): 222–228.

Herndon, C. M., Young, K., Herndon, A. D., and Dole, E. J. (2000) Parkinson's disease revisited. *Journal of Neuroscience Nursing*, **32** (4): 216–221.

Hofmann, N. (1999) Understanding the neuropsychiatric symptoms of Huntington's disease. *Journal of Neuroscience Nursing*, **31** (5): 309–313.

Nowak, R. (2000) Early warning for Parkinson's. *New Scientist*, **168** (2266): 14.

Quarrell, O. (1999) *Huntington's Disease, The Facts*. Oxford University Press, Oxford, UK.

Yang, J.-L., Weissman, L., Bohr, V., and Mattson, M. P. (2008) Mitochondrial DNA damage and repair in neurodegenerative disorders. *DNA Repair (Amst.)*, **7** (7): 1110–1120.

14 The ageing brain and dementia

- The hippocampus and memory
- The natural ageing brain
- The dementias
- Alzheimer's disease
- The molecular neurobiology of Alzheimer's disease
- Dementia with cortical Lewy bodies
- Pick's disease
- The drugs used in dementia
- Key points

The hippocampus and memory

The hippocampus is situated within the hippocampal fissure, close to the **parahippocampal gyrus**, part of the temporal lobes on both sides (see Chapter 1 and Figures 1.4, 9.1, 10.3, 10.4 and 10.5) (Blows 2000). This area is sometimes called the **hippocampal complex** or **hippocampal formation**, because several structures occur close together and have many interconnections with each other. The components of the complex are:

- the **dentate gyrus**, the innermost cell layer of the hippocampus;
- **Ammon's horn** (see Figure 10.3, Chapter 10), another part of the hippocampus, consisting also of a layer of neurons that can be subdivided into four areas, **CA1**, **CA2**, **CA3**, and **CA4** (where *CA* means *cornu Ammonis*, or 'Ammon's horn');
- the **subiculum**, also included in the hippocampus by some authors;
- the **entorhinal cortex**, which lies between the subiculum and the perirhinal cortex (see Figure 10.3);
- the **perirhinal cortex**, which lies between the entorhinal cortex and the parahippocampal cortex (Figure 10.3);
- the **parahippocampal cortex**, the outermost component of the complex (see Figures 9.1, 10.3).

The connections between these areas and with other parts of the brain are:

- afferent (incoming) pathways into the entorhinal cortex from the **cingulum**;
- afferent pathways into the entorhinal cortex from the major sensory association areas of the cortex, e.g. visual, auditory, **somatosensory** (i.e. from the body), and **gustatory** (taste) areas;

- the **perforant pathway**, from the entorhinal cortex to Ammon's horn and dentate gyrus;
- the **alvear pathway**, from the entorhinal cortex to Ammon's horn;
- the **mossy fibre pathway**, from the dentate gyrus to CA3 of Ammon's horn;
- the **Schaffer collateral pathway**, from CA3 to CA1 of Ammon's horn;
- efferent (outgoing) pathways via the **fornix** (the main axonal pathways leaving the hippocampus) to areas of the frontal cortex, thalamus, and the hypothalamus (especially the **mammillary bodies**).

The hippocampus has several important roles. These include the conversion of **short-term memory** to **long-term memory** (which is closely related to learning) and influencing thinking through connections with the frontal cortex. It also has a part to play in emotions, especially the regulation of **aggression**. It is closely linked to the adrenal hormone cortisol, regulating cortisol release via the hypothalamus and pituitary gland pathway. Cortisol is the hormone that is increased during stress, so the hippocampus is also part of the brain's normal stress response.

Memory

There are several ways of classifying memory, one way being the division into **long-term memory** and **short-term memory**, i.e. the difference between remembering events that took place 20 years ago and events that happened 20 minutes ago. Another way to classify memory is the division into **explicit memory** and **implicit memory**, i.e. the difference between memory that comes with *conscious thought* – for example, trying to remember Aunt Edith's telephone number – and *automatic* or *subconscious* memory – for example, finding the way from your bedroom to the bathroom at home. These classifications are roughly correlated, in that long-term memory is broadly implicit, whereas short-term memory is more likely to be explicit. The term *commit to memory* implies a shift of memorised facts or skills from explicit to implicit memory; that is, making the memory automatic or long term. This is achieved by *rehearsal* of the facts or skill, often many times, in much the same way as an actor memorises the lines of a play, a pianist prepares for a concert, or a tennis player practises for a match. There is no substitute for the rehearsal of facts; it is crucial for all implicit (or long-term) memory activities, such as taking examinations. It is the basis of the *learning process*, an essential ingredient of success for all aspiring actors, pianists, and tennis stars, as well as those hoping to pass examinations.

At a biochemical level, memory is the result of neurons producing and maintaining first a short-term memory, then in some cases creating long-term memory in the form of a **long-term potentiation (LTP)**. Initially, the sensory stimulus increases activity in the enzyme **adenyl cyclase (AC)**, which then increases the amount of available **cyclic adenosine monophosphate (cAMP)** (see Chapter 4, Figures 4.2 and 4.3). cAMP activates the enzyme **protein kinase (PK)**, which changes the electrical activity of the presynaptic membrane. This is the basis of a short-term memory. PK also enters the nucleus of the neuron and activates **cyclic AMP-responsive element-binding protein (CREB)**, which causes specific gene activation. These proteins then form new and stronger synapses. These are permanent (or at least semi-permanent) changes in the synapse that allow for enhanced impulse transmission between pre- and postsynaptic neurons both ways across the synaptic cleft, i.e. the basis of long-term memory. This means that the changes appear to allow for **retrograde** impulses to cross back from the postsynaptic to the presynaptic membranes. It occurs in the hippocampus and other parts of the brain as a result of increased levels of activation or repetition by a specific excitatory action potential (or stimuli). The formation of this LTP change, i.e. a state of heightened stimulation in the synaptic membrane that occurs each time a specific impulse arrives, also requires the function of glutamate acting on AMPA and NMDA receptors, and the presence of calcium. A similar, but depressive (inhibitory), effect on the synapse is called **long-term depression** (**LTD**, not to be confused with the disorder called depression). Between them, LTP and LTD may provide the synaptic mechanism for **declarative memory**, i.e. memory of facts and events.

The brains that are best suited to learning and memory are the brains of children (see Chapter 2). All the anatomy of the brain is in place at birth, but the nervous system is far from mature at that point. The development of the nervous system involves the formation of new synaptic connections; this continues throughout childhood until puberty, and learning is a major part of this process. The bulk of synaptic formation occurs during the childhood years, and this is exactly the time when the brain is best suited to forming the permanent proteins and synapses needed for memory. Adult brains are somewhat more resistant to this kind of change, although of course learning does take place at any age.

Long-term memory is not found in one place in the brain; many areas serve to store information that can be retrieved when required – the so-called **working memory**. However, the conscious working memory is primarily the role of the frontal lobes – the prefrontal cortex particularly. Here, memory and thought work together on matters that concern us at any particular moment. The prefrontal cortex is vital for the memory needed for spatial tasks, remembering objects, self-ordered tasks, and analytical reasoning. Input into this frontal lobe activity is via the hippocampus. With the retrieval of short-term memory at its disposal, and with the influence it has on thinking and emotions, the hippocampus is a powerful tool in the processing of thought. It is not surprising that problems arising with the hippocampus seriously disrupt not only memory, but also the whole ability to think properly.

Declarative memory is divided into **semantic memory**, i.e. the raw facts and figures, and **episodic memory**, the context in which these facts and figures occur. For example:

- **Semantic** = 9 is a number; **episodic** = 9 is the ninth numerate in a set sequence of numerates that start at 1.
- **Semantic** = fish have gills; **episodic** = fish have gills, which are part of a system by which these animals extract oxygen from the environment.

Hippocampal memory appears to be the result of LTPs in CA1, and to a lesser extent in CA3 of Ammon's horn. Damage to these cell layers appears to impair episodic memory and cause **anterograde amnesia** (i.e. memory loss occurring after some form of brain injury). To lose *all* declarative memory requires lesions of the brain that involve both the limbic areas of the medial temporal lobe and the hippocampus. In fact, lesions anywhere, from the hippocampus through the fornix to the mammillary bodies and anterior thalamus, can disrupt memory. It would appear that this circuit is critical in the formation and recall of memories (Figure 14.1).

The relevance of all this to dementia is that mild memory loss can be due to **mild cognitive impairment** (**MCI**), which increases the risk of that individual developing dementia. MCI can be either memory losses (called **amnestic MCI**) or losses of skills other than memory (called **non-amnestic MCI**). The pathology of MCI is complex, involving multiple factors, but significantly it includes neurofibril formations within the entorhinal cortex, hippocampus, and amygdala and excessive activity within the CA3

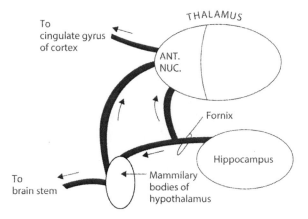

To
cingulate gyrus
of cortex

THALAMUS

ANT.
NUC.

Fornix

Hippocampus

To
brain stem

Mammilary
bodies of
hypothalamus

Figure 14.1 Connections of the hippocampus important in memory. Ant. Nuc. is the anterior nucleus.

cells of the hippocampus. Loss of the synapses and ultimately death of neurons adds to the problem, accelerating the sufferer further toward dementia. A single neuron can have hundreds of synapses, so the loss of key neurons in the brain is likely to interfere with memory significantly. This loss primarily affects short-term memory, as long-term memory is better preserved. During these early stages of dementia, patients can remember where they were in the Second World War, but can't remember what they had for breakfast that morning. Eventually, as dementia gets worse, long-term memory is affected. What education in childhood has created, dementia can ultimately destroy.

The natural ageing brain

Like all organs, the brain changes naturally as a result of the ageing process (Figure 14.2), but the functions of the brain can often be retained to extreme late age in many people. This shows the remarkable compensation the brain is able to undergo (known as **plasticity**), which demonstrates that dementia is not inevitable.

Age-related neuron losses vary not only between individuals but also between different parts of the brain in the same individual. Naturally occurring neuron loss can begin as early as 23 years of age, but this is very slow at first, increasing after 60 years of age. Rarely, the total losses of neurons could be, in the worst case scenario, as much as 40% – the equivalent of just less than half the brain lost – and yet good cerebral activity can be retained. The 40% figure is very rare, and the majority of people would sustain far less neuron loss than this. Whatever the losses, the retention of good brain function is the most important point. A very good example of excellent cerebral function in late age is the remarkable English composer Havergal Brian, who wrote *20 symphonies* between the ages of 81 and 92 years old – an amazing feat of late-age brain activity.

It was thought for many years that neurons were the type of cell that was incapable of replication after birth, so that losses could not be replaced. For the majority of neurons this is still the case. However, humans are now known to be capable of neuronal replication in a few brain locations, e.g. the dentate gyrus of the hippocampus, after birth. Where neuron losses do occur, this may be attributed to reduced blood flow to the brain caused by age-related

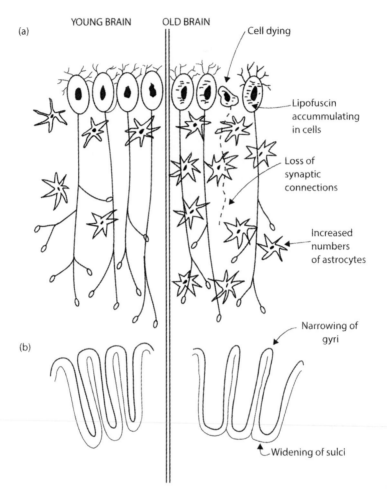

Figure 14.2 The brain gets old. (a) Left is the young brain, but on the right the brain shows cell losses with corresponding synaptic losses, increased astrocytes and lipofuscin deposits in the neurons. (b) Narrowing of the gyri and widening of the sulci is a gross anatomical change in the elderly brain.

changes in the arteries that supply the head. Neurons are sensitive to glucose and oxygen and will deteriorate and finally die when faced with a decline in the glucose and oxygen supply. Each neuron can have hundreds of synaptic connections, so one neuron lost can account for the loss of many synapses. Synapses are vital for memory and learning. The neocortex loses glutamate synapses from around the age of 23 onwards, with about 20% lost by the age of 70 years. Some 40% or so of the glutamate synapses could be lost from the hippocampus with age.

Sustaining good cerebral blood and oxygen flow reduces neuronal losses and improves the brain's ability to compensate for those losses that do occur. Therefore using the brain may be beneficial in preventing neuronal losses, since stimulated areas of the brain use and receive more blood and therefore keep the brain active until a late age.

Neuronal losses are part of the reason for the brain's loss of protein in old age. About 15% of the protein in the brain is lost between the ages of 35 and 70 years, and this is partly responsible for the reduction of brain weight with age, from about 1400 grams in a male aged 20 down to 1200 grams in the same male aged 80. In contrast, both the volume of extracellular water and the number of astrocytes in the brain *increase* with age, and the ventricles within the brain gradually enlarge. The cerebral cortex shrinks and shows a widening of the **sulci** and a narrowing of the **gyri** (see Chapter 1), with atrophy of the frontal lobes predominating. **Lipofuscin**, an age-related pigment derived from lipid, is deposited inside the ageing cells of the brain and elsewhere. The amount varies in different parts of the brain. Apart from lipids, lipofuscin contains sugars and several metals, including zinc, copper, aluminum, mercury, and iron. Several of these metals are known neurotoxic agents, notably mercury. The presence of lipofuscin deposits in tissues is not only related to age but is also linked to Alzheimer's disease (AD) and Parkinson's disease (PD). Several neuro-degenerative disorders, called **lipofuscinoses**, are also caused by lipofuscin, e.g. **Batten's disease**. This autosomal disorder starts slowly in childhood (between 4 and 10 years of age) with visual difficulties and fits. These children develop motor instability with stumbling and gradual loss of motor skills, resulting in immobility. The fits gradually get worse, cognitive abilities decline, and speech is slowly lost. Dementia and blindness are usually followed by an early death.

The brain's chemistry also changes with age; **noradrenaline** and **dopamine** concentrations slowly decline in some parts, and this has been linked to depression in some elderly persons. Some ageing cells, both neurons and astrocytes, can produce **free radicals** (also called **reactive oxygen species, ROS**) from their metabolism, and these chemicals, based on oxygen, damage cell membranes and other structures, including deoxyribonucleic acid (DNA). This process is called **cell senescence**, and these cells can export these dangerous chemicals, thus damaging other healthy cells nearby.

Factors affecting brain ageing and dementia

The following are some other good or bad factors that affect ageing of the brain, and dementia risk:

- Cognitive stimulation of the brain in the form of new learning retains good brain connections, preserves neurons (especially in the hippocampus), and strengthens pathways well into late old age. In fact, people exposed to new learning showed less amyloid plaque formation, a hallmark of dementia. 'Brain-training exercises' may be useful in this regard, but there is, so far, little evidence either way on these. Retirement is an ideal opportunity to seek out new sensory and learning experiences, e.g. new skills and subjects, and undertake projects that stimulate mental activity. But don't wait for retirement – new learning should be a lifelong endeavour. In this context, the age-old saying 'use it or lose it' really does apply.
- Maintenance of normal blood glucose is linked to preservation of good cognitive activity. High blood glucose concentration, especially in relation to **diabetes type 2**, is linked to cognitive decline (there are 3.2 million type 2 diabetics in the UK currently, and this number is rising). Poorly controlled diabetes causes brain ageing five times faster than in nondiabetics, and suffering diabetes over a 20-year period during mid-life can cause a 19% greater decrease in cognitive function than that seen in nondiabetics. Peaks and troughs in blood glucose concentrations have been shown to cause damage to the dentate

gyrus in the hippocampus, and thus affect memory. This all suggests that impaired insulin signalling though the insulin cell surface receptors in the brain damages neurons and results in their loss. A protein called **glucagon-like peptide-1 (GLP-1)** appears to be involved in both insulin receptor signalling and new neuron production, and a new experimental drug known as **(VAL8)GLP-1** promotes new neuron growth in the memory areas of the brain. The drug **liraglutide** binds to GLP-1 receptors, activating these receptors and causing increased insulin release while suppressing glucagon secretion. It is currently in use as a treatment for diabetes type 2 but has been found to reverse the symptoms of dementia by about 30%.

- People with high blood **cholesterol** (i.e. higher than 6 millimols per litre) have a 50% greater risk of AD compared with those having low blood cholesterol.
- Coffee, cocoa, and tea appear to be growing in importance as healthy drinks. They contain chemicals called **flavanols,** which improve blood flow to the hippocampus, especially the dentate gyrus. This reduces those forgetful moments (or so-called **senior moments**) and are said to have a protective role against age-related mental decline, which is caused by loss of synapses, not whole neurons. They may also help to protect against depression, AD (see page 315), and PD (see Chapter 13).
- **Resveratrol** is an antioxidant with anti-inflammatory properties found in grapes, red wine, and some berries. It appears to have neuroprotective, anticancer, and life-extending properties, but the full extent of these properties in humans has not been quantified.
- Smoking and alcohol drunk to excess are both linked to a faster than average decline in cognitive ability and is a serious risk factor for dementia in old age. Those indulging in these habits have shown that onset of dementia is, on average, about 8.5 years earlier than would otherwise have happened.
- The use of some drugs in **chemotherapy** (i.e. anticancer drugs) have sometimes caused a state of cognitive dysfunction often called 'chemo fog', or 'chemo brain'. This includes headaches, confusion, and impaired memory, which may last for years after the chemotherapy is stopped. Brain scans show microstructure damage to the white matter of the corpus callosum and several other brain pathways, and lower than normal levels of response from the prefrontal cortex (see Chapter 1) and parahippocampal gyrus (see Chapter 10) in postchemotherapy patients.
- Contrary to this, an anticancer drug called **bexarotene** has been shown to reduce the protein **amyloid** from animal brains with resulting cognitive improvement, and it may prove useful for humans.
- **Benzodiazepine** drugs (e.g. **diazepam** and **lorazepam**), which are commonly prescribed for insomnia, are now linked to a 50% increase in the risk of developing AD. This effect occurs if the drugs are taken for 3 months or more, which supports the concept that these drugs should be prescribed for short-term use only, i.e. 4 weeks maximum.
- **Meditation** (Luders et al. 2015) and exercise appear to have a brain preservation effect, reducing age-related cognitive decline and neuron losses. The reasons for this are not fully understood. Exercising at least twice per week in mid-life reduces the risk of dementia 20 years later, but even exercise during old age improves cognitive abilities. The result of this exercise is to increase brain activity and improve glucose uptake by neurons during memory-related tasks.
- Relaxation is also recommended as a means of retaining good cognitive function in older people, as stress-induced cortisol can shrink some brain areas with corresponding

loss of function. Those with a calm and relaxed approach to life have a 50% lower risk of developing dementia.

- Sleeping on your side may improve your brain function. This relates to the mechanism for removing toxic proteins from the brain during sleep (see Chapter 16). This position appears to be more efficient at removing unwanted proteins from the brain than laying on your back or front.

- High levels of the amino acid **homocysteine** have been found in the blood of AD sufferers and very high levels found in non-sufferers appear to increase their risk of developing the disease (Smith et al. 1998). Homocysteine is not obtained from the diet; instead it is regularly produced from the combination of another amino acid called **methionine** (which is derived from protein in the diet) with **adenosine** from **adenosine triphosphate (ATP)**, the high-energy molecule found all cells. Part of this combination is used in the metabolism of adrenaline and in the normal function of DNA. What is left is converted to homocysteine, a destructive amino acid that must be rendered harmless. The body does this by turning much of this homocysteine either back into methionine with the help of **vitamin B_{12}** (called **cyanocobalamin**) or into **cysteine** with the help of **vitamin B_6**. **Folic acid** (also called **folate**) is **vitamin B_9** and is also involved in this process. If the blood concentrations of these vitamins are low, homocysteine concentrations build up in the blood as its conversion declines. High homocysteine concentrations appear to be very toxic to nerve cells and blood vessels, increasing the risk of AD. Low concentrations of vitamin B_{12} and folate in the circulation suggests that there is a lack of these nutrients in the person's diet. Reducing the concentrations of homocysteine may be achievable by increasing the dietary intake of these vitamins. However, it is not entirely clear whether the high levels of homocysteine are a cause of AD or whether they are perhaps the effect of early AD before any symptoms occur (i.e. when it is asymptomatic). Evidence points more towards the former, but caution is urged before anyone considers taking any vitamin supplements. Excess vitamins can themselves be harmful, and a balanced diet would normally provide all the body's needs.

- A lack of **vitamin D (D_3 = cholecalciferol)** is now linked to two or three times faster cognitive decline in older adults compared with those having normal vitamin D concentrations. Those subjects with low vitamin D showed loss of episodic memory and decision-making abilities quite quickly, and demonstrated a decline in their general cognitive abilities. An appropriate diet rich in vitamin D, and regular vitamin D checks with prescribed supplementation if required, would be a useful strategy for everyone over 60 years.

- **Blood group AB** people carry an 82% greater risk than the other blood groups of developing age-related cognitive decline. The mechanism for this is currently unknown and requires further study.

The dementias

Dementia means 'loss of mind' and is one of two mind-destroying disorders, the other being schizophrenia. The cost of dementia in lives is already high, but it is destined to get higher. There are currently about 850,000 people with dementia in the UK, and 500,000 of them are women (approximately 62%). By 2025, the projected number of dementia sufferers in the UK is more than 1 million, and more than 2 million by 2050. The risk of developing dementia doubles every 5 years after the age of 65. Clearly, there is a great need to find answers to this devastating disorder, as it is reaching epidemic proportions.

314 The ageing brain and dementia

There are key risk factors for dementia, which include age, diabetes, smoking, midlife obesity, high blood pressure, and high serum cholesterol (see above). But dementia can also be caused by: brain damage from a head injury; cerebral infections; reduced blood flow to the brain; compression of the brain from a **space-occupying lesion** (**SOL**); or from a bio-chemical imbalance. Vascular disease caused by ageing arteries, which reduces the arterial blood supply to the brain (i.e. **cerebral ischemia**), often causes areas of cerebrum to die (i.e. **cerebral infarcts**), and accounts for about 15–25% of dementia cases. Starved of blood, the oxygen-sensitive neurons die and may be replaced with scar tissue. Trauma (head injury) accounts for only about 3% of dementias, but is important in relation to sports injuries. **Traumatic brain injury** (TBI) is a growing concern, in athletics, football, and boxing in particular, where the risk of repetitive head injuries is high. TBI can be anything from **mild traumatic brain injury** (**MTBI**, also known as **concussion**) to severe. But it is the repeti-tive nature of this type of injury that is most worrying. The person returns to their sport after recovery from a first injury only to sustain further subsequent injuries. Multiple repeated minor injuries are known to cause long-term neurological problems, resulting in a higher than expected risk of dementia, depression, and death at an early age.

At a molecular level some of the reasons why brain cells die, leading to dementia, are becom-ing evident. The **telomere** is a stretch of **DNA** that normally lies beyond the length of the genes at the end of a chromosome. Being outside the gene sequence, the telomere would appear to be of no genetic value. However, it was found that normally the telomere shortens with each cell division, and at a critical point it becomes so short that it triggers cell death. It also shortens in response to cellular stress. In patients suffering from non-Alzheimer's dementia, the telomere was shorter than people of the same age without dementia. Those with long telomeres suffered less cognitive decline than others of the same age with shorter telomeres.

As an indication of the variety of dementias occurring, a list of some types are included here:

- **attentional dementia** with some loss of arousal of the conscious mind;
- **intentional dementia** with loss of vigilance;
- **cognitive dementia** with a loss of remote memory;
- **amnestic dementia** with a loss of recent memory;
- **multi-infarct dementia**, caused by a number of minor strokes;
- **Binswanger's disease** (also called **subcortical arteriosclerotic encephalopathy**), a subcortical degeneration of the brain's white matter, which may be due to **hyperten-sion** (high blood pressure) in some cases, which causes vascular disease in the brain and white matter destruction;
- **dementia with cortical Lewy bodies** (**DCLB**) (about 10% of dementias);
- **Pick's disease**, dementia with characteristic cortical Pick bodies (see page 327);
- **Hashimoto's encephalopathy**, a rare autoimmune neuroendocrine disorder, in which antibodies attack the brain cells, causing a range of symptoms (e.g. confusion, short-term memory loss, disorientation) that can be misdiagnosed as other disorders, especially AD;
- **primary age-related tauopathy** (**PART**), similar to AD but with a pathology that affects the tau protein only, with no plaque involvement (see Alzheimer's disease, below) – symptoms are likely to be confused with AD, leading to a misdiagnosis;
- **Susac's syndrome**, a rare autoimmune disorder in which antibodies attack the inner lin-ing of blood vessels in the brain, inner ears, and retina of the eye – the result is acute confusion with memory loss, unusual behaviour, dizziness, blurred vision, and progres-sive deafness (Star et al. 2015);

- **posterior cortical atrophy**, a rare form of progressive dementia that causes deterioration of the visual cortex (occipital lobe) before affecting memory;
- **Alzheimer's disease (AD)**, a form of dementia with characteristic brain changes of plaques and tangles, which accounts for about 45% of dementias.

Alzheimer's disease

Alois Alzheimer (1864–1915) was a German psychiatrist who in 1906 described a dementia with two specific changes found in the brain after death. These changes were the presence of *extracellular* **plaques** and *intracellular* **neurofibrillary tangles (NFTs)** and these became the hallmarks of this disease.

Two main forms of AD are recognised: **early-age onset** AD (before 65 years) showing a family history of inherited genetic origin (i.e. **familial Alzheimer's disease, FAD**) and a **late-age onset** AD (after 65 years) of less genetic and more sporadic origin. This disorder has been, and still is, the subject of intensive research for several reasons. First, the pathology of AD is related to other brain-destructive disorders such as PD and Huntington's disease. Advances in the understanding of one of these disorders has provided valuable insights into the others (see mitochondrial DNA, Chapter 13). Second, there is a very interesting link between AD and **Down syndrome**. Third, the devastation caused by this disease, both to the patient and to the family, is catastrophic, as it usually occurs at a time of life when an ageing partner is ill equipped to care for a spouse with advanced dementia. It reduces formerly highly intelligent people to a pitiful state, with no hope of recovery. The fear that any of us could end our days in this manner drives research forward in an attempt to prevent the tragedy. Estimates put the number of AD sufferers in the UK at around 400,000, with this figure set to rise significantly with the ageing population.

Dementia causes memory losses and erosion of personality; relatives say that the patient is nothing like their former self. Mood changes with emotional blunting occur, with abnormal and inappropriate behaviour, especially restless wandering at any time of the day or night and getting lost in familiar places. Dementia sufferers ask the same questions and tell the same stories repeatedly. They rely on others to make decisions (Shurkin 2009). People with dementia develop a state of self-neglect and need everything done for them. One important form of self-neglect is that these people may suffer from a lack of adequate nutrition. Several factors combine to cause this, including memory losses (e.g. when to eat, how to prepare food), inadequate supervision by family carers or hospital staff, poor oral hygiene, and constipation. Carers can improve the person's overall state of health by effective interventions to maintain a healthy mouth and bowels, and by ensuring that nutritious meals are eaten by the patient daily (Biernacki and Barratt 2001).

Anything from 1 to 4 years prior to the diagnosis of AD, the individual goes through a period of *mild cognitive impairment*. This involves a range of problems, from occasional memory lapses to poor decision-making. Memory loss and confusion are perhaps the problems for which the more advanced stages of this disorder are best known. **Amnesia** (memory loss) at first is primarily short term. **Confusion** is not uncommon in the elderly in any case, and is often *acute*, i.e. relatively short-lived and caused by a physical problem that may be easily corrected, such as constipation, sleep loss, fever, or a drug side effect. Other, more difficult conditions that can cause confusion, especially in the elderly, are: cardiac, renal, or liver failure; blood glucose instability in diabetes; other endocrine and metabolic disorders, such as acidosis, epilepsy, vitamin deficiencies, malnutrition, or dehydration; post-anaesthetic or other drug withdrawal; head injury; brain tumours; or stress. Confusion that is persistent, after all the physical causes have been eliminated, may be a sign of dementia.

The molecular neuropathology of Alzheimer's disease

AD is a progressive deterioration of brain function associated with neuronal losses. Before the age of 65 about 1% of the population are sufferers, and by the age of 85 the figure is 10% of the population. The devastating effects of the disease on the individual and their family, together with a proportional increase in the elderly population resulting in greater numbers of people suffering from the disease, makes it a major mental health problem. After years of difficulties, much progress has now been achieved in understanding the pathology of AD, and it is expected that research will continue to make strides towards prevention of its worst effects.

The plaques

The plaques described by Alzheimer are made from the central core of an abnormal **amyloid** protein called **beta-amyloid (Aβ42**, which is 42 amino acids long). Normally **Aβ42** exists in very small quantities in the brain, but it accumulates in large amounts in AD, hence the abnormality. Amyloid levels in the brain fluctuate according to a circadian rhythm (i.e. a cycle of amyloid production taking about 24 hours to complete), which is controlled by **orexin** (see also eating disorders, Chapter 9) (Kang et al. 2009). The cycle causes higher levels of amyloid to occur when awake and lower levels when asleep, leading to speculation that abnormalities in orexin or its production may lead to insomnia, which could increase the risk of AD (see also Factors affecting brain ageing and dementia, on page 311, and Chapter 16).

A large gene on chromosome 21 called the *APP* gene (Figure 14.3) codes for the normal **amyloid β precursor protein (APP)**. The primary function of APP is in synaptogenesis and synaptic repair after damage. Other functions have been suggested but supported by only limited evidence. In the cell body, APP is found associated with the **endoplasmic reticulum (ER)** of the neuron, where it normally undergoes cleavage (i.e. being cut by enzymes) into the **Aβ40** and **Aβ42** forms (**Aβ40** has 40 amino acids long, i.e. a shorter chain version than the **Aβ42**) (Figure 14.4). Cleavage of APP is carried out by two enzymes, **beta-secretase** and **gamma-secretase. Presenilin 1 (PSEN1** or **PS1)** and **presenilin 2 (PSEN2** or **PS2)** are the APP cleavage components of the enzyme **gamma-secretase**. The genes for coding the PS1 and PS2 proteins are on chromosome 14 (PS1) and chromosome 1 (PS2). More is known about PS1 than about PS2. PS1 attaches across the ER membrane, influencing APP cleavage within the ER. PS2 may bind to APP and affect its cleavage by this means.

One further gene involved is the **17-beta-hydroxysteroid dehydrogenase X (***HSD17B10***)** (formerly the *ERAB* gene, abbreviated from **endoplasmic-reticulum associated binding protein)** on chromosome X (Xp11.2). It codes for a mitochondrial **dehydrogenase enzyme** that catalyses (i.e. breaks down) a wide range of fatty acids, alcohol, and steroids as part of energy production. This enzyme is overproduced in neurons during AD and interacts with beta-amyloid. In AD, it also relocates to the plasma membrane and is probably involved in the export of amyloid from the cell into the plaques.

In **FAD**, mutations within the *APP* (chromosome 21), *PSEN1* (chromosome 14), *PSEN2* (chromosome 1), and *HSD17B10* (chromosome X) genes cause errors in the proteins that these genes code for, leading to mistakes in the way these proteins function. Mutations are

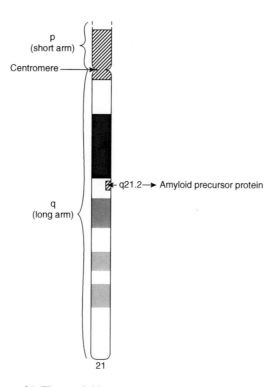

Figure 14.3 Chromosome 21. The amyloid precursor protein (*APP*) gene is at 21q21.2.

abnormal changes in the DNA within the chromosome, thus creating abnormal proteins. In the case of the *APP* gene the mutation results in excessive APP protein, whereas mutations in the *PSEN1* and *PSEN2* genes cause errors in the cleavage of APP, causing excess of the abnormal Aβ42 form. The combination of all three mutations results in large accumulations (**plaques**) of the **Aβ42 protein oligomers** (molecules of low molecular weight made from no more than five monomer units) collect around neurons and white matter. This Aβ42 must find its way out of the neuron to become extracellular plaques. Mutations of the *HSD17B10* gene may be involved in this process. Once accumulated between the neurons, Aβ42 plaques allow for the development of abnormal glial cell production and accumulation (called a **gliosis**, mostly of **astrocytes**), especially around blood vessels (**perivascular gliosis**). If the astrocytes identify that too much beta-amyloid is coming from a neuron the astrocytes can kill that neuron with a deadly combination of two substances, **ceramide** and the protein **prostate apoptosis response-4 (PAR-4)**, packaged together in lipid-coated vesicles. The plaques disrupt the ion channels in neuronal membranes, and therefore interfere with sodium, potassium, and calcium movements involved in nerve impulse conduction (see Chapter 3). Beta-amyloid plaques are linked to lower than normal levels of **acetylcholine**, which is the neurotransmitter used by neurons involved in learning and memory. Current drug treatment (see below) is aimed at restoring this loss of acetylcholine.

An enzyme called **12/15-lipoxygenase** influences the function of another enzyme, **beta-secretase** (see above), which is involved in beta-amyloid production. In AD, 12/15-lipoxygenase

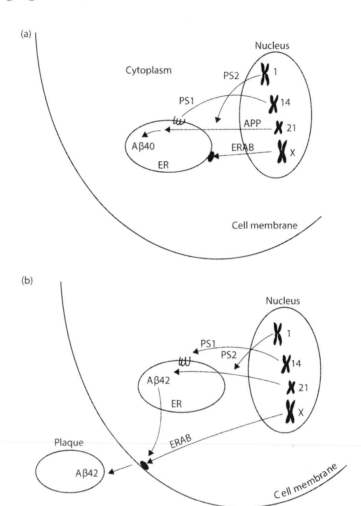

Figure 14.4 (a) Normal amyloid protein production, and (b) amyloid plaque formation outside the cell
in Alzheimer's disease. ER is the endoplasmic reticulum.

is overactive, resulting in excessive beta-amyloid production. Future drugs may include
compounds that block the activity of 12/15-lipoxygenase, thus restoring normal function of
beta-secretase (Chu et al. 2012).

The spread of beta amyloid plaques through the brain is a major developmental process of AD, and it appears that these plaques start in one place, the **epicentre**, and spread
to neighbouring neurons that have connections to the epicentre. This suggests that normal beta-amyloid in contact with abnormal beta-amyloid plaques gets converted to the
abnormal type and goes on to produce plaques. The abnormality in the protein involves
misfolding, i.e. the protein folds in an abnormal manner. It then becomes an agent capable
of causing misfolding of neighbouring proteins, and this process spreads slowly through

the brain. This is very similar to the spread of abnormal proteins called **proteinaceous infectious particles (prions** for short) in **Creuztfeldt–Jakob disease (CJD)**, in which prions
recruit other proteins to become prions when in contact with them. Eventually this process
spreads and large parts of the brain get involved. The patient goes into intellectual decline
and it finally leads to their death. In AD, the pathology is very similar. Some of the drugs
in development now are aimed at halting this conversion of normal amyloid into abnormal
beta-amyloid 42 and therefore preventing the spread of this disease across the brain (see
Future drugs on page 329).

The neurofibrillary tangles

The tangles inside the neurons described by Alzheimer are made from an abnormal form
of **tau protein**. A normal tau protein is a **microtubule-associated protein (MAP)**, which
interacts with the protein **tubulin**, the main component of the cell microtubules. Tau is
essential for the assembly and stabilisation of the cell cytoskeleton. Microtubules are also
vital for functions such as axonal transport, and abnormal tau may also be partly responsible for disruption of this process. The abnormal form of tau accumulates as tangles
(Figure 14.5).

In AD, the neurons of the temporal and frontal lobes, and also of the hippocampus, lose
up to 70% of a particular enzyme called **choline acetyltransferase (ChAT)** (not be confused with another enzyme, *acetylcholinesterase*, or *AChE*, which is involved in the drug
treatment of AD). The role of ChAT is to combine **choline** (derived from the diet) with
acetyl-CoA to form the neurotransmitter **acetylcholine (ACh)**. A loss of ChAT causes a
reduction in the choline and ACh content of these cells. The result is an adverse effect on
APP cleavage, leading to an increased amount of Aβ protein inside the cell. These higher
levels of Aβ protein contribute to a process called **oxidative stress** within the cell, involving an increase in the production of **reactive oxygen species**, highly reactive chemical
agents based on oxygen that damage cellular processes. A mechanism for this has been
identified, whereby Aβ protein binds two metals, iron and copper, and in the process these
metals donate electrons to oxygen. The negatively charged oxygen then reacts with hydrogen to form **hydrogen peroxide (H_2O_2)**, a highly reactive and damaging compound. In
this case, the damage is disruption of the normal **phosphorylation–dephosphorylation
cycle** of proteins in the cell. The phosphorylation, i.e. adding of a **phosphate (PO_4^{3-})** to
proteins, and dephosphorylation, i.e. removal of a phosphate from proteins, is a mechanism
for activating or deactivating proteins. The disruption of this process as a result of oxidative
stress causes **hyperphosphorylation** of tau, i.e. tau becomes saturated with phosphate and
thus accumulates as tangles (called **tau inclusions**). Similarly, **acetylation** (the adding of
an **acetyl group, C_2H_3O**) to tau protein reduces its microtubule function and promotes its
aggregation as tau inclusions. The absence of normal tau causes tubulin to fail in its role of
microtubule formation (Figure 14.5).

Two other proteins are apparently involved in AD. The first, called **ubiquitin**, attaches to
the abnormal tau at a late stage during tangle formation. Ubiquitin has a range of functions,
but its most important role is to attach to, and therefore label, those proteins that are destined
for destruction by proteolytic enzymes. This is possibly the function of ubiquitin in tangle
formation, although the destruction does not appear to happen. The second is a protein called
the **AMY antigen**, which is produced along with beta-amyloid as an amyloid-associated

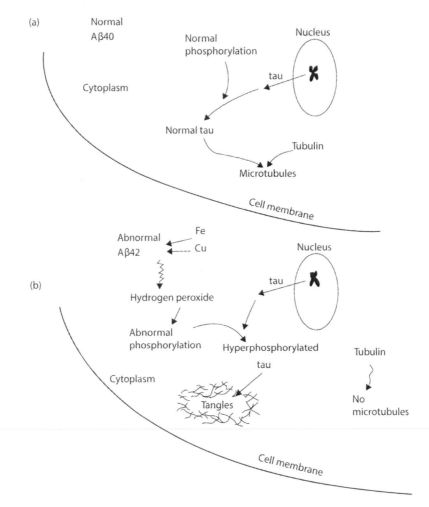

Figure 14.5 (a) Normal tau synthesis and (b) abnormal tau tangles in Alzheimer's disease. Fe and Cu
are the chemical symbols for iron and copper, respectively.

antigen. It coexists with beta-amyloid in plaque lesions found in both sporadic and familial
AD and in adult Down syndrome patients.

The genetics of AD

As noted before, the *early-age onset* form of the disease (beginning before 65 years of age)
is more often genetically inherited than the *late-age onset* form (beginning after 65 years
of age). Familial AD studies, especially in the early-age onset group, often show multiple
mutations in the three major autosomal dominant genes identified already, namely the *APP*
(chromosome 21), *PSEN1* (chromosome 14), and *PSEN2* genes (chromosome 1). In the
over-65 age group, the genetic evidence is less compelling, but 20–40% of people in this
group show a genetic error on the **apolipoprotein E (*ApoE*)** gene on **chromosome 19**.

Three forms of the *ApoE* gene have been found in studies of the Northern European indigenous population; *ApoEε-2* (8% of the population), *ApoE-e3* (77% of the population), and *ApoEε-4* (15% of the population). Within the human population as a whole, the percentage of allele combinations of *ApoE* are approximated as follows:

$$\varepsilon-2/\varepsilon-2 = 1-2\%, \ \varepsilon-2/\varepsilon-3 = 15\%,$$
$$\varepsilon-2/\varepsilon-4 = 1-2\%, \ \varepsilon-3/\varepsilon-3 = 55\%,$$
$$\varepsilon-3/\varepsilon-4 = 25\%, \ \varepsilon-4/\varepsilon-4 = 1-2\%$$

It is the *ApoEε-4* version that increases the risk for late-age onset AD by 8–10 times more than the other variants. *ApoE-ε-4* at one allele is the risk of AD starting in the *late* sixties and seventies age group, while the gene present at both alleles doubles the risk of developing the disease and brings the onset age to the *early* sixties. Apolipoprotein E is a protein that binds with fats (lipids) to form lipoproteins. These package cholesterol and other fats for transport through the blood. Apolipoprotein E is an important component of **very low-density lipoproteins (VLDLs)**. The *ApoEε-4* gene adds to the accumulation of Aβ42 in plaque formation, although the mechanism remains unclear. It is possible that apolipoproteins normally break down beta-amyloid, but the *ApoEε-4* variation is the least efficient of the three alleles at carrying out this process, and therefore allows beta-amyloid to accumulate. *ApoEε-4* also increases the substance **cyclophilin A**, which causes breakdown of the endothelial cells lining the blood vessels in AD patients. This loss of endothelial integrity effectively reduces the **blood–brain barrier**, the system of cells lining the blood vessels that normally prevents unwanted substances (e.g. toxins) from entering the brain. This barrier is highly efficient at a young age, but becomes less efficient with increasing age. The build-up of cyclophilin A in these cells renders the blood vessels leaky, resulting in the loss of neurons caused by both the toxic effects of unwanted substances entering the brain and a reduction of blood flow through the brain. At the same time, the problems with the blood–brain barrier cause an inability to allow the removal of amyloid-beta protein from the brain, adding to its accumulation between neurons. Cyclophilin A also creates an increase in the inflammatory substance **nuclear factor-kappaB (NF-κB)**. This substance boosts production of **matrix metalloproteinases (MMPs)**, enzymes that damage blood vessels and reduce blood flow (Figure 14.6). NF-κB in the hypothalamus has low activity at a young age, but increases in activity in old age. This older age increase was linked to a reduction of **gonadotrophin-releasing hormone (GnRH)** production and to early death. Blocking NF-κB with drugs, and/ or replacing the concentrations of GnRH showed intellectual and cognitive improvement and promoted new neuron growth. Trials in human subjects may lead to the development of new drugs that block the action of NF-κB. Some existing chemical agents already show promise in this area and could become more widely used to treat age-related mental decline.

An interesting twist to the story of the *ApoEε-4* gene is the fact that *young people* with this gene variation appear to be intellectually brighter than those without the gene variant. They gain higher levels of education and have better attention spans and memory abilities. It appears that all the versions of *ApoE*, including *ApoEε-4*, produce apolipoproteins that help to remove unwanted amyloid from the brain. This process gradually malfunctions with increasing age, but the malfunction is significantly earlier for the *ApoEε-4* variant.

Apolipoprotein J (ApoJ, also called **clusterin)** is another apolipoprotein under investigation. The clusterin protein, coded for by the *CLU* gene at 8p21, is involved in the clearance of cell debris and cellular **apoptosis (programmed cell death)**. Mutations of the gene have

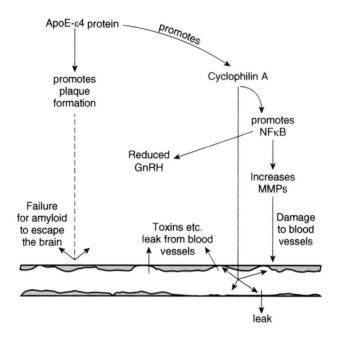

Figure 14.6 The *ApoEε-4* and cyclophilin A pathway in Alzheimer's disease.

been linked to AD. The normal protein has been shown to protect the brain against the toxic effects of beta-amyloid build-up, reducing inflammation and blood vessel lesions. This provides another avenue of research to find a drug based on normal ApoJ.

Expression of a gene called **mesenchyme homeobox 2** (*MEOX2*), found in blood vessel endothelial cells, is low in AD. Low levels of the protein from this gene results in a failure to form a blood supply because the endothelial cells could not develop, and therefore died. Restoring gene expression in the brain was shown to stimulate new blood vessels with improvement to the brain's microcirculation blood supply. This could become another new approach to future therapy.

Another gene that may have a part to play in AD is the **cholesterol ester transfer protein** (*CETP*) gene. This gene codes for a protein that controls the size of cholesterol particles. A mutation of this gene, in which the amino acid **isoleucine** is replaced by the amino acid **valine**, results in a protein that causes a slower cognitive decline, especially in memory. How this mutation becomes protective to neurons is not fully understood. Lipid levels and functions are becoming important in our understanding of brain activity and decline, partly because the brain houses 25% of the body's cholesterol, and high blood cholesterol is a risk factor for dementia. Drugs that alter *CETP* gene function to replicate this mutation are in development.

Also under investigation in relation to AD is **phosphatidylinositol binding clathrin assembly protein** (**PICALM**), coded for by the *PICALM* gene at 11q14.2. This protein is involved in synaptic function, and gene mutations have recently been associated with late-age onset AD.

A particular mutation involved in AD is a rare variant of the *TREM2* gene, which normally codes for receptors expressed on the surfaces of immune cells, notably **microglia** (see Chapter 3). These cells are **phagocytic** in the brain, helping to clear away waste proteins, including amyloid. *TREM2* mutations are linked to a three-fold increased risk for AD, probably because the mutation downgrades this role of the microglia, allowing the accumulation of plaques. Microglia affected by the *TREM2* mutation also release toxic and proinflammatory chemicals that damage cells and promote amyloid production.

A specific mutation of the gene **KL-VS** increases the amount of a protein called **klotho**. Normal concentrations of klotho improve kidney and heart function, but the higher concentrations from the gene variant create a large **right dorsolateral prefrontal cortex (rDLPFC)**. The raised concentrations also improve cognitive abilities and reduce mental decline in old age, slowing down the onset of dementia. This one gene variant can add about 3 years to a person's life-span. Approximately 3% of the population carry the beneficial *KL-VS* mutation, but raising klotho levels in those at risk of AD, if that becomes possible, is likely to be beneficial in delaying the onset of the dementia.

The gene **PCDH11X** codes for the protein **protocadherin**, a molecule important for communication between neurons in the brain. The gene is on the X chromosome, of which women have two but men have only one. Those women with a variant of the gene on both their X chromosomes carry a high risk of dementia, because protocadherin appears to be broken down by an enzyme linked to AD. The gene variant on only one of the X chromosomes in women, or on the singe X of men, carries a much lower risk. This may go some way to account for there being twice as many women with dementia than men over 65 years of age.

Mitochondrial DNA mutations may also have a role to play in some dementias, notably AD (see Figure 12.6 in Chapter 12). The relationship between mitochondrial gene errors and AD is not clear and is controversial. Mitochondrial genes were discussed in Chapter 13 in relation to PD and Huntington's disease, and a similar pathogenesis may apply to AD.

AD could also involve the accumulation of beta-amyloid protein damaging the mitochondrial membrane, which then disrupts membrane permeability. The change in membrane ionic permeability causes oxidation and other forms of damage to the mitochondrial DNA and failure of cellular energy. This would result in neuronal cell death, called **apoptosis**, if these genes become faulty. Mitochondrial DNA mutations, including point mutations and deletions, may play a more important role in the sporadic (i.e. non-inherited) forms of the disease.

Epigenetics is the study of changes affecting DNA without altering the base sequence of the gene. These changes include **methylation**, a natural mechanism the body uses to switch genes on or off by adding or removing a **methyl group** to the DNA. In those areas of the brain most affected by dementia, notably the cerebral cortex and hypothalamus, one particular gene, *ANK1*, was found to be **hypermethylated**, i.e. excessive amounts of methyl groups attached. Methylation is normally reversible, and given the hypermethylation appears to happen early in the disease, it seems reasonable to suggest that a medication can be developed to restore *ANK1* to normal.

Immunity and inflammation in AD

The immune system and the brain share a closer relationship than previously thought. Several new discoveries shed more light on this:

- Lymphatic vessels, a major transport route for immune cells such as **T-cell lymphocytes**, actually penetrate the meninges and drain the brain of fluid, an aspect of anatomy not previously realised. This brain lymphatic network moves fluid to the lymph nodes of the neck called the **deep cervical nodes**.

- A physical communication between the brain and immune system occurs across the **choroid plexus**. The choroid plexus is composed of tiny tufts of blood vessels inside the ventricles of the brain from which **cerebrospinal fluid (CSF)** is produced (see Chapter 1). This is the **blood–CSF barrier**, which normally allows only suitable substances to pass from the blood into the CSF. People who carry the *ApoEε-4* gene develop leaky blood vessels, which allow toxics substances to pass from the blood into the brain (see Genetics, above).
- A protein molecule of the immune system called **interferon-beta (IFN-β)** appears to become harmful to the brain in old age. Certain chemicals, which could become the basis of future drugs, block the action of INF-β and help to restore some cognitive function as well as stimulate the production of new neurons in the hippocampus.
- The bacterial composition of the digestive system changes with age, and there are indications that those changes may have some impact on the ageing process of the brain. There is growing interest in a potential lifelong gut–brain interaction mediated through the immune system, and changes in one-half of this interaction must somehow affect the other half.

Observations have identified that those patients taking steroids for any condition have a low incidence of AD. The anti-inflammatory effect of the steroids apparently dampens an immune reaction (called the **inflammatory response**) in the brain caused by the destructive factors listed below. This increase in the inflammatory response by immune cells can, itself, cause neuronal cellular damage.

The following is a list of the mechanisms that suggest an inflammatory component in the cause of cell destruction in AD (Figure 14.7):

- the excessive production of **prostaglandins** by the enzyme **cyclooxygenase (COX)**, which increases the level of the neurotransmitter **glutamate**, leading to glutamate-induced neuronal cell death;
- the neuronal damage (in particular DNA damage) caused by oxidation from **free radicals**;
- the phagocytic cells of the brain, called **microglia**, which normally clear away the debris that occurs in the brain, but in AD appear to produce toxic **cytokines** such as **interleukin-6 (Il-6)** (see Genetics, above);
- the increased release of an inflammatory protein called **tumour necrosis factor (TNF)**, which induces the vagus nerve to promote an inflammatory response against brain cells that are in a state of chronic inflammation;
- the release of soluble toxins called **amyloid beta derived diffusible ligands** from beta-amyloid breakdown, which may become important in cell destruction;
- the protein **prostate apoptosis response-4 (Par-4)**, which occurs in higher than normal levels and may contribute to neuronal destruction, especially if combined with **ceramide** in vesicles produced by astrocytes.

From this stems the idea that anti-inflammatory drugs may slow the progress of the disease. Not everyone should take steroids, of course, but other **nonsteroidal anti-inflammatory drugs (NSAIDs)** may benefit the AD patient, or could even be given as a preventative measure. The drug **prazosin**, an alpha-blocker and vasodilator, has been shown to have both anti-inflammatory and astrocyte-boosting properties, and may prove to be useful in preventing memory decline in humans.

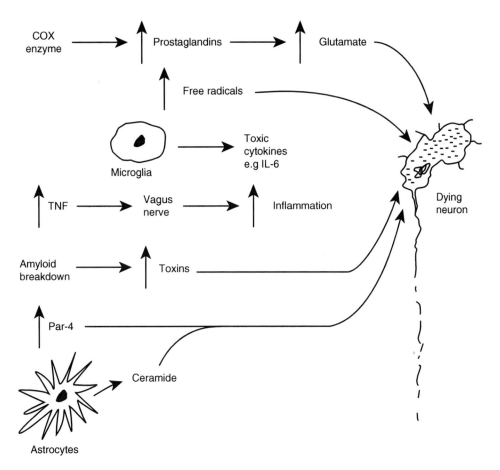

Figure 14.7 The inflammatory response in Alzheimer's disease. Arrow pointing up = increased.

Inflammation is often, but not always, caused by an infectious organism, and some postmortem brain samples taken from late-age onset AD patients have revealed the presence of the bacterium ***Chlamydia pneumoniae (Chlamydophila pneumoniae)*** in some, and the virus ***herpesvirus 1 (HSV1)*** in others. The *intracellular* organism *Chlamydia pneumoniae* was located to the temporal lobes and hippocampus, just the areas affected most by this disease. This does not, of course, prove that the organism is the cause of AD; rather it may increase the risk of developing the disorder. Microglia and astrocytes appear to be the main cells in which this organism survives, and the fact that it also lives *inside* the neuron makes it more difficult to treat. It is suspected that people with the mutant *ApoEε-4* gene allele are more susceptible to these infections.

Association of AD with Down syndrome

Down syndrome is a **trisomy 21** (three copies of chromosome 21 instead of two). Chromosome 21 is the site of the *APP* gene, which means that Down syndrome sufferers carry three copies of this gene in every cell. Two interesting correlations have been found to link AD with Down syndrome:

- Down syndrome sufferers develop Alzheimer-like dementia at 30+ years and have been found to have multiple, diffuse plaque formation up to 10 years before dementia symptoms arise.
- Elderly AD sufferers were found on average to have had a higher than expected number of Down syndrome children earlier in their lives.

Those affected with Down syndrome express five times more APP in the brain than normal owing to the 50% extra APP present. The risk of developing AD is proportional to the amount of APP produced by the three copies of the gene present.

Detecting AD

Diagnosis of AD is based on symptoms, and the disease was previously confirmed only at postmortem. Now there have been advances in detecting AD early in the disease, even before symptoms arise, when treatment is most effective:

- A blood test is being developed based on 10 proteins, called **biomarkers** (i.e. biological markers) which, when present, indicate the presence of the disease. These proteins appear in the blood of mild cognitive impairment (MCI) patients and trials of the test show about 87% accuracy in predicting which of those with mild memory loss will develop AD within a year. It could be available for widespread use anytime between 2016 and 2020.
- Another blood test looks at the activity of 150 key genes by analysing the blood **ribonucleic acid (RNA)** concentrations. Those with high RNA concentrations (thus high gene activity) had better cognitive health than those with lower scores. It could be helpful in screening older people for the early signs of dementia.
- **Amyloid imaging** involves the use of a radioactive tracer called **Pittsburgh compound B (PiB)** injected into a vein. This locks onto amyloid accumulating in the brain, and being mildly radioactive it emits a signal that can be detected by a **positron-emission tomographic (PET)** scanner. The brain areas affected by amyloid accumulations create very bright areas on the brain picture obtained, showing exactly where, and by how much, amyloid is replacing brain tissue. Given the battery of new therapies that are under development, including a large number of new and exciting drug treatments awaiting final clinical trails (see The drugs used in dementia, page 328), early detection of plaque accumulation using PiB and PET technology will be very beneficial in allowing very early medical intervention to slow the course of the disease.
- A new scanning technique uses a chemical marker to show up serotonin receptor density in the hippocampus. These receptors are particularly vulnerable in those people developing AD as the hippocampus suffers cell losses and shrinks. The researchers recorded reduction of serotonin receptor densities in the hippocampus during the early stages of AD and as the disease progressed.

Dementia with cortical Lewy bodies

In 1912, Frederic Lewy (1885–1950) discovered abnormal intracellular aggregates of protein in cells dying from PD. **Lewy bodies**, as they became known, are rounded microscopic deposits of the protein **alpha-synuclein** that are found in deteriorating nerve cells. They can be present in the basal ganglia in PD, and in the cortex of AD. Dementia with cortical Lewy bodies (DCLB) accounts for about 10% of all dementias, but about 20% of AD patients also have cortical Lewy bodies (i.e. they have a combination of AD with DCLB, and DCLB may be a variation of AD). About 2% of the normal elderly population also have Lewy bodies. The proposed difference between AD, AD with DCLB, and DCLB is shown in Table 14.1. The symptoms of DCLB are very similar to those of AD but with greater emphasis on motor symptoms such as extrapyramidal tremors and walking difficulties. Some additional psychiatric symptoms can occur, such as hallucinations and delusions, and a reduction in cognitive ability includes alternating periods of alertness with periods of confusion and unresponsiveness.

Pick's disease

Pick's disease, also called **frontotemporal dementia (FTD)** or **frontotemporal lobar degeneration (FTLD)**, was described in 1892 by Arnold Pick (1851–1924), earlier than the description of Alzheimer's disease (1906). It is rarer than AD, with few patients showing familial inheritance. This indicates that genes are not a powerful influence in this disease. The cause remains unknown. The onset of symptoms mostly occurs at about 50 to 60 years of age, affecting women more than men. The early symptoms show a predominance of social and personality changes, rather than memory and intellectual deterioration as in AD. This is due to the neuropathology that is characteristic for this disease. The brain shows a significant atrophy (a loss of superficial neurons) in the anterior *cortical* aspects of the frontal and temporal lobes. The atrophy is rare and less severe in the parietal lobe and extremely rare in the occipital lobe and cerebellum. This is very much a disease of the front half of the brain. Astrocytes proliferate in these areas of atrophy, with **gliosis** (glial cell proliferation) and fibrous tissue deposited. Neurons in the affected areas become swollen and oval in shape, with an absence of Nissl bodies. In place of the Nissl bodies, abnormal **Pick bodies** fill the cell cytoplasm, pushing the nucleus to one side. Pick bodies are rounded inclusions of neurofilamentous proteins similar to typical neurofibrillary tangles (but different in many respects) and, like neurofibrillary tangles, they disrupt the cell's internal cytoskeleton. However, the typical neurofibrillary tangles and the plaques seen in AD are both missing in this disease. **Hirano bodies**, another form of intraneuronal inclusion found mostly in the hippocampus, are present in many cases. These are made from deranged cytoskeletal components. Another feature is the extensive loss of myelination within the white matter coming from the affected cortical areas.

Pick's disease causes changes in the personality and social behaviour patterns in the patient during its early stages. The deterioration of social habits may include inappropriate sexual

Table 14.1 The distinction between Alzheimer's disease (AD) and dementia with cortical Lewy bodies (DCLB)

Dementia type	Plaques	Tangles	Lewy bodies
AD	Present	Present	Absent
AD with DCLB	Present	Present	Present
DCLB	Present	Absent	Present

or criminal activities, the patient showing a loss of normal inhibitions and a lack of insight. Changes in mood may be characterised by either apathy or a state of euphoria. As the disease progresses, the patient suffers speech and language difficulties and in the later stages memory and intellect decline.

A particular gene mutation, the **progranulin (*GRN*)** gene, is often associated with FTD. Mutations of this gene cause defects in a cell signalling pathway called the **Wnt pathway** (see Chapter 10, Figure 10.1). This pathway is important in neurodevelopment, and the gene mutation prevents this pathway from functioning as it should, so neurons cannot develop normally. Future drugs designed to inhibit this pathway may help to restore normal cortical neuron development.

Variations of this disease have been noted, such as **Pick's disease type II**, where severe gliosis (predominance of glial cells) occurs within the *subcortical* white matter, nuclei, brain stem, and parts of the spinal cord. The cortex is less affected, with shrunken cells (not swollen) and mild gliosis. Another type of Pick's disease is the **behavioural variant FTD (bvFTD)**, in which the early changes include abnormal personality and emotional symptoms.

The drugs used in dementia

Donepezil, galantamine, and **rivastigmine** are reversible **acetylcholinesterase inhibitors**, used as a treatment of the symptoms of mild to moderate AD. They have little effect on patients with advanced disease. These drugs work by blocking the action of **acetylcholinesterase**, the enzyme that breaks down acetylcholine, thus increasing the level of acetylcholine in brain circuits devastated by a lack of this neurotransmitter. Donepezil reduces the rate of cognitive deterioration in about 40% of cases but has no effect on dementias caused by failure of cerebral circulation. These drugs can induce unwanted dose-related cholinergic side effects, which include nausea, vomiting, diarrhoea, dizziness, insomnia, and rarely **syncopy** (fainting). Acetylcholinesterase inhibitors should be prescribed only by consultants specialising in the treatment of dementia. Prescribing a drug treatment is based on careful assessment of the patient's cognitive abilities and behaviour, including their ability to provide for themselves a suitable level of self-care. Assessments should be repeated every 6 months. The patient's carer should be included in the assessment process and in any decision to prescribe a drug, with administration routine, dosage, and side effects fully explained to them. This is because cognitive decline in the patient may lead to poor drug compliance, and therefore supervision of medication by a responsible carer can become essential. After initial specialist assessment, drugs may continue to be prescribed by the patient's own doctor under a shared-care protocol.

These drugs are well absorbed from the gut so they are suitable for oral use. They are metabolised in the liver and are excreted via the kidneys. Donepezil has a 100% oral bioavailability and a long-half life (70 hours), and is usually given at night. Galantamine also has 100% oral bioavailability, but a much shorter half-life (5 to 7 hours). Rivastigmine has a 40% oral bioavailability due to **first pass metabolism**, and a very short half-life (1 hour).

Memantine is an NMDA glutamate receptor antagonist that reduces the damaging overactivity of glutamate within nerve cells. It also has antagonistic activity at the serotonin 5-HT3 and nicotinic acetylcholine receptors, and an agonistic effect on dopamine D_2 receptors. It has become a treatment for moderate to severe dementia, although its high cost has limited its use in the UK.

Future drugs for dementia

It is unfortunate that we have not had any drugs that can actually halt or even reverse dementia, but this is about to change. New drugs hold great promise of preventing the slow decline seen with AD.

There are many clinical trials going on testing new treatments and diagnostic procedures for AD. A large number of these are new drug treatments for dementia in various stages of development. Some could be in clinical use within a few years. Among these new drug studies there are:

- inhibitors of the enzymes that produce beta-amyloid, including 12/15-lipoxygenase (see above);
- blockers of beta-amyloid aggregation;
- drugs that combat hyperphosphorylated tau production and accumulation;
- agents that protect neurons against death and promote brain cell health;
- vaccines or antibodies that clear away accumulated beta-amyloid;
- memory-boosting drugs;
- drugs that prevent normal amyloid conversion to abnormal beta-amyloid and therefore halt the spread of the disease across the brain;
- compounds that block the clumping together of tau and beta amyloid oligomers.

New drugs based on **monoclonal antibodies (mAb**, or **moAb)** are being developed. Antibodies are natural proteins of the immune system that are produced by **B-cell lymphocytes**. There are five classes of antibody (also called **immunoglobulins**, or **Ig**). These classes are **IgA**, **IgD**, **IgE**, **IgG**, and **IgM**. They attack foreign proteins (called **antigens**) and render them susceptible to destruction by components of the immune system. Monoclonal antibodies are specific to a single protein and are all derived (or cloned) from a single unique parent cell, and therefore they all attack one protein type. The drug **solanezumab** (the ending -*mab* = 'monoclonal antibody'), is an IgG directed to attack the mid-domain component of the soluble amyloid protein, and promote their removal before they accumulate. The drug has been shown to slow down the cognitive decline seen in AD by about 34%. It works best during the early stages when the disease is mild, and has shown to be remarkably safe for use in humans. Further trials of this, and other drugs of this type (e.g. **aducanumab**, **crenezumab**, and **gantenerumab**) are underway. The efficacy of these drugs during the early stages of disease highlights the need for early detection (see Detecting AD, on page 326). Now antibody therapy targeted at the **tau** protein found in the tangles is under development.

Salsalate is another drug that targets tau protein by preventing the formation of tangles. It blocks **acetylation,** i.e. it blocks the enzyme that adds an **acetyl group** to normal tau (see The neurofibrillary tangles, page 319), and this helps to prevent tangle formation. Salsalate is a non-steroidal anti-inflammatory agent that is already in clinical use for treating pain in osteoarthritis and rheumatoid arthritis. It has a good safety record, and if clinical trials go well in humans it could quickly be available for the treatment of dementia.

Ampakines are a class of drugs that improve memory by a different mechanism (Figure 14.8). They prolong the memory by stimulating glutamate binding to **AMPA receptors**. Increased AMPA receptor activity then promotes the function of NMDA receptors and thereby establishes improved LTP in the postsynaptic membrane. However, there is a down side to memory-boosting drugs. Growing evidence indicates that memory is closely associated

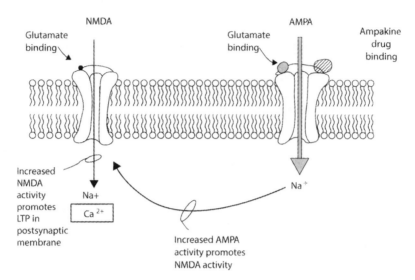

Figure 14.8 Ampakine drug action. By binding to AMPA receptors, these drugs increase glutamate activity at that receptor. The increased sodium entry here promotes NMDA receptor activity in the same cell membrane, resulting in a large calcium influx, which boosts memory.

with pain, both the memory and the sensation of pain (Day 2002). Boosting memory with drugs may have the adverse effect of increasing pain sensitivity, so everything that hurts normally would hurt even more with these drugs. It is a stark choice for the elderly with dementia: improve your memory but suffer more pain, or live in comfort and memory loss. It may be possible, however, to target the drugs to different areas of the brain, i.e. to the areas that process memory and not to the areas that process pain. In addition, other drugs that block pain-related enzymes in the spine may reduce the sensation of pain in persons taking these drugs (Day 2002).

Rember was a drug in development containing a form of methylene blue, which proved to be an inhibitor of tau protein aggregation, i.e. it prevented the formation of tangles in AD. The 2008 trials showed an 81% improvement in patient cognitive ability for those taking 60 mg three times a day for nearly a year. It is now replaced by a second-generation drug, based on Rember, called **LMTX**. This has been shown in trials to stop the progression of **Pick's disease**. It not only prevents a tau aggregation, it also releases previously aggregated tau as a soluble form that can easily be cleared from the brain. Other drug initiatives are in progress, and these are some of them:

- **Luminescent conjugated polythiophenes** are showing promise as agents that halt the spread of prions throughout the brain, as a possible treatment for Creutzfeld–Jakob disease (CJD). They may also prove of value in preventing the spread of beta amyloid through the brain (see The plaques, page 316).
- Another approach is to find drugs that interfere with the production or processing of APP. Ten proteins were developed to bind with APP, and of these one (**P8**) was found to prevent APP cleavage. This results in far less beta-amyloid production, and therefore less plaque formation. It is hoped that human trials will give good results.

- An experimental agent called **VAR-10303** has been shown to improve cognitive abilities and increase production of **neurotrophic factors** (e.g. **brain-derived neurotrophic factor** and **nerve growth factor**) and to improved hippocampal synaptic plasticity. Neurotrophic factors have neuronal protective and regeneration properties.

New cells for old!

Stem cells are undifferentiated cells, i.e. they are cells that have not yet been designated as any particular cell type. Now stem cells derived from primary fibroblasts taken from skin tissue provided by two AD sufferers have been artificially manipulated to form neurons. As they come from AD patients, they contain the gene mutations linked to AD, e.g. the **progranulin (*GRN*)** mutation (see page 328). These new neurons will be used to test new drugs in the laboratory, and perhaps one day they could possibly be used to replace missing cells in dementia, after replacing the gene mutations with normal genes, and thus restore brain function. Already, a very small brain, with the start of a tiny spinal cord has been produced using this method. It contains 99% of all the genes normally found in the human brain, but no blood vessels. It could, one day, contribute towards rebuilding a damaged mind, but the research is at a very early stage, and is therefore a potential treatment for the future.

Key points

The hippocampus and memory

- The hippocampal complex consists of the dentate gyrus and Ammon's horn, which is further divided into areas CA1, CA2, CA3, and CA4.
- The subiculum, the entorhinal cortex, the perirhinal cortex, and the parahippocampal cortex are all areas of the temporal lobe linked to the hippocampus.
- Memory is based on the formation of long-term potentiation (LTP) at the synapse.
- Damage to Ammon's horn CA1 and CA3 areas, the fornix, the mammillary bodies, and the anterior thalamic nucleus can cause memory loss.

The ageing brain

- Naturally occurring neuron loss can begin as early as 23 years of age, but is insignificant during these early years. It is likely to increase after the age of 60.
- Neuron losses may be attributed to reduced blood flow to the brain caused by age-related changes in the arteries that supply the head.
- Neurons are sensitive to oxygen and glucose and will not function when faced with a decline in the oxygen and glucose supply.
- Synapses are vital for memory and learning.

Alzheimer's disease

- AD is a dementia with the presence of extracellular plaques and intracellular neurofibrillary tangles.
- Early-age onset AD is more genetically based than late-age onset AD.
- The plaques have a central core of abnormal beta-amyloid protein (Aβ42).

- Familial Alzheimer's disease (FAD) usually has mutations of the *APP* (chromosome 21), *PSEN-1* (chromosome 14), *PSEN-2* (chromosome 1), and *HSD17B10* (chromosome X) genes.
- The tangles inside the neurons are made from an abnormal form of tau protein.
- People in the over-65 age group have an increased risk of dementia if they have the *ApoEε-4* (apolipoprotein E) gene variation on chromosome 19.
- AD appears to have an inflammatory component due to an inflammatory response to beta amyloid.
- AD is linked with Down syndrome through chromosome 21.

The drugs used in dementia

- Donepezil, galantamine, and rivastigmine are reversible acetylcholinesterase inhibitors.
- Ampakines are future drugs that are being investigated for improvement of memory.
- There are many other possible future drugs that improve cognitive abilities in AD, and some of these should be available for clinical use by 2020.
- AD patients often require supervision by carers during drug administration to ensure patient safety and compliance.
- Carers should also be alert to drug side effects.

References

Biernacki, C. and Barratt, J. (2001) Improving the nutritional status of people with dementia. *British Journal of Nursing*, **10** (17): 1104–1114.

Blows, W. T. (2000) The nervous system, part 2. *Nursing Times*, **96** (40): 45–48.

Chu, J., Zhuo, J.-M., and Pratic, D. (2012) Transcriptional regulation of beta-secretase-1 by 12/15 lipoxygenase results in enhanced amyloidogenesis and cognitive impairment. *Annals of Neurology*, 57. DOI: 10.1002/ana.22625.

Day, S. (2002) Painful memories. *New Scientist*, **173** (2332; 2 March): 29–31.

Kang, J. E., Lim, M. M., Bateman, R. J., Lee, J. J., Smyth, L. P., Cirrito, J. R., Fujiki, N., Nishino, S., and Holtzman, D. M. (2009). Amyloid-beta dynamics are regulated by orexin and the sleep-wake cycle. *Science*, **326** (5955): 1005–1007.

Luders, E., Cherbuin, N., and Kurth, F. (2015) Forever young(er): potential age-defying effects of long-term meditation on gray matter atrophy. *Frontiers in Psychology*, 5. DOI: 10.3389/fpsyg.2014.01551.

Shurkin, J. N. (2009) Decoding dementia. *Scientific American Mind*, **20**: 56–63.

Smith, D., Clark, R., Jobst, K. A., Sutton, L., Ueland, P. M., and Refsum, H. (1998) Hyperhomocysteinemia: an independent risk factor for histopathologically-confirmed Alzheimer's disease, *in* Homocysteine: a possible risk factor for Alzheimer's disease, online at: http://www.sciencedaily.com/releases/1998/05/980504125421.htm.

Star, M., Gill, R., Bruzzone, M., De Alba, F., Schneck, M. J., and Biller, J. (2015) Do not forget Susac syndrome in patients with unexplained acute confusion. *Journal of Stroke and Cerebrovascular Diseases*, **24** (4): e93–95. DOI: 10.1016/j.jstrokecerebrovasdis.2014.11.028.

15 Learning, behavioural, and developmental disorders

- Introduction
- Learning disorders
- Communication disorders
- Behavioural disorders
- Developmental disorders
- Intellectual disabilities
- Obsessive-compulsive disorder and tic disorders
- Key points

Introduction

The learning and developmental disorders generally begin during childhood and have a range of symptoms that are likely to vary from child to child, and in severity. They also have a combination of causes, i.e. often with a genetic basis interacting with social, psychological, and environmental factors. These are referred to as having a polygenic aetiology.

A classification of such disorders includes the following:

- learning disorders (dyslexia, dysgraphia, and dyspraxia);
- communication disorders (expressive language disorder, stuttering);
- behavioural disorders (attention deficit hyperactive disorder);
- developmental disorders (autism, Asperger's syndrome, Rett syndrome);
- intellectual disabilities (phenylketonuria, Tay–Sachs disease, fetal alcohol syndrome);
- obsessive-compulsive disorder (OCD) and tic disorders (e.g. Tourette's syndrome).

Learning disorders

Dyslexia

Dyslexia is a reading/writing disorder (*dyslexia* = 'faulty reading') in which any three of the following four symptoms may be present:

1   words or letters being reversed during reading after the age of 8 years;
2   deterioration of writing;

3   difficulty with hearing;
4   difficulty with learning by rote.

A poor level of literacy, where reading skills lag behind what is expected for the child's age, in combination with any of the symptoms above is called **developmental dyslexia (DD)**. Between 5% and 10% of schoolchildren have significant deficits in their reading skills. Reading begins with the understanding of the phonics (sounds) of words, or different parts of words, and this is learnt first from the spoken language. After this, the child must learn to associate the phonic sounds with the written symbols of the language as printed on the page, so reading becomes a translation (in two stages) of the written symbols into spoken sounds. Sufferers of dyslexia appear to find this difficult to varying degrees, although in all other respects they are usually intellectually well developed. It may be that a child has problems with either fast identification the written form of the language (**rapid automatised naming**, or **RAN**), or the spoken sounds of the language (**phonological impairment**). Either of these on their own is **single deficit**, or problems with both at the same time is **double deficit**. A child with double-deficit dyslexia will show much greater problems with reading skills than a child with single-deficit dyslexia (Norton et al. 2014). RAN deficits occur as a result of problems with the **right cerebellar lobule VI**, and phonological defects are the result of problems with the **left inferior frontal** and **parietal lobes**.

Developmental dyslexia appears to be familial, suggesting a genetic basis to the disorder. The concordance rate for developmental dyslexia in **monozygotic (MZ, or identical)** twins is 84–100%, and for **dizygotic (DZ, or non-identical)** twins is 20–35%. The difference indicates a genetic basis for the disorder.

Multiple genes have been identified as associated with dyslexia (Williams and O'Donovan 2006):

- *DYX1* (dyslexia specific 1) found at 15q21, a gene strongly linked to single-word reading and spelling; disorder of this gene results in both spelling and reading difficulties, and this provides a biological basis for the linkage between these two skills.
- *DYX2* (dyslexia specific 2) found at 6p21.3, a gene strongly linked to the awareness of phonics in the spoken word.
- *DYX3* found at 2p15-16, *DYX4* found at 6q13-16, *DYX5* found at 3p12-q12, *DYX6* found at 18p11.2, *DYX7* found at 11p15.5, *DYX8* found at 1p34-p36, and *DYX9* found at Xq27.3 are all susceptibility genes, meaning that if mutations of these are inherited they increase the risk of this disorder. Strong genetic linkage is evident with *DYX3*, *DYX6*, and *DYX8;* more moderate linkage is associated with *DYX4*, *DYX5*, *DYX7,* and *DYX9*.

Most of these genes are normally involved in brain development, and mutations are likely to be involved in causing developmental errors, in particular disruption of brain cell migration before birth (see Chapter 2). Disorganised cell layers in part of the thalamus known as the **lateral geniculate nucleus (LGN)**, have been found in dyslexia. This area of the thalamus is the relay point for visual stimuli from the retina of the eye to the visual cortex within the occipital lobe of the cerebrum (the area of the visual cortex involved in reading is the left **fusiform gyrus**). The thalamic cells that are disrupted are those of the **magnocellular layers** (Figure 15.1), i.e. large cells that convey sensory impulses relating to visual depth of field and the visual perception of movement to the visual cortex. They respond if the

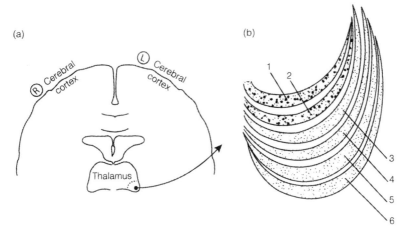

Figure 15.1 The magnocellular layer (layers 1 and 2) of the lateral geniculate nucleus of the thalamus, which are disrupted in dyslexia. Layers 3 to 6, the parvonuclear layers, are unaffected.

words being read move away from the most light sensitive parts of the retina, the **fovea**, due to unintended eye or head movements, and bring the focus back onto the fovea. Other thalamic cells within the LGN, the **parvocellular layers**, which convey colour and fine detail impulses to the cortex, are unaffected by the disorder. Pathways from the magnocellular layers of the LGN activate the part of the visual cortex called V5, which functions in the event of movement within the visual field. In dyslexia, V5 activation by the sensory input from the LGN magnocellular layers appears to be disturbed. Reading is affected, possibly because sufferers have unsteady binocular visual fixation, i.e. as they stare at the words, letters appear to the reader to move around on the page and become jumbled due to uncontrolled head or eye movements. This is a common complaint made by those with dyslexia. They transpose letters within a word, and this causes them to misread words; for example, the written word *dog* may be read as *god*. The poor visual fixation on the word to be read (i.e. the eyes wander slightly from the word) and the magnocellular layers somewhat distorting the visual image of words results in poor reading skills (Stein 2001). Movement involves space, and other symptoms associated with dyslexia show disturbance to movement and space-related skills, including poor handwriting, difficulties with balance (e.g. when riding a bicycle), delayed walking skills, and slowness in learning how to tell the time. These skills require visual input and the difficulties found in dyslexia suggest problems associated with the development of the posterior occipital lobe, i.e. the primary visual cortex, or its input from the visual pathways via the LGN.

Dyslexic people also seem to have part of their upper temporal lobe, the **planum temporale**, equal in size on both sides. Normally, the left planum temporale is larger than the right (Figure 15.2). Only 11% of the population have a right planum temporale larger than the left. The fact that they are more or less symmetrical in dyslexia is significant. This region contains Wernicke's area, the language area, and this has led to speculation that the planum temporale is normally larger and more dominant on the left because it is involved in language and speech perception.

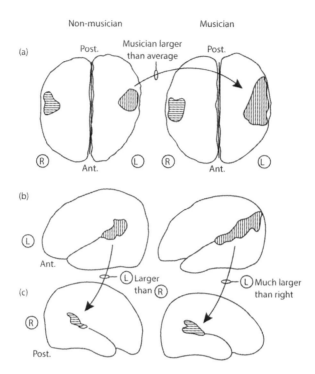

Figure 15.2 The planum temporale in (a) superior, (b) left lateral, and (c) right lateral views. Normally, the left planum temporale is larger than that on the right in most people. In musicians, especially those with perfect pitch, the left planum temporale is considerably larger than the right. In those with dyslexia the planum temporale tends to be of equal size on both sides.

Dysgraphia and dyspraxia

Dysgraphia is a disorder of writing, causing problems with spelling, in two main forms.

- **Phonological dysgraphia** is the inability to write words phonetically, or according to the sounds of words. This disorder is thought to be caused by neuronal damage to the superior temporal lobe. The ability to write whole words is retained.
- **Orthographic dysgraphia** is the inability to write and spell visually based irregular words. Here the ability to write whole words is poor, while phonetic writing is preserved. This disorder is thought to be caused by neuronal damage to the inferior parietal lobe.

Writing is a function primarily of that half of the brain dominant for speech, the left hemisphere of the cerebral cortex in most people. It is here that the twin speech areas are located, Wernicke's area for language construction and Broca's area for the motor organisation of the muscles for speech.

Dyspraxia is a disorder of movement (*praxis* = 'to do or to act') in which specific motor skills cannot be carried out despite there being no evidence of paralysis. It is the speed of movements that appears to be impeded. Speech is affected in some cases (**verbal dyspraxia**) because speech involves rapid, skilled movements of the jaw and tongue. In normal speech we are capable of producing as many as 15 sounds every second. Sufferers of dyspraxia may also have some degree of difficulty with reading (an overlap with dyslexia) or with purposeful movements, thus appearing clumsy (sometimes called **motor dyspraxia**). Swallowing and sucking movements remain normal. The term *developmental dyspraxia* is used frequently, as the disorder appears to be a failure to correctly organise the motor (or movement) pathways in the brain during brain development.

Communication disorders

Children with expressive language disorder find problems in expressing themselves verbally, due to limited vocabulary and difficulties in learning new words. They may also have problems retrieving words from memory and find it hard to apply correct grammar. Two main forms of this disorder are recognised: (1) the *developmental* form, where symptoms start sometime after birth as the child grows and the cause is unknown; (2) the *acquired* version that occurs after a stroke or head injury later in life. The child's ability to understand others' spoken language is unimpaired. Those children who do fail to understand language that is spoken to them have a variation of the disorder call receptive-expressive language disorder.

Stuttering (or **persistent developmental stuttering, PDS**), is the interruption to normal fluent speech by the reiteration of single sounds or word syllables, or by prolonged delays. It affects about one million adults worldwide (1–2% of the adult population). It affects more adult males than females; a ratio ranging from 3 males to 1 female up to 5 males to 1 female. About 15% of 4- to 6-year-old children are affected, but many will grow out of the problem.

The cause of stuttering is now becoming clearer. Excess dopamine in circuits of the brain, especially within the basal ganglia, has been indicated because dopamine antagonist drugs help to prevent stuttering, but they do cause side effects that prevent them from being a first-line treatment. Normally the left hemisphere of the brain is used in fluent speech. Brain scans reveal a dysfunction in the left hemisphere during stuttering, with a compensatory overactivity of the same areas in the right hemisphere. Also, in normal speech, the left frontal lobe (involved in language planning) is activated moments before the central cortex (involved in speech execution). The frontal lobe activity is absent, or even comes after the central cortex activity in those who stutter. This is a timing error between the left frontal lobe and the central cortex. Further studies revealed a structural defect in the pathways that link the frontal lobe with the central cortex, and it appears that the right hemisphere activation may be trying to bypass this defect. Females lateralise their speech skills less than males (see Chapter 2 for lateralisation). This is possibly the reason why boys that stutter have four times less chance of recovery than girls.

Another abnormality occurs in **Broca's area**, the speech motor area of the frontal lobe (Brodmann 44 and 45; see Chapter 1), where abnormal grey matter development is seen in those who stutter. Normally, the thickness of this grey matter gets thinner with age, a process that is in keeping with increased efficiency in the functions of Broca's area. To remain quite thick indicates that this area has problems maturing.

Several gene mutations have been linked to stuttering. The **GNPTAB** gene, the **GNPTG** gene, and the **NAGPA** gene are all involved in lysosomal activity (lysosomes contain digestive enzymes that break down unwanted cellular components). The **GNPTAB** gene, at 12q23.3, codes for a protein that helps in the breakdown and recycling of cell components inside the lysosomes of the cell. The **GNPTG** (16p) and **NAGPA** (16p13.3) genes code for proteins that are also important for enzyme activity related to lysosomal metabolism. The link between these proteins and the problem of stuttering is not yet clear. **Stuttering familial persistent 1 (*STUT1*)** at 18p11.3-11.4, ***STUT2*** at 12q24.1, ***STUT3*** at 3q, and ***STUT4*** at 16q are further genes associated with stuttering.

Behavioural disorders

Attention deficit hyperactive disorder

The two related conditions, attention deficit disorder (ADD) and attention deficit hyperactive disorder (ADHD) affect learning by disrupting the child's ability to raise attention and concentrate on any specific subject. The difference between these two disorders is solely the degree of additional hyperactive disruptive behaviour, which becomes a dominant feature of the condition in ADHD. Some authors consider them to be different degrees of the same disorder, and others even suggest that ADHD is not a 'real disease' but more of a description of symptoms we all go though at some point in our lives, although the discovery of genes and related pathology may contradict this assessment. The full debate is beyond the remit of this book.

The symptoms of ADHD include severe impulsive, disruptive, and even aggressive behaviour, restlessness, and inability to concentrate on a subject. It affects approximately 3% of the population, mostly children. The cause and the associated pathology are not fully understood, but recently there have been some interesting test results suggesting that these children lack some of the systems in the brain that inhibit impulsive and aggressive behaviour (Taylor 1999). Such an inability to block disruptive behaviour would result in acting without thinking or realising the consequences.

Genes are a key factor in about 75% of ADHD patients, and an autosomal dominant inheritance pattern can be found in families with this disorder. The mutations involved are mostly centred on dopamine and serotonin receptor genes. The D_4 receptor gene (***DRD4*** at 11p15.5) mutation may account for about 30% of the genetic risk of this disorder. ADHD is often inherited along with other conditions, which further complicate the picture. ADHD is regularly associated with substance abuse, for example alcoholism, and with depression. One gene in particular, found at locus 5p15.3, is strongly implicated in the condition. Called ***DAT1***, this gene codes for a protein that transports the neurotransmitter dopamine across the cell membrane, but it is not clear how this is involved in the condition.

The brains of sufferers show little gross difference from normal brains. There is some reduction in brain volume, in particular the prefrontal cortex, especially in those children with two copies of the *DAT1* gene mutation (Fernandez-Jaen et al. 2015). Grey matter volume reduction is caused by changes in synapses, and white matter reduction is caused by changes in myelination due to pathology of the oligodendrocytes (Bennet and Lagopoulos 2015). The lateral prefrontal cortex, dorsal anterior cingulate cortex, caudate nucleus, and putamen all appear to be involved in this disorder, but the changes are not physically obvious. The most important differences are disturbances in the biochemistry of the brain in ADHD. There appears to be an overall reduction in dopamine, and an 8% reduction in glucose metabolism in the premotor cortex and prefrontal cortex (both parts of the frontal lobe of the cerebrum).

The treatment of ADHD may include prescription of drugs, which, under specialist supervision, may be required for some years, sometimes even into adulthood. These drugs include the amphetamines **dexamfetamine** and **lisdexamfetamine mesilate**, a prodrug of dexamfetamine, and those drugs related to amphetamines such as **methylphenidate hydro-chloride (Ritalin)** and **atomoxetine.** Dexamfetamine and lisdexamfetamine are used when methylphenidate or atomoxetine fail to achieve the desire effect. They are stimulants of the central nervous system with increasing levels of dopamine, improving alertness, and con-centration. These drugs remain controversial because they can produce side effects such as nervousness, loss of appetite, insomnia, headaches, dizziness, and, rarely, hallucinations. The controversy is also fuelled by the growing debate centred on whether society should be medi-cating children. The concern is about what possible long-term harm this may be doing to our children at a time of important brain development. Methylphenidate can also affect the rest of the body, causing possible growth failure, damage to heart muscles, and low blood cell counts. Some parents of affected children taking Ritalin have claimed remarkable transformations in their children in terms of better behaviour and concentration. However, other parents have said that this drug has not been beneficial, causing additional behavioural problems. In either case, there is clearly a need for a comprehensive treatment plan for all sufferers from ADHD, in which drugs such as methylphenidate may or may not form part of the therapy, based on a joint decision between specialist medical staff and the child's parents (Scott 2000).

Developmental disorders

Autism spectrum disorder

Autism spectrum disorder (**ASD**) is a group of developmental disorders so called because affected children appear to withdraw from normal social interactions, including parental rela-tions, and prefer their own company in isolation (*auto* = 'self'). They also show restricted, stereotypical, and ritualised patterns of interests and behaviour. They fail to develop the skills necessary for normal human interactions; notably, communication skills are lacking to varying degrees, or even absent. The social isolationism is akin to that seen in schizophrenia, a disorder to which autism is linked. Social interactions with other people were found to improve when a low dose of **oxytocin**, a hormone from the hypothalamus via the pituitary gland (see Chapter 5), was administered. This suggests that the hypothalamic oxytocin cells were not functioning adequately, and that oxytocin may reverse some emotional and social symptoms of ASD.

Because of developmental links between the face and the brain, genetic disorders of the brain may cause facial deformities. In ASD, these are very subtle, but appear to be a broad upper face with wider eyes, a short middle region of the face (cheeks and nose), and a wider mouth and **philtrum** (the depression in the centre of the upper lip).

ASD encompasses a number of disorders, including:

* **autistic disorder**, defined as the severe symptoms that meet nearly all the diagnostic criteria for autism;
* **Asperger's syndrome**, a mild form of autism affecting mostly boys;
* **pervasive developmental disorder (not otherwise specified) (PDD-NOS)**, intermediate in severity between Asperger's syndrome and autistic disorder;
* **childhood disintegrative disorder (CDD)**, a rare but most severe form of autism (see below);
* **Joubert syndrome**, which includes autistic symptoms (see below);
* possibly **Rett Syndrome** (see below);

- possibly **fragile X syndrome** (see Chapter 6 and below);
- **Timothy syndrome (TS)**, a rare autosomal dominant congenital disorder that includes severe autistic symptoms as well as physical deformities; the mutation occurs on the *CACNA1C* gene at 12p13.33, which codes for a subunit of a calcium channel; affected children die at an early age (average 2.5 years), but may live long enough to develop the autistic symptoms.

ASD is also sometimes associated with other conditions, notably epilepsy, Down syndrome, various single-gene defects, infections (e.g. congenital rubella, or German measles), some temporal lobe tumours, and hydrocephalus (Rapin 1998). Hydrocephalus is excessive water around the brain due to a build-up of cerebrospinal fluid (CSF), which can cause extensive brain damage.

ASD shows various degrees of severity, from mild at one end of the spectrum through to severe at the other end. The cause of autism appears to be multifactorial, and there are now many genes strongly linked to the disorder, and many of these same genes also underpin intellectual disability (see below). ASD affects about 1 in 250,000 infants (0.0004%), with boys being more often affected than girls.

Genetics

At least some forms of autism are genetically inherited in families. Twin studies offer the best evidence of this. If one monozygotic (identical) twin has autism, the other twin has up to 96% chance of having autism; that is, there is a concordance rate of 96%. In a case of concordance, both twins develop the disorder, whereas in a case of discordance, one does but the other does not develop the disorder. In dizygotic (non-identical) twins the concordance rate is about the same as for ordinary siblings with the disorder (i.e. 2–3%). Even 2% is a much higher chance of developing the disorder than the 0.0004% recorded for the population as a whole, indicating that the figures for twins and sibling relationships is strongly influenced by inherited genetic factors. Understanding of the genes themselves has grown, with perhaps as many as 1000 gene mutations now linked to autism. Sixty of these mutations show very strong linkage to the disorder. The important genes (and their gene loci) are *AUTS1A* (7q36), *AUTS1B* (7q31), *AUTS2* (3q25-q27), *AUTS3* (13q14), *AUTS4* (15q11-13), *AUTS5* (2q), *AUTS6* (17q21), *GLO1* (6p21.3), *AUTSX1* (Xq13), *AUTSX2* (Xp22.33), *AUTSX3* (Xq28), and *SPCH1* (7q31), a gene involved in speech. Some of the genes on the X chromosomes that are known to be mutated in ASD are regulated by **fragile X mental retardation protein (FMRP)**, which is produced by the X-linked gene **fragile X mental retardation 1 (*FMR1*)**. This gene is mutated in **fragile X syndrome** (see Chapter 6), and this causes the FMRP protein to be malformed. This creates a link between fragile X syndrome and ASD genes, and a possible explanation for the autistic-like symptoms seen in fragile X syndrome.

Two genes on chromosome 5 code for proteins that help to bind cells together and therefore influence neuronal connections. Mutations in one of these, *CDH10*, was found in 65% of patients with autism.

A deletion (Chapter 6) of part of the **trimethyllysine epsilon (*TMLHE*)** gene may be involved in mild ASD. The gene is at Xq28, the same as the *MECP2* that causes Rett syndrome (see below) because Xq28 contains 183 different genes. The *TMLHE* gene codes for the first enzyme (**trimethyllysine dioxygenase**) in a process that leads to the production of **carnitine**, which is necessary for the transportation of fatty acids into the mitochondria for the early stages of energy production from fats. Loss of this enzyme due to the gene deletion can cause carnitine deficiency, and this would limit the use of fatty acids as an energy source. However, carnitine is acquired mostly from the diet (75% comes from eating meat), and the body only has to make up any dietary shortfall (e.g. in vegetarians, and especially vegans). The link between this gene mutation and mild ASD is not strong, and the presence of this particular deletion is not currently recognised as an important risk factor.

Environment

About 3% of childhood neurobehavioural disorders, including ADHD and ASD, are caused by environmental factors, with a further 25% caused by an interaction between environmental factors and genetics. Ten top environmental suspects are lead, methylmercury, **polychlorinated biphenyls (PCBs)**, **organophosphate pesticides**, **organochlorine pesticides**, endocrine disruptors, automotive exhaust, **polycyclic aromatic hydrocarbons (PAHs)**, **brominated flame retardants**, and **perfluorinated compounds** (Landrigan et al. 2012).

Perhaps as many as nine out of ten children with ASD have some degree of gastrointestinal problem, e.g. inflammatory bowel disease. This can cause the bowel to leak its contents into the bloodstream to varying extent. The normal gut **flora** (healthy bowel bacteria) may become abnormal in ASD, e.g. fewer healthy and more harmful organisms derived from the environment, and it is possible that these harmful bacteria could leak into the blood and influence brain function.

Exposure to fine articulate pollutants, less than 2.5 micrometres in size, present in the air during pregnancy may also increase the risk of ASD in the fetus. This particularly applies to exposure to fine particulates during the third trimester of the pregnancy.

Children born prematurely have part of their third trimester outside of the uterus. The third trimester of pregnancy is a period of rapid brain development when connections between various brain components are being established. Preterm babies must make some of these developments in a very different environment outside the uterus instead of the natural environment inside the uterus. This affects the way these connections are made, and it is known that preterm delivery increases the risk of developing ASD and ADHD. The most important of these affected connections is the **salience network** (see Chapter 1), where the thalamus, prefrontal cortex, and insular and interior cingulate regions are inadequately connected. Children with ASD and ADHD were found to have poor connections in this pathway. These connectivity problems persist into adulthood.

Asperger's syndrome (AS)

Some individuals are considered to have a mild form of autism called **Asperger's syndrome (AS)** (or **Asperger disorder**), named after Hans Asperger, an Austrian physician. It affects males three times more than females. Sufferers demonstrate varying degrees of the following symptoms:

- an inability to respond to normal social interactions with other people;
- restricted interests and behavioural patterns, often linked to one object or topic;
- an inability to form peer relationships;
- poor reciprocal emotional abilities;
- abnormal nonverbal gestures.

This behaviour tends towards the isolationism also seen in autism, but in AS verbal communication, and cognitive and intellectual development are normal (Sadock et al. 2009).

Childhood disintegrative disorder

One type of autism is **childhood disintegrative disorder** (**CDD**, or **Heller's syndrome**) where the child starts developing normally after birth but then from about aged 2 years the child mentally regresses, losing social, language, motor, and intellectual skills. They develop autistic-like abnormal communication and behavioural symptoms, with repetitive motor mannerisms. It is very rare, occurring in less than 2 children per 100,000 with ASD, mostly boys. They never regain the lost skills. Investigations have shown that mothers of children with autism, particularly of CDD, may have **immunoglobulin G** (**IgG**) antibodies in their blood, which are specific to fetal brain cells. By crossing the placenta, these antibodies get into the fetal circulation and brain, where they can disrupt brain development. IgG and complement proteins are sometimes found in the digestive system of autistic children. These are normally blood plasma immune proteins, and are not expected to be found inside the bowel. Their presence outside the blood is similar to conditions seen in autoimmune disorders.

Pervasive developmental disorder (not otherwise specified)

Children who do not meet all the required criteria for a diagnosis of autistic disorder, but are more severe than Asperger's syndrome, are sometimes classified as having **pervasive developmental disorder (not otherwise specified)** (**PDD-NOS**). The children in this category vary in their symptoms widely, with no two children being the same. Generally they have impaired social interaction skills, some language difficulties but not as severe as in autistic disorder, fewer repetitive behavioural mannerisms, and have a later age of onset.

Joubert syndrome

The cerebellum in autistic sufferers may also be affected, showing a poorly developed **vermis** (Figure 15.3). The cerebellar vermis is a median lobe (i.e. it runs along the midline) that appears worm-like (*vermis* = 'worm'). The cerebellar vermis is also poorly developed, and sometimes missing in an autosomal recessive disorder called **Joubert syndrome**. Children with this condition have **ataxia** (unsteady movements), **hyperpnoea** (abnormal breathing), abnormal eye and tongue movements, and fits, and they show the symptoms of autism, suggesting that the cerebellar vermis is involved in the cause of some aspects of autism. Genetics appear to be involved as well, with at least 20 genes (*JBTS1–JBTS20*), known to be linked to this disorder. Joubert syndrome is one of a series of disorders called **ciliopathies**, i.e. abnormalities of the cell **cilia** structure and function. How this affects neurons to cause Joubert syndrome is not fully understood.

Brain changes in ASD

Some of the biological changes that have been identified in ASD are as follows.

- The visual cortex of the occipital lobe processes impulses from the eyes concerning facial recognition by assigning this task mainly to part of the fusiform gyrus and a few

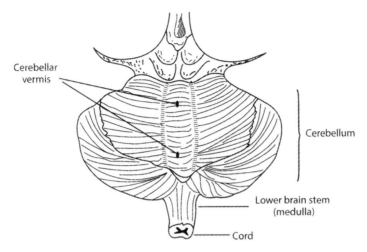

Figure 15.3 The cerebellum – dorsal view showing the vermis (the central ridge) – the malformation of which is becoming important in mental health.

other areas nearby. In some patients with autistic disorder, the fusiform gyrus has fewer and smaller neurons than normal, and as a result the area is hypoactive. This would account for autistic children having difficulties with social interactions with other people, since these interactions are dependent on identification of people, and that, in turn, relies on facial recognition (van Kooten 2008).

- **Mirror neurons** occur in the premotor cortex, part of the frontal lobe, and their purpose is to allow individuals to copy the actions of others. Copying is a vital component of learning, and these neurons not only perform this task but are apparently involved in higher cognitive functions related to copying, including language and understanding others' intentions. These mirror circuits were first found in monkeys, and were called 'monkey-see, monkey-do neurons'. In ASD, these neurons appear only to respond to what the individual does, but not to what they see others do. This is thought to be partly responsible for the lack of social skills related to learning and people interactions that are seen in ASD.
- Another important factor in ASD is possible damage to the central nervous system of the fetus during or shortly after pregnancy. The highest incidence occurs if fetal brain development is disturbed during the early stages of pregnancy (see IgG in CDD, above).
- Children with ASD appear to have inadequate synaptic pruning, resulting in an excess of synapses in the brain. Many of these excess synapses are damaged, but the cells responsible for removing these dead or damaged structures (a process called **autophagy**, carried out by phagocytes such as **microglia**) failed to clear away the debris. This was due to the overactivity of a gene called **mechanistic target of rapamycin (*mTOR*)** at 1p36.22, which normally has a strong influence over autophagy. The overactive gene in ASD stopped the process of autophagy, and future drugs that reduce *mTOR* activity and are now under development may be useful in correcting some of the symptoms.
- Another problem is closely linked to these excess synapses. Synapses often occur at the ends of tiny branches on dendrites called **dendritic spines**. An enzyme known as **UBE3A** is normally involved in brain development. It is usually switched off when not

required by adding a phosphate molecule to the enzyme (a process called **phosphoryla-tion**). An ASD-linked gene mutation prevents this phosphorylation of UBE3A, and the enzyme becomes overactive. The result is excessive production of dendritic spines. So the ASD child has excessive numbers of both dendritic spines and synapses. Some compounds that reduce UBE3A activity are under development.

* **Antidiuretic hormone (ADH, or vasopressin)** is the hypothalamic hormone released from the **posterior pituitary gland** (see Chapter 1), and it is essential for control of water loss through the kidneys. However, it does have other functions, and a greater emphasis is now placed on research into its relationship with mental health. It is linked (with **oxytocin, OT**) to social bonding of children with their parents, one of the social skills not well developed in autism. Both hormones share a close structural relationship, and also share a receptor (called the **OT receptor**), which binds OT and ADH. In addition, vasopressin binds to three other receptors (**V1a, V1b,** and **V2**). The V2 receptor is found in the kidney and is involved in the fluid balance control function of ADH. V1a is found in the liver, and V1b is found in the anterior pituitary, where is has influence over **adrenocorticotrophic hormone (ACTH)** release, and thus ultimately **cortisol** release from the adrenal cortex (see Chapters 1 and 9, and see HPA axis in Chapter 11, Figure 11.5). ADH affects the sensory aspects of the brain, i.e. sensory processing, in ways that are not fully understood. Low ADH is thought to inhibit bonding by causing inadequate sensory processing, thus allowing the sensory system to become overloaded, a state the child then tries to avoid. Research is in progress to see if delivering ADH via nasal spray improves the autistic child's ability to bond with those he or she knows. OT delivered via nasal spray to autistic children has also proved to be beneficial. Research showed that it allowed the children to socialise more; in particular they became able to distinguish between people being mean or nice, a task they could not achieve otherwise. The research found that autistic children had fewer OT receptors than normal (Lange and McDougle 2013).

Savantism

Linked with autism is the contradictory and puzzling phenomenon known as savantism. About 30% of autistic people have an extraordinary talent in one particular skill, usually focused on music, mathematics, art, or memory. These people are known as **savants**. There is some debate as to how or why a selection of people with a disability such as autism can excel to such an advanced degree in one specialised subject. Their particular skill does involve exceptional practice, especially in music, but the question remains: are these talents 'built in' to the brain from birth, and does the practice serve to sharpen these skills to a very high level? The attention to detail demonstrated by savants is amazing, and it is this that sets them apart from others in the same field of talent. Some brain differences have been found in savants, e.g. they may show an increase in the brain size in those areas involved in their particular talents, but they equally show thinner than normal areas in other parts of the brain. However, this brain thickening could result from the large amounts of practice they carry out for their skill. The notion of brain thickening as a result of persistent practice is becoming better understood as part of plasticity, i.e. the brain's ability to adapt to changes in circumstances. So savantism may therefore be a question of motivation, i.e. it may be that some autistic children become highly motivated to develop one particular skill in which they then develop to an amazingly high standard. Perhaps if this level of motivation was found more often in non-autistic children they could equally develop similarly amazing talents and skills.

Rett syndrome

Rett syndrome is another condition that involves the clinical symptoms of autism, although it is not always regarded as part of ASD. The disorder, affecting almost entirely girls, is very rare, occurring in about 1 in 10,000–15,000 girls. Sufferers develop normally for about the first few months of life, but then further development is arrested at about 12–18 months of age, followed by a serious decline in growth and development. This rapid decline includes autistic symptoms with dementia, and these may be the first clinical signs of this disorder. The symptoms progress to include motor problems such as abnormal hand movements and failure to walk, failure of head growth leading to **microcephaly** (a small head), and some-times a slight increase in the level of ammonia in the blood (**hyperammonaemia**). Rett syndrome is caused by mutations of the gene **methyl CpG binding protein 2** (*MECP2*) on the X chromosome at Xq28, a region that contains 183 genes (see TMLHE, above). Such mutations result in loss of noradrenaline from the **locus coeruleus**, and low levels of noradrenaline in the brain generally, which is a pathological feature of this disorder. Mutations of another gene called *SYN1* (found at Xp11.23) may be involved in Rett syn-drome. The normal gene codes for the protein **synapsin I**, which is one of several proteins called **synapsins** that are critically involved in synaptogenesis (the formation of synapses) and in the modulation of neurotransmitter release at the synapse. Exactly how this gene mutation causes the symptoms is not yet clear, but neuronal developmental problems have been found on brain examination. Affected brain cells show membrane-bound **inclusions** (abnormal structures within the cell body) in both neurons and oligodendrocytes, with small cell size, reduced ability to generate action potentials, and a loss of dendrites with concur-rent loss of synaptic connections.

Intellectual disability

Intellectual disability is characterised by a below-average intellectual ability involving cog-nitive deficits over a wide range of skills. These skill deficits include those related to the standard skills required for normal daily living, such as communication, self-care, inter-personal skills, and academic ability. Intellectual disability can be regarded as a spectral phenomenon, i.e. being very mild at one end of the spectrum to very severe (or profound) at the other end of the spectrum. Intellectual disability may cause varying degrees of language development problems, various motor deficits causing movement problems, weak academic performance, and poor social skills.

The biological causes are numerous, ranging from genetic through to environmental factors. Chapter 6 identifies a number of intellectual disability syndromes of genetic and chro-mosomal origin, specifically of the X chromosome (see Figure 6.13 and Table 6.3). Other causes include toxins, infections, brain trauma, and metabolic and nutritional disorders.

Some genetic causes of intellectual disability

Phenylketonuria (**PKU**) is an autosomal recessive gene disorder that affects about 1 in 20,000 children worldwide. In this disorder the *essential* dietary amino acid **phenylalanine** cannot be metabolised fully owing to a recessive gene error found at 12q22-q24.1, the gene coding for the enzyme **phenylalanine hydroxylase** (Figure 15.4). This enzyme converts phenylalanine to tyrosine, which is the precursor to dopamine and noradrenaline.

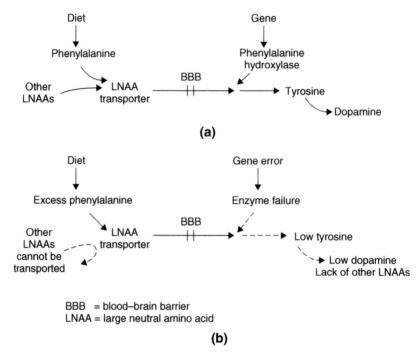

Figure 15.4 Phenylalanine hydroxylase action, (a) normally and (b) in phenylketonuria.

As a result of the failure of the enzyme, phenylalanine builds up in the blood and the brain. Phenylalanine has to be transported across the blood–brain barrier by a protein, the **large neutral amino acid (LNAA) transporter**. This transporter protein is also essential for carrying other LNAAs across the blood–brain barrier. In the event of excessive phenylalanine in the blood, the transporter is swamped and works only on phenylalanine. Therefore, a shortage of the other LNAAs in the brain causes brain damage, leading to intellectual disability (Figure 15.4). The severity varies from mild to profound, sometimes with microcephaly, mood disorders, and behavioural problems. A simple test can detect the problem early, and this can allow sufferers to reduce the complications with a low phenylalanine diet (allowing just enough for tissue growth and repair) and sometimes medication with **sapropterin**. This drug is a synthetic form of the dietary nutrient **tetrahydrobiopterin**, which acts as a cofactor necessary for the function of **phenylalanine hydroxylase**. Occasionally, it is an absence of this cofactor that is the reason why phenylalanine hydroxylase fails, and phenylalanine builds up, causing PKU.

Tay–Sachs disease is a recessive inherited disease more common in the Jewish population than in other populations. The children with this disorder initially develop normally from birth, but between 3 and 6 months old they suffer a progressive degeneration of the central nervous system (CNS). The CNS degeneration causes blindness, fits, paralysis, intellectual disability, and usually death between 2 and 6 years old. The **HEXA** gene, found at 15q23-q24, codes for a subunit of the enzyme **beta-hexosaminidase A**. The gene can have any of the 120 or more mutations that have been found in Tay–Sachs disease. Beta-hexosaminidase A is an enzyme found in the lysosomes of neurons. It breaks down a fatty waste called

GM2 ganglioside, which is then normally excreted from the cell. Failure of this subunit, due to one of the many gene errors, results in this waste accumulating within the neuron, which then subsequently dies. Although every generation carries the faulty gene, the disease is recessive and may skip one or more generations.

Other genetic causes of a small percentage of intellectual disability are mutations of the **thyroid hormone receptor interactor 8 (*JMJD1C*)** gene at 10q21.3. This gene controls the activity of other genes, as part of **epigenetics**, i.e. DNA not coding for proteins directly but influencing other genes.

Some teratogenic causes of intellectual disability

Fetal alcohol syndrome (FAS) occurs when women drink too much alcohol during pregnancy (Figure 15.5). The alcohol acts as a teratogen, which is an agent that crosses the placenta and harms the developing fetus. A teratogenic agent may be living (e.g. a virus) or nonliving (e.g. a chemical or drug, such as alcohol). As a result of excessive alcohol consumption during pregnancy, the child may show signs of intellectual disability along with multiple physical abnormalities, such as low birth weight, facial and skeletal abnormalities, and nervous system damage. They have low to average intellectual skills, including poor judgement and difficulties in learning from experience. As an older child they are unlikely to demonstrate anything higher than an average performance at school, and they have problems following directions. The worst problems result from drinking alcohol during the earliest stages of pregnancy, when embryonic development is taking place. There is probably no safe level of alcohol drunk during pregnancy, as even low prenatal consumption is shown to cause learning, memory, and growth problems in schoolchildren. A similar problem occurs with illicit drugs taken by mothers during pregnancy. '**Crack babies**' are born to cocaine abuse mothers who took the drug during pregnancy. These children are less alert than normal with poor emotional and cognitive responses. They also have disturbed sleep patterns, irritability, and possible intellectual disability. Cocaine causes constriction of blood vessels supplying the fetus, resulting in low oxygen supply, which in turn restricts growth and development.

Nicotine is another teratogen that affects the fetus if the mother smokes during pregnancy. Nicotine has the effect of narrowing blood vessels (much like cocaine) and this reduces the blood supply to the fetus. In addition, the carbon monoxide in cigarette smoke binds tightly to the hemoglobin, preventing oxygen from binding, so the maternal and fetal blood both carry less oxygen than normal. Embryonic and fetal growth requires a good oxygen supply, and this is exactly what is lacking when nicotine and carbon monoxide are introduced into the maternal blood by smoking. Intellectual disability is due to the reduced oxygen supply to the fetal nervous system. In addition, most of the other 4000 or more toxic chemicals found in cigarette smoke, such as the poison **cyanide** and the neurotoxic metal **lead**, will enter the maternal blood and cross as teratogens into the fetal blood. The results of this chemical assault on the fetus is catastrophic, including more than doubling the risk of losing the baby through stillbirth. Babies born live to mothers who smoked during pregnancy are of low birth weight and may be born premature. Low birth weight usually means that the vital organs are underdeveloped and therefore do not perform as well as they should for a newborn child. The brain is chief among these organ deficits. The fetal neural damage caused by maternal smoking has a lifelong effect on the child's brain, causing poor intellectual development, learning difficulties, and behavioural problems (e.g. increased risk of ADHD). Motor and sensory deficits are more common in babies born to smoking mothers (Figure 15.6).

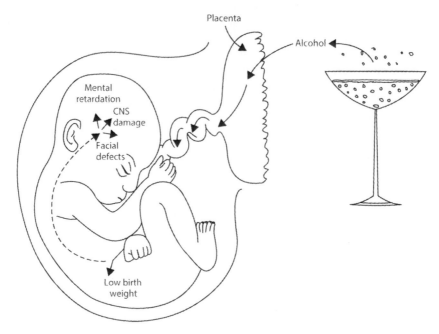

Figure 15.5 Fetal alcohol syndrome (FAS). Alcohol and other drugs are teratogenic, i.e. they cross the placenta and have serious adverse effects on the embryo or fetus.

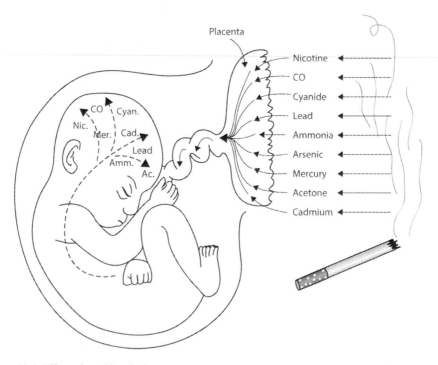

Figure 15.6 Effect of smoking during pregnancy.

Obsessive-compulsive disorder and tic disorders

Obsessions are repeated thoughts, ideas, or phrases, and **compulsions** are irresistible repetitive activities, such as repeated handwashing, which the patient must go through in order to prevent some degree of fear and anxiety. Both of these together in the same patient make up **obsessive-compulsive disorder (OCD)**. If these activities are stopped or prevented in some way, the person concerned may quickly go into a panic attack. About 2% of the population will suffer from OCD at some point in their life; about 1 million people in the UK.

OCD is associated with increased activity of several brain areas, notably a loop extending from the **orbitofrontal cortex**, through the **cingulate gyrus, caudate nucleus, globus pallidus**, and the **thalamus**, then back to the cortex (Insel 2010). Two pathways, an excitatory and an inhibitory pathway, pass from the caudate nucleus through the globus pallidus to the thalamus. The excitatory pathway is said to facilitate previously learnt and automatic behaviour, while the inhibitory pathway reduces it, thereby allowing the individual to move on to new behaviours. Brain scans show that in OCD much of this loop is overactive, notably the caudate nucleus, thalamus, and orbitofrontal cortex. The globus pallidus is underactive, and that allows the thalamus to become overactive, which causes an imbalance that keeps the patient locked in a cycle of repetitive behaviour (Figure 15.7).

Higher than average level of activity in the orbitofrontal cortex, in particular the medial area, which is normally involved in making moral decisions, means that ODC sufferers are more sensitive than expected to moral dilemmas. They can become more anxious about moral decisions and their outcome.

Interrupting this loop is one approach to treatment. One surgical technique under development involves using lasers to burn out a very small patch of the anterior cingulum (the surgery is called an **anterior cingulotomy**). Results of trials show sustained improvements in some patients up to 5 years after surgery.

An alternative view is that a reduction of serotonin and an increase in noradrenaline in the diffuse modulatory systems may be involved in this disorder (see Chapter 11 for a discussion of these systems). Together the diffuse modulatory systems help to control the loop function, but an imbalance between serotonin and noradrenaline could cause an increase in loop activity. This is supported by the fact that treatment with antidepressant drugs called **selective serotonin reuptake inhibitors (SSRIs)**, which increase the concentration of serotonin in the brain, helps to reduce the symptoms. Neurosurgery has also been used successfully to reduce the symptoms of OCD in cases that fail to respond to drugs. This involves cutting through some of the pathways that pass from the frontal lobe to the limbic parts of the brain (Ron 1999).

There is some evidence to suggest that OCD may have a genetic susceptibility, as a higher than average incidence can be demonstrated in some families. Relatives of those with OCD have a six-times greater risk of developing OCD than families without OCD. Monozygotic (MZ) twins have a concordance rate of 80–87% for OCD, while dizygotic twins have a 47–50% concordance rate. People with OCD also have a higher risk of depression and anxiety than the general population. The **catecholamine-*O*-methyl-transferase (*COMT*)** gene codes for the enzyme that breaks down the neurotransmitters dopamine, adrenaline, and noradrenaline, and *COMT* gene errors are suspected to be part of the cause, as it was discovered that this gene is underexpressed in OCD.

Body dysmorphic disorder (BDD) is a similar and related problem to OCD. Here, the sufferer believes their body, often their face, is in some way the wrong shape, and they may spend many hours before a mirror trying to correct or hide the so-called problem. It may

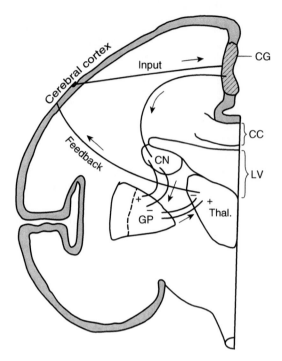

Figure 15.7 The loop extending from the orbitofrontal cortex to the cingulate gyrus (CG), through the striatum (caudate nucleus, CN) to the globus pallidus (GP), then to the thalamus (Thal.) with feedback to the orbitofrontal cortex again. Either excitatory or inhibitory pathways influences learning and automatic behaviour. In OCD, excessive function of the CN reduces activity in the GP, which allows overactivity in the thalamus to cause excessive stimulatory feedback to the orbitofrontal cortex.

even prevent the individual from leaving their home as they do not want to be embarrassed by the problem in public. It may affect between 1% and 2% of the population, but about 15% of people seeking cosmetic surgery may be individuals with BDD. It could be thought of as a 'body obsession'. People with BDD also show an inability to detect negative facial emotions because they concentrate on small facial features (e.g. the lips or eyes) rather than the whole face. But remarkably, BDD sufferers have the ability to identify famous people from an upside-down facial image, a task non-BDD individuals would normally find difficult.

Obsessive-compulsive personality has features in common with OCD, but differs by the individual being rigid and dogmatic, with blunted emotions. They work continuously, finding little or no time to maintain friendships or indulge in leisure. Obsession with perfectionism and following rules dominates their activities. They may be seen as dominating and authoritarian to their subordinates. As much as 7% of the population may have obsessive-compulsive personality, affecting men more than women.

Gilles de la Tourette syndrome (or **Tourette's syndrome, TS**) is characterised by motor and vocal **tics**, i.e. uncontrollable and repetitive muscle twitches of the head and shoulders particularly, and involuntary abnormal vocal sounds (e.g. grunts, barks, whistles). These tics are associated with abnormal behaviour, such as pulling hair and self-mutilation, and especially the compulsion to utter obscene words (**coprolalia**) and to repeat words many times (**echolalia**). The symptoms of the condition begin between the ages of 2 and 15 years, and about 75% of the patients are male. The gene mutations involved in the aetiology of this disorder are multiple, complex, and not fully understood. The genes that have been studied so far are:

- **BTB/POZ domain-containing protein 9 (*BTBD9*)** at 6p21 (a mutation of this gene is also linked to another neurological condition called restless legs syndrome). This gene error appears to be responsible for the 'pure' form of the disorder, i.e. without any additional signs of the other conditions that sometimes accompany it, notably OCD and ADD. *BTBD9* normally codes for a protein in the amygdala, caudate nucleus, cerebellum, and the hippocampus, although the function of this protein is unknown.
- **Histidine decarboxylase (*HDC*)** at 15q21-22, which codes for the enzyme **L-histidine decarboxylase**, which is essential for the production of **histamine** from **histidine**. Histaminergic neurons occur in the posterior hypothalamus, and radiate out to other brain areas (see Chapter 4, Figure 4.19). Disruption to histamine production results in tics of the type seen in TS, but the reason is not clear.
- Other genes linked to this disorder have been located to 11q23 and 13.q31. However, the numbers of TS cases linked to these genes are very small (about 1%) and the genes themselves are still under investigation.

Tic disorders have been categorised as simple tics, complex tics (a combination of tics with obsessive repetitive behaviour), and OCD (i.e. without tics, see above). From what is known currently, the pathology of the brain in TS appears to be centred on the same pathways as OCD:

- **The basal ganglia:** dopaminergic systems of the basal ganglia appear to be involved as dopamine receptor antagonists, particularly D_2 antagonists such as haloperidol, have reduced symptoms significantly, whereas drugs with a dopamimetic action (i.e. mimicking dopamine) make the symptoms worse. The basal ganglia is implicated in the disease because of its motor function and because some discrepancy in the symmetry of both the **putamen** and the **lentiform nucleus** have been identified in some sufferers (Breedlove et al. 2010). In addition, the caudate nucleus shows some reduction in a particular cell type known as the *parvalbumin-positive* cells (Kalanithi et al. 2005). These cells have a regulatory control function on the basal ganglia circuits routed through the caudate nucleus. A new treatment, deep brain stimulation, appears to improve the symptoms in the few cases where the treatment was tried. It consists of electrodes implanted deep into the brain to stimulate brain activity. This treatment is still in the trial stages and the long-term consequences of this approach are unknown.
- **The cerebral cortex:** increased volumes of the dorsal prefrontal and parieto-occipital cortex and thinning in the frontal, sensorimotor, and parietal areas have been noted in a number of patients studied. This thinning correlates well with the severity of the tics, and supports the classification of these disorders into complex, simple, or no tics (OCD). White matter shows changes in various subcortical areas. The corpus callosum shows changes in volumes and in microstructure. Tics are generated in association with the supplementary motor area, and biochemical changes occur mostly in prefrontal cortex.
- **Thalamus and brain stem:** unfortunately, the findings in the thalamus are not consistent and unreliable. They centre on the volume of the thalamus, found to be above normal in some studies and below normal in others. Some increase in the midbrain grey matter in TS sufferers has been reported.

Key points

Dyslexia

- Nine genes have been identified associated with dyslexia, dyslexia specific 1 (*DYX1*) through to dyslexia specific 9 (*DYX9*).
- The brains of dyslexia sufferers may show disorganised cell layers within part of the thalamus, called the lateral geniculate nucleus (LGN), part of the visual pathway.

Dysgraphia and dyspraxia

- Dysgraphia is a disorder of writing and spelling, in two forms: phonological dysgraphia and orthographic dysgraphia.

Attention deficit hyperactive disorder

- A gene called *DAT1*, found at locus 5p15.3, may be one factor causing attention deficit hyperactive disorder (ADHD). It codes for a protein that transports dopamine across the cell membrane.

Autism

- Autistic children appear to withdraw from social interactions, including parental relations, and become isolated (*auto* = 'self').
- Autism is caused or influenced by multiple genes.
- Autistic spectral disorder (ASD) is used to indicate a number of different disorders with common symptoms at various degrees of severity.
- The cerebellum in some autistic sufferers is also affected, showing a poorly developed vermis.
- A milder form of autism is called Asperger's syndrome.

Rett syndrome

- Rett syndrome also involves the clinical picture of autism, the sufferers being almost always girls.
- The main gene causing Rett syndrome is methyl CpG binding protein 2 (*MECP2*) at Xq28.

Phenylketonuria

- Metabolism of the essential dietary amino acid phenylalanine fails owing to a recessive gene mutation.
- The gene codes for the enzyme phenylalanine hydroxylase.
- As a result of the failure of the enzyme, phenylalanine builds up in the blood and in the brain, causing mental retardation.
- A phenylalanine-free diet can allow normal mental development.

Tay–Sachs disease

- Children with this disorder develop normally from birth, but between 3 and 6 months old they suffer a progressive degeneration of the central nervous system.

- The CNS degeneration causes blindness, fits, paralysis, intellectual disability, and usually death between 2 and 6 years old.
- The gene for Tay–Sachs disease is the *HEXA* gene.

Fetal alcohol syndrome

- Too much alcohol consumed during pregnancy acts as a teratogen and affects the fetus.
- The result is a mix of both physical and mental abnormalities.
- There is no safe level of alcohol consumption during pregnancy.

OCD and Tourette's syndrome

- Obsessions are repeated thoughts, ideas or phrases; and compulsions are irresistible repetitive activities.
- Obsessive-compulsive disorder is associated with increased activity of a loop consisting of the orbitofrontal cortex, the cingulate gyrus, the caudate nucleus, the globus pallidus, and the thalamus.
- Tourette's syndrome is characterised by motor and vocal tics, i.e. uncontrollable and repetitive muscle twitches of the head and shoulders, and involuntary abnormal vocal sounds (e.g. grunts, barks, whistles).
- The main gene involved in Tourette's syndrome is probably *BTBD9* at 6p21.

References

Bennett, M. R. and Lagopoulos, J. (2015) Neurodevelopment sequelae associated with gray and white matter changes and their cellular basis: a comparison between Autism Spectrum Disorder, ADHD and dyslexia. *International Journal of Developmental Neuroscience*, **46**: 132–143. DOI: 10.1016/j.ijdevneu.2015.02.007.

Breedlove, S. M., Watson, N. V., and Rosenzweig, M. R. (2010) *Biological Psychology: An Introduction to Behavioural, Cognitive and Clinical Neuroscience* (6th edition). Sinauer Associates, Sunderland, MA.

Fernández-Jaén, A., López-Martin, S., Albert, J., Fernández-Mayoralas, D. M., Fernández-Perrone, A. L., de La Peña, M. J., Calleja-Pérez, B., Rodríguez, M. R., López-Arribas, S., and Muñoz-Jaeño, N. (2015) Cortical thickness differences in the prefrontal cortex in children and adolescents with ADHD in relation to dopamine transporter (*DAT1*) genotype. *Psychiatry Research*, **233** (3): 409–417. DOI: 10.1016/j.pscychresns.2015.07.005.

Insel, T. R. (2010) Faulty circuits. *Scientific American*, **302** (4): 28–35.

Kalanithi, P. S. A., Zheng, W., Kataoka, Y., DiFiglia, M., Grantz, H., Saper, C. B., Schwartz, M., Leckman, J. F., and Vaccarino, F. M. (2005) Altered parvalbumin-positive neuron distribution in basal ganglia of individuals with Tourette's syndrome. *Proceedings of the National Academy of Sciences of the United States of America*. Online at: http://www.pnas.org/content/102/37/13307.full-aff-1

Landrigan, P., Lambertini, L., and Birnbaum, L. (2012) A research strategy to discover the environmental causes of autism and neurodevelopmental disabilities. *Environmental Health Perspectives*, **120** (7): a258–a260. DOI: 10.1289/ehp.1104285.

Lange, N. and McDougle, C. J. (2013) Help for the child with autism. *Scientific American*, October 2013, 58–63.

Norton, E. S., Black, J. M., Stanley, L. M., Tanaka, H., Gabrieli, J. D. E, Sawyer, C., and Hoeft, F. (2014) Functional neuroanatomical evidence for the double-deficit hypothesis of developmental dyslexia. *Neuropsychologia*, **61**: 235–246.

Rapin, I. (1998) What a neurologist would like to know about autism and doesn't. *Neuroscience News*, **1** (4): 6–13.

Ron, M. A. (1999) Psychiatric manifestations of demonstrable brain disease, *in* Ron M. A. and David A. S. (eds), *Disorders of Brain and Mind*. Cambridge University Press, Cambridge, UK.

Sadock, B. J., Sadock, V. A., and Ruiz, P. (2009) *Kaplin and Sadock's Comprehensive Textbook of Psychiatry* (9th edition). Lippincott, Williams and Wilkins, Baltimore, MD.

Scott, S. (2000) Bad behaviour. *New Scientist*, **166** (2239): 44–45.

Stein, J. (2001) The magnocellular theory of developmental dyslexia. *Dyslexia*, **7** (1): 12–36.

Taylor, E. (1999) Early disorders and later schizophrenia: a developmental neuropsychiatric perspective, *in* Ron M. A. and David A. S. (eds), *Disorders of Brain and Mind*. Cambridge University Press, Cambridge, UK.

van Kooten, I. A. J., Palmem, S. J. M. C., Cappeln, P., Steinbusch, H. W. M., Korr, H., Heinsen, H., Hof, P.R., van Engeland, H., and Schmitz, C. (2008) Neurons in the fusiform gyrus are fewer and smaller in autism. *Brain*, **131** (4): 987–999.

Williams, J. and O'Donovan, M. C. (2006) The genetics of developmental dyslexia. *European Journal of Human Genetics*, **14**: 681–689. DOI: 10.1038/sj.ejhg.5201575.

16 Sleep

- Introduction
- Why we sleep
- Physiology of normal sleep
- The neurological control of sleep
- Dreams
- Effects of sleep loss on health
- Sleep disorders
- Sleep medication
- Key points

Introduction

Among all the functions of the brain, sleep is possibly one of the most bizarre. After 16 hours or so of being awake, the brain appears to shut down and fall asleep for an average of about 8 hours. No other organ does this. It clearly serves a vital purpose, because sleep is inevitable; the brain itself will eventually overcome all attempts to stay awake and will induce a state of sleep. And sleep impinges heavily on health. Insufficient sleep is a major factor both in the cause and the symptoms of mental health and physical disorders. Sleep pattern disturbances are seen in several disorders, e.g. depression and anxiety states, and management of sleep disorders is an important component of treatment.

Why we sleep

Sleep has remained a mysterious phenomenon since humans began thinking about it. It does seem illogical for humans and animals to spend a large part of their lives sleeping when they could be doing other things, not to mention that during sleep humans (and animals) are significantly less able to protect or defend themselves against attack. There have been many theories about why we spend approximately a third of our lives in this activity. It had been assumed that sleep was the time for the brain to rest, but sleep researchers have known for some time now that this is not true. Quite the opposite, in fact – the brain is very active during sleep. Neurons fire impulses almost as frequently while asleep as they do when awake. Sleep may offer rest for the body, but not for the brain, which remains active day and night for a lifetime.

Now, much clearer insights into the purposes of sleep are becoming available. There appears to be a number of activities that are promoted during sleep, the important ones being:

- consolidation of cognitive functions, in particular memories (Stickgold and Walker 2007);
- cleansing the brain of metabolic waste (Xie et al. 2013);
- increasing the activities of genes that are involved in the production of oligodendrocytes (myelin-producing cells; see Chapter 3) (Bellesi et al. 2013);
- possibly weakening of synaptic connections, restoring their baseline levels of strength and conserving energy, the 'synaptic homeostasis hypothesis' (Tononi and Cirelli 2006, 2013).

Memory consolidation

Consolidation of memories requires a good degree of brain plasticity (see Chapter 1) and an understanding of the different types of memory (see Chapters 2 and 14). It is not just about learning (or memorising) new information, but the ability of the brain to integrate that new information into the older information that is already stored, thus updating it. So important is sleep in this process that researchers refer to it as 'sleep-dependent memory consolidation'. Modification of old memories to be updated by new information requires, on the micro scale, plasticity down to protein molecular level. Memory integration on the macro scale appears to involve modification of entire memory systems and networks, i.e. building new memories into multiple pathways and synapses. Such complex macro and micro processes are apparently better done during sleep as a function of slow-wave sleep (see Physiology of normal sleep, page 358). Parts of the brain that are actively storing memories during sleep generate more 'slow-wave' activity.

Cleansing the brain

In the second function on the list, metabolic toxic waste is removed from brain cells and tissues by the cerebrospinal fluid (CSF). When awake, CSF and tissue fluid (or extracellular fluid, ECF) around the cells for the most part remain separate. CSF remains mostly within the ventricles and subarachnoid spaces. Glial cells occupy the spaces between neurons (called **interstitial space**), and they control the flow of CSF into and out of the brain through channels. During sleep these glial channels expand by 60%, increasing the flow of CSF into the brain. This allows for all the wastes, especially beta-amyloid protein that accumulated during the previous day in the ECF, to be washed out by the CSF for excretion. The lymphatic system is responsible for functions of this kind in all the other body tissues, and these microscopic channels opening during sleep allow CSF to carry out the same function in the brain. This sleeping 'lymphatic-like' function was called the **glymphatic system** by researchers. During sleep, removal of wastes such as beta-amyloid protein occurs twice as quickly than when awake. This protein is a problem seen in Alzheimer's disease, where it accumulates as extracellular plaques (see Chapter 14). What is still uncertain is why we need to be asleep for this function to take place, i.e. Why do these channels open only when asleep? And is the need to clean out wastes from the ECF part of the process of inducing the onset of sleep? It is possible that this 'brain washing' function and being awake are, for some reason, incompatible.

The glymphatic drainage of the brain was shown to be more efficient at clearing the brain of toxic waste when sleeping on the side (i.e. the lateral position) rather than on the back (supination) or the front (prone).

Increased activity of genes

Genes involved in the creation of **oligodendrocytes** show heightened activity during sleep compared with when awake. Sleep therefore results in additional oligodendrocytes, and therefore extra myelin production. This allows myelin restoration and repair to take place more efficiently. Sleep deprivation not only removes this benefit, but also causes raised activation levels in genes linked to cellular stress and death. However, the benefits of this gene activation (myelination repair), happen over a long period (i.e. weeks or months), not during the space of a few nights' sleep.

The synaptic homeostasis hypothesis (SHY)

During waking hours, many synapses are strengthened as a result of use, i.e. dealing with environmental stimuli or cognitive processes such as learning. This synaptic strengthening is a reinforcement of those networks processing that data, including memory storage. If left like that, synaptic strengthening would accumulate daily to the point at which brain plasticity would be severely reduced, i.e. the brain would reach saturation point in synaptic strengthening, similar to a computer running out of memory. During slow-wave sleep (NREM stages 3 and 4), these strengthened synapses are downgraded to a more basal level of strength, which is energy sustainable, allows brain plasticity to continue, improves grey matter efficiency, and is beneficial for learning. This reduction of synaptic strengthening may also include loss of unwanted synapses or dendritic spines by the process of synaptic pruning (see Chapter 2). This downgrading process preserves the variation of individual synaptic strengths, and therefore the patterns of learning achieved prior to sleep, i.e. memories are preserved (Figure 16.1). On awakening, the brain, now restored to a baseline homeostatic condition, is ready to begin the processing of new information coming in from the senses.

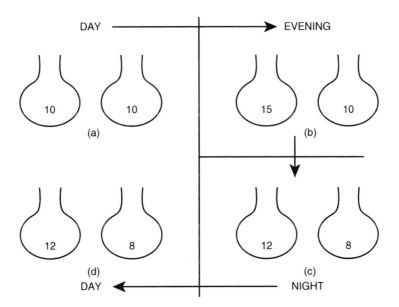

Figure 16.1 Synaptic homeostasis hypothesis (SHY). (a) Both synapses are equal strength at the start of the day (total = 20). (b) The left synapse has increased strength during the day. (c) During sleep, the two synapses readjust to 20 again, but still with the left synapse stronger, ready for (d) the next day.

Physiology of normal sleep

Sleep is one of our **circadian rhythms** (*circa* = 'about', *dian* = 'a day'); i.e. the full sleep–wake cycle takes about one day to complete, with sleep occupying approximately one-third of that time in adults. It is, however, a very complex phenomenon, with much still to learn about it.

Two types of sleep are recognised: (1) rapid-eye movement (**REM**) sleep; and (2) non-rapid eye movement (**NREM**) sleep.

REM sleep

REM sleep is identified by the rapid movement of the eyes beneath the closed lids, and appears to be the lightest form of sleep. It occurs soon after falling asleep and returns regularly throughout the course of the night (Figure 16.2).

During REM sleep, the muscles of the body are in a state of **atonia**, a type of paralysis. This is to prevent the sleeping person from acting out their dreams. They are said to have 'an active mind in a paralysed body'. The pathway involved (called the **peribrachial pathway**) passes down the spinal cord, starting from the **magnocellular nucleus** of the **peribrachial area** (within the brain stem) to the **lower motor neurons** (**LMNs**) that control the muscles. Activation of this pathway inhibits these motor neurons, causing inhibition of the body's skeletal muscles (Figure 16.3).

During REM sleep, the heart rate, blood pressure, and respiratory rate are all raised but irregular. Cerebral blood flow and brain oxygen consumption are increased in REM sleep. A person in REM sleep can be woken quite easily and may report dreaming. The brain waves produced during REM sleep, as seen from **electroencephalogram** (**EEG**) recordings, are desynchronised and mostly **beta waves** (14 or more Hz) with some **theta wave** activity (4–7 Hz). This is similar to the waking state, which is also beta wave activity, accompanied by alpha waves (8–13 Hz) when in the relaxed state (Figure 16.4). REM sleep is often referred to as '**paradoxical sleep**' because of the similarity of EEG recordings with those taken when awake.

REM sleep is divided into two stages: (1) phasic, during which the eye movements and muscle twitches occur; (2) tonic, the periods between phasic REM. REM is characterised by

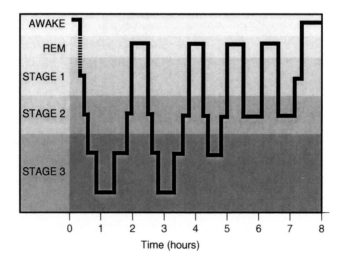

Figure 16.2 The 8-hour sleep cycle.

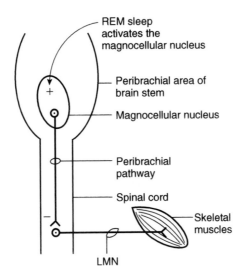

Figure 16.3 Atonia during REM sleep.

cerebral desynchronisation of brain waves seen on EEG. **Synchronisation** means that brain waves add up to a significant amplitude (as measured in Hz). **Desynchronisation** means that brains waves do not add up; therefore the amplitude is low.

The peribrachial area initiates all the activities related to REM sleep, including skeletal muscle atony, jerky eye movements, and cortical desynchrony via the thalamus. During REM sleep, the eyes appear to be following events taking place in the dreams beneath the closed lids. These rapid eye movements are maintained by acetylcholine neurons from the peribrachial area to the **tectum** at the back of the brain stem. Two small bumps on the tectum are the **superior colliculi**, which are important in visual tracking of moving objects while awake. It would appear that they may be involved in tracking false visual objects during dreams.

NREM sleep

NREM sleep is characterised by synchronised wave patterns on EEG, regular heart rate, respiration, and blood pressure, reduced oxygen consumption, and lower body temperature. NREM is divided into four stages, according again to the EEG recordings.

Stage 1

The 'lightest' of the four stages, identified by the presence of **theta waves** (4–7 Hz). This stage lasts typically 5 to 15 minutes.

Stage 2

This stage is 'transitional' sleep between light and deep sleep, identified by the presence of 'sleep spindles' and 'K complexes' on the EEG (Figure 16.4). It lasts about 20 minutes. **Sleep spindles** (or **sigma waves**) occur in two forms: slow (11.13 Hz) and fast (13–15 Hz).

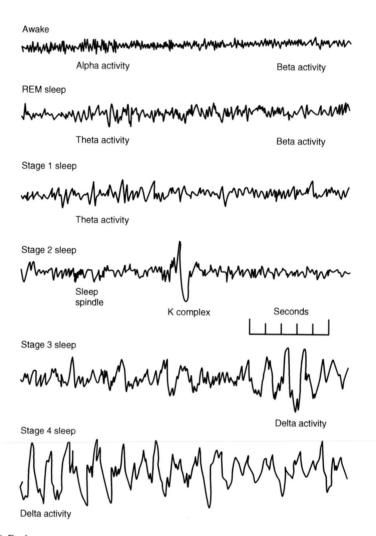

Figure 16.4 Brain waves.

They last for at least 0.5 seconds and are generated in the reticular nucleus of the thalamus. They appear to indicate an interaction going on between the thalamus and the cortex (i.e. **thalamocortical rhythms**). This kind of activity maintains tranquility in the sleeping subject during otherwise disruptive external noise. They are also important in the integration of new information into previously existing knowledge, i.e. the more sleep spindles there are the better the memory. They show a good correlation with levels of intellect, and therefore may serve as a possible measure of intellectual ability (Fogel and Smith 2011). In schizophrenia, there is often a lack of the normal pattern of slow and fast sleep spindles.

   K complexes are more commonly seen in the NREM cycles occurring early in the night. They are widely generated across the cortex but are seen more often over the frontal lobes, and are related to two functions: (1) aiding sleep-based memory consolidation; (2) suppressing arousal of the sleeping subject in response to stimuli that the brain has considered to be harmless and unimportant. In individuals with **restless leg syndrome** (see below), the K complexes coincide with the leg movements. Benzodiazepine drugs have been shown to reduce K complexes by increasing GABA (inhibitory) activity.

Stages 3 and 4

This stage is the 'deepest' form of sleep, identified by the presence of **delta waves**. These stages are often referred to as '**slow-wave sleep**' because of the delta wave pattern on the EEG recording (1–3 Hz). The differences between stage 3 and stage 4 are seen in Figure 16.4 (i.e. stage 3 = 20–50% delta waves; stage 4 = more than 50% delta waves), but they are not always accepted as two separate stages by everyone, in which case they are both regarded as stage 3 (Figure 16.4).

The normal sleep pattern over an 8-hour period is seen in Figure 16.2. On falling asleep, the subject passes through REM first, then NREM stages 1 to 4 in order. After about 60 minutes in NREM 3 to 4, the subject returns to REM, repeating these events several times throughout the night. Notice in Figure 16.1 that the NREM cycles get lighter each time, with no stages 3 and 4 in the last third of the night, and REM gets slightly longer with each cycle, ending the sleep with a short REM period.

Sleep requirements and patterns

Newborn babies need about 16 hours of sleep in 24 hours, of which 50% is REM and 50% is NREM (mostly stage 2). Adults need between 7 and 9 hours per 24 hours, split into about 25% REM to 75% NREM. The elderly need less than 20% REM, the rest NREM, but the overall amount of sleep decreasing with age to about 6 hours in 24 hours.

Infants have **polyphasic** (many phases per 24 hours) sleep, i.e. five or six alternate sleep/ wake periods in 24 hours. **Monophasic** (one phase per 24 hours) sleep comes at the same time as loss of both night feeds and daytime sleeping. The elderly may revert back to a poly-phasic sleep pattern by taking short afternoon sleeps and sleeping less at night. There is some evidence now that lunchtime napping for working adults improves their afternoon cognitive abilities (Lovato and Lack 2010).

Sleep patterns have changed over time. The standard number of hours sleep expected for adults is 7 to 9 (average of 8) per night. But questions are now being raised about the validity of having 8 hours' sleep in one session. Historically, our ancestors had 12 hours 'sleep' bro-ken after 3 or 4 hours with 3 hours awake time, then the rest as a second sleep period (known as **segmented**, or **bimodal**, **sleep**). This appears to be the natural way for humans to sleep, but they were forced into one sleep period during the Industrial Revolution. This may be the reason why people sometimes wake in the middle of the night and have difficulty getting back to sleep (known as **sleep maintenance insomnia**). However, this splitting of the 8-hour sleep period into two parts with a few hours awake in the middle is not really something to worry about, and simply the brain remembering its natural bimodal sleep pattern, but it is unfortunate if the individual has to rise early to get to work.

The neurological control of sleep

The neural control of the sleep–wake cycle is complex and not fully understood. Several apparently separate brain activities cause both sleep and the waking state to occur alternately, with no single overall mechanism in command. To complicate the issue further, a number of natural brain chemicals are also involved: in particular orexin, serotonin, melatonin, and histamine.

The awakened state

The waking state is regulated by areas of the brain situated in the brain stem, hypothalamus, and the basal region of the forebrain. On EEG, the brain shows a more *unsynchronised* pattern of electrical activity (Figure 16.4).

Orexin (also called **hypocretin**) is an important promoter of the waking state and appetite (see Chapter 9). Neurons that use orexin are active in the lateral hypothalamus, and their effects extend to many parts of the brain and spinal cord. During the waking periods, these neurons are active, but their activity is reduced significantly when asleep, i.e. when orexin concentrations are low. Another chemical that promotes being awake is **histamine**, which is mostly active as a neurotransmitter during the day but significantly less active during NREM sleep, and at its lowest activity level during REM sleep. Histamine pathways extend from the hypothalamus to many other parts of the brain (see Figure 4.19 in Chapter 4). Antihistamine drugs cause drowsiness because they block the activity of histamine at the **H1 receptor**, and this stops histamine's function of promoting arousal. **Gamma-aminobutyric acid (GABA)** prevents histamine activity. This inhibitory neurotransmitter acts as a braking mechanism to reduce the action of histamine and therefore prevent overexcitement of the brain. Low GABA results in a mania-like state with restlessness and sleeplessness.

Acetylcholine and **noradrenaline** both promote brain alertness. Increased levels of acetylcholine (see Figure 4.18) in the **reticular activating system (RAS)** of the brain stem (see Chapter 1) occurs during the day and in REM sleep, stimulating activity in the cerebral cortex. Levels fall during NREM sleep. Neurons that use acetylcholine in the **peribrachial area** of the pons appear to initiate REM. These neurons are sometime referred to as 'REM-on' cells. They activate about 80 seconds before REM begins. 'REM-off' cells in the midbrain appear to terminate REM sleep, 'REM-on' and 'REM-off' cells being mutually inhibitory (Lu et al. 2006). 'REM-off' cells themselves act in response to excitatory input from serotonin, noradrenaline, and orexin to induce waking (Figure 16.5). Noradrenaline (Figure 4.6) appears to be different from acetylcholine during REM, i.e. high concentrations during the day, but low concentration in both REM and NREM sleep.

The sleeping state

For sleep to occur, those brain areas that promote wakefulness need to be disengaged from the cerebrum, or inhibited in some way. This is done by the **thalamus**, which governs the stimuli that pass to the cortex. It is mostly the thalamus that is responsible for the *slow-wave* component of sleep seen on EEG in NREM sleep (Figure 16.4). In addition, a chemical called **adenosine** increases in the brain gradually during the day, and increases even more during the evening. Adenosine is found in **adenosine triphosphate (ATP)**, the cellular high-energy molecule. Brain energy storage, in the form of glycogen, gradually gets used during the day, and extracellular adenosine accumulates. Sleep provides the opportunity to remove this build-up of adenosine and replenish the glycogen stores. During the evening, adenosine inhibits many of the brain's activities that promote wakefulness, thus promoting sleep. Levels of adenosine gradually fall as REM sleep becomes more frequent, and this eventually allows the areas that promote wakefulness to take over. **Caffeine** blocks adenosine receptors (see Chapter 8), and

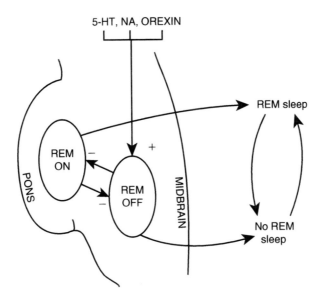

5-HT, NA, OREXIN

Figure 16.5 Peribrachial area, REM-on, REM-off. 5-HT = serotonin, NA = noradrenaline.

therefore the sleep-inducing adenosine cannot exert any influence on the brain, and the wakeful state is sustained.

Areas that promote sleep include the **ventrolateral preoptic nucleus (VLPN)** in the **anterior hypothalamus** (Figure 16.6). This area has adenosine receptors, and has a reciprocal GABA inhibitory effect on other areas of the brain that promote the awakened state. Thus, if the VLPN is active, those areas that promote being awake (i.e. the brain stem and forebrain arousal areas) are inhibited, and the reverse is true when awake (the brain stem and forebrain arousal centres inhibit the VLPN) (Figure 16.6).

The **suprachiasmic nucleus (SCN)** is also in the hypothalamus, just above the **optic chiasma** (where optic nerves carrying retinal impulses partially cross the midline). The SCN receives about 10% of the impulses induced by light falling on the retina. These impulses travel from the retina to the hypothalamus via the **retinohypothalamic pathway**. Behind the hypothalamus is a small gland – **the pineal gland**, which has connections with the SCN (see also Seasonal affective disorder, Chapter 11, Figure 11.8). This gland uses serotonin as a substrate for the production of the hormone **melatonin**. The cells of the gland **(pinealocytes)** concentrate the serotonin, which is first converted to **N-acetyl-serotonin**, and then converted further to melatonin.

The level (or intensity) of light falling on the retina causes the SCN to have different responses. In daylight (or bright light) conditions, the intense impulses from the retina cause the SCN to fire rapidly. The SCN impulses that pass to the pineal gland are inhibitory, and shut down melatonin production. In low light levels (i.e. in darker conditions), the SCN firing rate is reduced, and this allows the pineal gland to produce melatonin. The SCN also influences the function of the VLPN (see above and Figure 16.7). The SCN, VLPN, and the pineal gland receive no light directly. Their response to light is based on light intensity on the retina. In this way, external light is able to act as a **zeitgeber** (German for 'time giver'), which is defined as any external stimulus that is used by the brain to control a circadian rhythm. The form of light that suppresses melatonin the most is **blue light** (460–480 nanometres

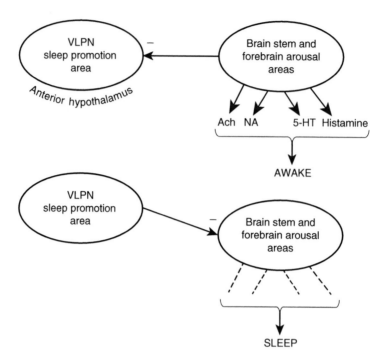

Figure 16.6 The ventrolateral preoptic nucleus (VLPN). Ach = acetylcholine, NA = noradrenaline, 5-HT = serotonin.

in wavelength) and this light is the dominant form given off by electronic screens. Watching televisions, computer screens, or any other form of electronic screen during the evenings and late at night exposes the viewer to excessive blue light just at the time when melatonin should be increasing in order to trigger sleep. The resulting blue light exposure suppresses melatonin and therefore disturbs sleep. One way around this (if screens cannot be avoided during the evening) is to wear specific orange-tinted glasses that are designed to filter out the blue light, especially for the final hour of screen use before retiring to bed. These glasses are said to improve both the length and quality of sleep.

Serotonin (5-hydroxytryptamine, or 5-HT) promotes being awake by increasing cortical arousal, prolongs the time it takes to get to sleep, and reduces REM sleep. Serotonin is at a low level during REM sleep. Cell bodies of serotonergic neurons (i.e. those using serotonin as the neurotransmitter) occur in the **raphe nucleus** of the brain stem (see Biochemistry, Chapter 11), and extend to many parts of the brain (see Figure 4.7 in Chapter 4).

Dreams

Two centres that are responsible for dreams have been located in the brain.

1   The deep fibre **mesocortical** and **mesolimbic dopaminergic pathways** within the frontal lobe, just above the eyes. These pathways link the frontal lobe with the limbic system and the brain stem. Any damage to these pathways results in the inability to dream. Because they are dopaminergic pathways, drugs such as **levodopa** can induce and increase dreams

by adding additional dopamine to this pathway (see Parkinson disease, Chapter 13). The normal function of this pathway during waking hours is to drive motivation of the individual towards interacting with the real world in order to satisfy internal biological needs.

2 The grey matter situated at the junction of the parietal, temporal, and occipital lobes (the **PTO** area). This area carries out high-level processing of all kinds of sensory information, including the formation of abstract thinking and mental imagery based on that information. It also prepares this information for its storage as memories (Figure 16.8).

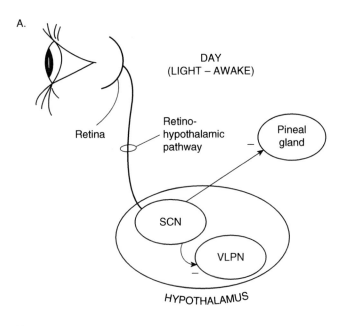

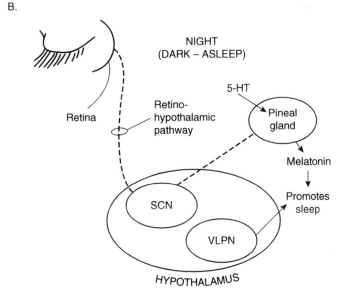

Figure 16.7 SCN and blue light impulses from retina in light and dark.

Although dreaming has been linked to REM sleep, dreams can also occur in NREM. This is because REM is controlled by a centre in the pons (see REM, page 358), and the two dream centres function separately to this. The rapid eye movements have been thought to be following events in the dream, but this has never been proven because there was no way of finding out what the eyes were following during sleep. Now, electrodes placed inside part of the brain called the **medial temporal lobe** have recorded neuronal signals immediately (about 0.25 of a second) after an eye movement. This part of the brain is not the vision area, but it is linked to vision and responds to pictures. The 0.25 of a second signal from the medial temporal lobe is similar to signals identified after eye movements made in response to real images seen when awake. However, given that the eyelids are closed during REM and the eyes are therefore actually seeing nothing, it would appear that the 'pictures' seen by this brain area are being generated by the brain itself.

Dreams also need two other functions to occur: deactivation (or blocking) of the motor functions of the forebrain, which is linked to atonia (Figure 16.3), and a sensory trigger.

Lucid dreaming describes when dreamers have the ability to recognise that what is happening is a dream and they can choose to continue or to wake up (dependent on the nature of the dream). If the dreamer chooses to continue, they can manipulate events in the dream according to their wishes. Those people who never have lucid dreams have a fundamentally different brain from those who do. Lucid dreamers have greater volumes of grey matter in the **frontopolar** region of the cortex (linked to evaluation of thoughts and feelings) than non-lucid dreamers, with greater levels of thought monitoring activity in this grey matter area. Other areas involved are the **dorsolateral prefrontal cortex** (linked to self-assessment) and the **precuneus** (linked to self-perception). Within seconds at the start of a lucid dream activity in these areas rises sharply.

Nightmares are bad dreams, often frightening and threatening. They appear to be a stable trait, i.e. if they are present as a child they are likely to be present into adulthood, although the frequency may gradually reduce. Nightmares are most often linked to REM sleep, although they do occur in NREM as well. REM is accompanied by an overall reduced **autonomic nervous system** (ANS; see Chapter 1) activity when compared with other sleep stages, although in the nightmare itself there may be '**ANS storms**', i.e. moments of ANS overactivity. REM activity during a nightmare is uninhibited and excessive. The central nucleus of the **amygdala** (see Figure 9.2 in Chapter 9) also appears to be involved. This has a regulatory function over emotional states such as fear and aggression (Chapter 9). In nightmares, this central nucleus becomes very sensitive and overreactive, and the excessive REM activity pushes the amygdala central nucleus into a state of nightmare, i.e. creating unreal threats and causes of fear. This is called **REM-related activation of the amygdala**. The **limbic cortex** is also activated (see Chapters 1 and 9) and the **prefrontal cortex** (Chapter 1) is deactivated in a nightmare, thus removing all rational analysis and interpretation of the dream. Recurring nightmares are sometimes seen in some seizures, notably those fits starting in the temporal limbic system, which has connections with the frontal lobe.

Effects of sleep loss on health

The longest anyone has stayed awake, under official observation, is 11 days. Longer periods have been claimed by some, but they cannot be verified.

Loss of sleep in the short term (i.e. a few nights of sleep loss) causes irritability, inability to concentrate, blurred vision, physical fatigue, some memory loss, poor cognitive ability,

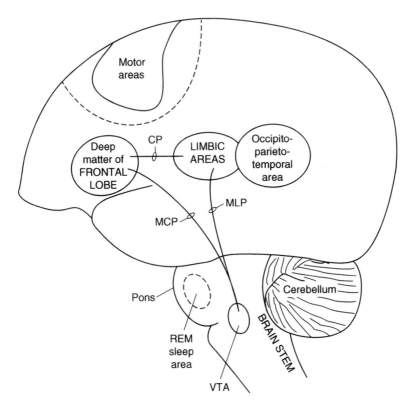

Figure 16.8 Dreams and nightmares. MCP = mesocortical pathway, MLP = mesolimbic pathway, CP = connecting pathways, VTA = ventral tegmental area.

reduced alertness, hormonal imbalance, raised blood pressure, mood disturbance, and poorer attention spans with corresponding reduction in task performance levels. There is also an increased risk of accidents (e.g. when driving). At about 17 hours of sleep loss, an individual's cognitive and motor skills are on a par with those seen with excessive alcohol consumption. Recovery from short-term sleep loss is not usually a problem when a normal sleep pattern is restored.

Chronic, long-term sleep loss can cause a large number of serious medical problems, including hypertension, cardiac failure, strokes, depression, cognitive impairment, child growth retardation, and poor quality of life, with increased mortality risk (in those with less than 6–7 hours' sleep per night). Severe insomnia triples the mortality risk in elderly men (one Chinese man died in his sleep after 11 days awake).

Even some seemingly unrelated conditions, including diabetes and cancer, are increased as a result of long-term sleep loss. The gene *ABCC9* codes for the protein **SUR2**, a potassium ion channel component, and genetic mutations of this gene have previously been linked to heart disease and diabetes. This gene is also one of the factors that determines how long an individual sleeps. People with two copies of one common variation of the gene slept for significantly less time than those with two copies of a different variation. The fact that this gene is linked to both diabetes (a metabolic disorder) and sleep duration provides a link between diabetes and sleep loss.

Over time, prolonged sleep loss also causes problems with the immune system, reducing the body's ability to fight infections. People who sleep fewer than 6 hours per night have a 4.2 times greater risk of developing the common cold than those who had 7 hours or more sleep per night (Table 16.1) (Prather et al. 2015).

Night workers accumulate a lot of sleep loss because, contrary to popular belief, the brain's regulatory clocks do not adapt to sleeping during the day and being awake at night. Night work ages the brain. After 10 years of night shifts the brains of some night workers had aged 6.5 years more than what they would have done working during the day. They had poorer memory and slower cognitive processing speed than those on day work. They also suffered from a lack of attention and had multiple 'microsleeps' (falling asleep for brief moments, such as dosing). **Microsleeps** are accompanied by reduced thalamic activity and increased activity in the grey matter area that deals with sensory processing (see Dreams on page 364). In the long term, the lost sleep accumulated during night work leads to excessive fatigue, hormonal changes, irregular eating habits including snacking, resulting in weight gain, and higher risk of diabetes due to the pancreas failing to produce enough insulin.

Long periods of sleep loss may cause brain cell losses (as observed in animal models). The **locus coeruleus** is vulnerable to this type of permanent damage when subjected to sleep deprivation. This area of the brain stem is the seat of noradrenergic activity (see Chapters 4 and 11). A protein called **sirtuin type 3 (SirT3)** has been found to protect the locus coeruleus from damage by sleep loss, although this may not be produced naturally in sufficient quantities. Finding ways to boost SirT3 production may be useful in preventing this form of brain damage.

Teenagers are particularly vulnerable to sleep loss problems. Each hour of sleep lost increases teenagers' risk of developing depression by 38%, increases their risk of suicide by 42%, and increases their risk of substance abuse by 23%. Teenagers with sleep deprivation find it more of a struggle to cope with self-control and judgement issues (Table 16.2).

Loss of sleep creates a 'sleep debt', which the brain tries to pay back with additional sleep when possible. As little as 1 week of building a sleep debt adversely alters the activity of 700 genes. Further sleep debt beyond 1 week changes the activity of nearly 5000 genes. Many of these genes are involved in controlling metabolism, immunity, and the response to stress. Sleep loss therefore lowers the body's ability to manage stress. Just 1 night of sleep deprivation alters the epigenetic DNA of the key metabolic genes that regulate the body's circadian cycles, and these alterations can be found in shift workers. The genes *BMAL1*, *CLOCK*, *CRY1*, and *PER1* become either **hypermethylated** (i.e. too much methyl group attachment to the DNA) or had their gene expression altered (Cedernaes et al. 2015).

Table 16.1 Sleep and the risk of catching the common cold

Hours asleep	More than 7	6 to 7	5 to 6	Less than 5
Risk of catching common cold (%)	17.2	22.7	30	45.2

Table 16.2 Teenage sleep loss in America, UK, Korea, and Japan

Country	USA	UK	South Korea	Japan
Average hours of sleep per night (teenagers)	7 hours 8 minutes	7 hours 38 minutes	5 hours 47 minutes	5 hours 47 minutes

Sleep loss may also be an early warning sign of a mental or physical disorder, and therefore investigation of the cause of sleep disturbance is important, rather than simply prescribing sleep medication.

Three steps to getting improved benefits of sleep may be by:

- not using electronic screens late at night, or by wearing orange-tinted glasses for at least the last hour of screen use before getting to bed (see page 363);
- retiring to bed at the same reasonable hour every night with the aim of sleeping the full 8 hours;
- sleeping on one side rather than on your back or front and not becoming stressed if you wake in the night for an hour or two; simply occupy these waking hours with quiet simple activities that help to induce sleep, keeping light levels low and not using electronic screens of any kind.

Sleep disorders

There are several types of sleep disorder.

- **Insomnia disorder** is the inability to sleep (see below).
- **Somnolence** is excessive daytime sleeping, but the term is not appropriate for feeling tired during the day.
- **Hypersomnolence (hypersomnia)** is excessive sleeping, during the day as well as at night. Daytime naps provide no relief from the desire to sleep. Waking up is a struggle. Causes include **encephalitis** (inflammation of the brain), metabolic and toxic conditions, excessive alcohol or drug use, withdrawal from stimulant drugs, and previous sleep deprivation.
- **Narcolepsy** is the occurrence of sudden sleep attacks (see below).
- **Obstructive sleep apnoea** or **hypopnoea syndrome** is a collection of symptoms, including snoring, snorting or gasping for air, with multiple short periods of apnoea (complete pauses in breathing for about 10 seconds or more) per hour during sleep. It may be caused by **central sleep apnoea** (see below), or it may be a temporary partial obstruction of the upper airways blocking airflow. Each episode of apnoea causes arousal, thus disturbing sleep. This condition is coupled with symptoms of fatigue, depressed mood, and sleepiness during the waking hours. It can affect anyone, but the elderly and obese are especially vulnerable.
- **Central sleep apnoea** is characterised by an absence of the brain stem stimulus to breathe, therefore all breathing efforts stop briefly. This causes the individual to wake up short of breath and gasping for air. It can happen five or more times per hour, and results in excessive daytime sleepiness.
- **Primary alveolar hypoventilation** is identified by multiple short episodes (10 seconds or more) of shallow breathing during sleep, linked to reduced arterial oxygen saturation and frequent waking up.
- **Circadian rhythm sleep–wake disorders** involve disturbance to the 24-hour clock that controls our sleep–wake cycle, and include the following.

    o **Advanced** or **delayed sleep phase syndrome**, where the circadian rhythm control of sleep is set earlier or later than expected for the time of day. In the advanced form, instead of feeling sleepy at about 11pm, this is moved forward to perhaps 7pm.

Equally, the time to wake up is moved forward to the early morning, e.g. 3am. This is seen more often in the elderly and is linked to **seasonal affective disorder (SAD**; see Chapter 11). In the delayed form, the circadian clock's time to rise is set later than expected, and the sufferer does not wake at the correct time in the morning.

o   **Irregular sleep–wake type**, when the circadian rhythm is disorganised in a manner that is variable within the 24-hour period, e.g. sleeping between 5pm and 2am for one cycle, between 8pm and 4am for another cycle, and so on.

o   **Non-24-hour sleep–wake** (or **free-running**) **type**, when the sleep period of the cycle drifts with each cycle, often later and later, so they don't fit within the 24-hour pattern. It may affect some blind people who don't have the light and dark cues that regulate the internal sleep–wake cycle.

o   **Situational circadian rhythm sleep disorder**, where the circadian rhythm control of sleep is disturbed by one's situation, e.g. **jet lag** or **night shift** work (for night workers see Effects of sleep loss on health on page 366). Jet lag is caused by a rapid change (over a few hours) of time zone. The traveller brings their circadian rhythm set at their departing time zone into a new and probably very different time zone. It will take several days for their internal clock to readjust to the new settings. Meanwhile they suffer varying amounts of fatigue, sleep loss, or excessive sleep, which is dependent on their age, the number of time zones involved, and the direction of travel.

- **Rapid eye movement sleep behaviour disorder** is where there are repeated episodes of wakening during sleep associated with complex speech or motor activity which, in some cases, may cause injury to the sufferer or their partner. These motor activities have arisen from REM sleep, and therefore fall mainly where REM occurs on the 8-hour nocturnal sleep pattern (look back at Figure 16.2). REM is linked to dreaming, and these speech or motor activities are sometimes said to be the result of the sufferer 'acting out their dreams'.

- **Restless legs syndrome (RLS)** is a situation in which sleep is disturbed by a constant need to move the legs rhythmically in order to prevent the onset of unpleasant sensations. These sensations include burning, tingling, aching, or itching of the affected leg. Movement prevents or relieves these symptoms. It mostly affects the middle-aged in the evenings or during the night, and there may be a family history of the syndrome.

- **Parasomnia sleep disorder** is when abnormal movements, emotions, or behaviours occur during the very early stages of sleep.

- **Disorders of arousal** include sleep (or night) terrors, sleepwalking, and confusional arousals.

   o   **Night terrors** are not to be confused with nightmares (see Dreams, page 364). Night terrors cause sudden wakening with screaming, intense fear, and hyperactivity of the **sympathetic nervous system** (with all the accompanying effects of tachycardia, rapid breathing, and sweating). It is more common in young children, and up to 6% of children have the problem, more boys than girls. It is less often seen in adults.

   o   **Sleepwalking** (or **somnambulism**) involves the individual leaving their bed when asleep and wandering about. It is more frequent during the earliest one-third of the night, usually in NREM stages 3 or 4. The sleepwalker has no memory of the event after waking. Since they are asleep during the sleepwalking episode they do not respond as usual, and can be difficult to wake up. It usually affects about 10% of children and mostly linked to a physical factor such as stress, fever, or medication. Most children grow out if it by the time they reach their teens.

o **Confusional arousals**, or **sleep inertia**, is when the individual wakes confused, drowsy as if not fully awake, with impaired motor activity and weakness, and with a desire to go back to sleep. It can last for up to 30 minutes or more. It occurs mostly when woken from deep NREM slow-wave sleep. It may be due to some remaining accumulation of adenosine that has not been fully removed.

- **Kleine Levin syndrome** is characterised by recurrent periods of excessive sleep (more than 11 hours per day) for between 2 days and 4 weeks per episode, with at least one episode per year. Sometimes during the waking period of an episode, the sufferer shows abnormal cognition, unreality, confusion, and unusual behaviour, such as excessive eating or hypersexuality. Between episodes, the sufferer shows normal alertness, cognition, and behaviour.

Insomnia

Insomnia (the inability to sleep) is the most common sleep disorder. Loss of sleep is due to many factors (Table 16.3), and requires investigation to find the cause. The patient is preoccupied with getting to sleep, and becomes frustrated and distressed. Insomnia can be transient, short term, or persistent.

- **Transient insomnia** is often the result of some form of temporary anxiety. It is unlikely to be serious and may not need any treatment. The brain is good at catching up with short periods of sleep loss.
- **Short-term insomnia** may be related to another physical or mental disorder. It lasts a few weeks and may benefit from medication prescribed for 1 week or so (but not longer than 3 weeks).
- **Persistent** (or **chronic**) **insomnia** is a symptom of a group of conditions linked by the difficulty in getting to sleep caused by two intertwined problems: (1) an anxiety state that may not always be obvious; (2) a conditioned associative response, i.e. an insomnia linked to certain conditions found at home, or perhaps when away from home, and the subject may sleep well when not faced with these conditions.

In some cases there is a genetic basis to insomnia, and this is linked to depression, i.e. the same gene or genes may be the cause of both disorders. These genes may include those that code for noradrenaline or serotonin, or their receptors, as both of these neurotransmitters are involved in the sleep–wake cycle and mood regulation. Both insomnia and sleep apnoea have been linked to depression, and there is evidence to show that treating the sleep problem significantly improves mental health (Levine 2012).

Long-term insomnia carries all the health risks associated with chronic sleep loss (see page 366), especially hypertension, depression, diabetes, and substance abuse.

Narcolepsy is a loss of the brain's control over the normal sleep–wake cycle. This causes disturbance of nighttime sleep with frequent waking, fear of sleeping at night due to nightmares, nighttime feeding with weight gain, excessive sleep taken during the day (often sudden 'sleep attacks'), fatigue, poor concentration, difficulty with short-term memory, **cataplexy** (sudden loss of muscle tone, with varying degrees of weakness, possibly leading to collapse), sleep paralysis (muscle paralysis during the waking or getting to sleep phase), and hallucinations of any sensory system at the transient moment of falling asleep (**hypnagogic**

Table 16.3 Some common causes of insomnia

Post-traumatic stress disorder (PTSD)
Depression
Schizophrenia and bipolar disorder
Brain disorders (e.g. tumours)
Pain and discomfort
Drugs (abuse, interactions, side effects, and withdrawal can all cause insomnia)
Fear, anxiety, and worry
Confusion
Infections
Strange or noisy environments
Any disturbance to the sleep–wake cycle (e.g. travel to a different time zone)

hallucinations) or waking up (**hypnopompic hallucinations**). There are an estimated 31,000 people affected by this condition in the UK alone, and the number of young people with this disorder is growing in the UK and the rest of Europe, for reasons that are not fully understood.

Sleep medication

Drugs that are used to treat insomnia are the **hypnotics**, divided into:

- benzodiazepines (**nitrazepam, flurazepam, loprazolam, lormetazepam**, and **temazepam**);
- non-benzodiazepine so-called '**Z-drugs**' (**zaleplon, zolpidem**, and **zopiclone**);
- **chloral hydrate**;
- **clomethiazole**;
- **antihistamine (promethazine hydrochloride)**;
- **melatonin**.

Drugs used to treat narcolepsy are:

- **sodium oxybate**;
- **modafinil**.

Benzodiazepines act at the gamma-aminobutyric acid (GABA) receptor known as the $GABA_A$ receptor (at the BDZ site), and promotes GABA to open the chorine channel (see Figure 4.13, Chapter 4). The additional influx of Cl^- causes prolonged resting membrane potential (Figure 3.3, Chapter 3), creating a state of inhibition (i.e. blocking action potentials). In the case of insomnia, this inhibitory effect of benzodiazepines sedates the brain and induces sleep. Benzodiazepines should not be prescribed for longer than 3 weeks, and preferably for only 1 week, to reduce the risk of dependence.

The non-benzodiazepines (Z-drugs) also act at the $GABA_A$ receptor as GABA agonists, promoting GABA activity. Zolpidem is an **imidazopyridine** drug with a half-life of 2–6 hours. Side effects include gastrointestinal disturbances, dizziness, drowsiness, headache, agitation, and the potential for dependence. Zopiclone is a **cyclopyrrolone** drug with a half-life of 4–6 hours. Side effects are similar to those for zolpidem, but also include disturbance of taste. Zaleplon is a **pyrazolopyrimidine** drug with a very short half-life of 1–1.5 hours.

Side effects include amnesia, drowsiness, and **dysmenorrhoea** (painful periods). These drugs are used to treat insomnia in the short term; a maximum of 2 weeks for zaleplon, and a maximum of 4 weeks for zolpidem and zopiclone.

Chloral hydrate was originally widely used as a night sedation, even in children. Now, the use of hypnotics in children is considered unjustified, and the use of chloral hydrate in the elderly has been shown to be of little value. As a result, and in the presence of much better drugs, chloral hydrate is now very rarely used as night sedation.

Clomethiazole is used for both insomnia and to prevent the symptoms of alcohol withdrawal. It is structured similarly to **vitamin B$_1$ (thiamine)**, but acts similarly to the benzodiazepines at the GABA$_A$ receptor, promoting the opening of the chlorine channel. It has a half-life of about 3.5–5 hours. Side effects include excessive nasal and pharyngeal secretions, headache, and irritation of the conjunctiva.

Promethazine hydrochloride is an antihistamine, i.e. it is an antagonist at the H1 histamine receptor in the brain. By blocking the H1 receptor it stops histamine from binding, and this prevents the histamine from carrying out its role in maintaining the waking state, so sleep is induced. It has a half-life of between 5 and 14 hours. Side effects include drowsiness, headache, urinary tract retention, dry mouth, and gastrointestinal disturbance.

Melatonin is the naturally produced hormone from the pineal gland of the brain (see The sleeping state, page 362). However, it can be given as a drug to induce sleep 1–2 hours before retiring to bed if necessary. Side effects are not common, but they include gastrointestinal disturbance, dry mouth, headache, dizziness, restlessness, and weight gain.

Sodium oxybate is the sodium salt of **gamma hydroxybutyrate (GHB)**, which is a central nervous system (CNS) depressant. It is both a natural substance produced in the brain from GABA, and is also used as a drug in narcolepsy. It binds to two different types of receptor in the brain, the GABA$_B$ and the specific excitatory GHB receptor. It acts as an agonist at the GHB receptor and as a weak agonist at the GABA$_B$ receptor. It is a scheduled drug that is used illegally (see Chapter 8). Its use in narcolepsy is mainly to prevent daytime sleeping, especially if linked to cataplexy. This is probably achieved by its action on GHB receptors, which promotes release of **glutamate**, an excitatory neurotransmitter. The depressant effects are through its action on the inhibitory GABA$_B$ receptors (see Chapter 4). The half-life of sodium oxybate is very short (30–60 minutes), so it requires repeated administration in two divided dosages, approximately 4 hours apart, in order to cover a nighttime sleeping period. Because of this complicated administration regime, and the fact that it is potentially a drug of dependence, it should only be prescribed under specialist supervision. Side effects include gastrointestinal disturbances, headache, dizziness, confusion, and a range of sensory and motor symptoms.

Modafinil is a CNS stimulant used to treat narcolepsy, with or without cataplexy. It increases histamine from the hypothalamus and increases dopamine in various parts of the brain, including the **nucleus accumbens** (see Figure 8.3, Chapter 8). It is therefore an amphetamine-related drug (see Figure 8.6). The dopamine increase is due to the drug's inhibitory function on **dopamine transporter (DAT)** (Figure 8.3). Half-life is 10–12 hours, and side effects include gastrointestinal disturbances, dry mouth, tachycardia, headache, and dizziness.

The CNS stimulant **dexamfetamine** is also used occasionally to treat narcolepsy, although is currently unlicensed for this purpose.

Drugs used to induce sleep, i.e. to treat insomnia, have to have short half-lives because it is necessary to clear the drug from the body by the time the waking day begins. Drugs with long half-lives would cause excessive and unwanted daytime sleeping. It is also necessary to keep insomnia treatment to as short a period as possible, to prevent dependence on the drug. Insomnia drugs should be prescribed for a period not exceeding 4 weeks, but preferably for only 1 week. If these drugs continue for more than 4 weeks there is a real risk that the patient will not be able to sleep without them. This is because the brain elevates its activity levels to compensate for the sedation by the drug. When the drug is then stopped, the brain remains overactive at night, causing insomnia. This is better prevented by limiting the period of prescription, but if it did happen, the drug would need to be reduced gradually over a period of weeks. The purpose of the medication, therefore, is to give the patient short-term urgently needed relief from the insomnia while the cause of the problem is investigated and other forms of treatment applied.

The use of hypnotics in children is now recognised as unjustifiable, and in the elderly they should be avoided if possible. This is due to the reduced excretion rate of the drug from the body, which then prolongs the drug's half-life, and this then causes daytime drowsiness and a high risk of injury from falls.

Key points

Why we sleep

- We sleep in order to consolidate cognitive functions, especially memories, to clean the brain of metabolic waste, to increase the activity of genes, and to restore synaptic baseline levels of strength to conserve energy.

Physiology of sleep

- Sleep is one of the circadian rhythms.
- Two types of sleep are recognised: rapid eye movement (REM) sleep and non-REM (NREM) sleep.
- There are three or four stages of NREM.

Neurological control of sleep

- Sleep is caused by complex interactions of brain areas (e.g. thalamus, suprachasmic nucleus, hypothalamus, pineal gland), neurotransmitters, and hormones (e.g. histamine, adenosine, orexin, melatonin).

Dreams

- Dreams are most often linked to REM sleep but can occur in NREM sleep.
- There are two main areas of the brain involved in generating dreams.

Effects of sleep loss on health

- Adequate and good quality sleep is essential for well-being.
- Sleep loss causes a wide range of short- and long-term problems with health.

Sleep disorders

- Insomnia is the inability to sleep, a common sleep disorder. It requires investigation to find the cause.
- Insomnia can be transient, short term, or persistent.
- Narcolepsy is a loss of the normal sleep–wake cycle. It causes frequent waking at night and excessive sleep during the day, often as sudden 'sleep attacks' and cataplexy.

Drugs

- Hypnotics have short half-lives to prevent excessive daytime sleeping.
- Hypnotic treatment should be kept short, i.e. not exceeding 4 weeks, but preferably for only 1 week.
- The use of hypnotics in children cannot be justified.
- Hypnotic use in the elderly should be avoided if possible.

References

Bellesi, M., Pfister-Genskow, M., Maret, S., Keles, S., Tononi, G., and Cirelli, C. (2013) Effects of sleep and wake on oligodendrocytes and their precursors. *Journal of Neuroscience*, **33** (36): 14288–14300 (4 September 2013).

Cedernaes, J., Osler, M. E., Voisin, S., Broman, J.-E., Vogal, H., Dickson, S. L., Zierath, J. R., Schioth, H. B., and Benedict, C. (2015) Acute sleep loss induces tissue-specific epigenetic and transcriptional alterations to circadian clock genes in men. *Journal of Clinical Endocrinology and Metabolism* **100** (9): E1255–E1261. DOI: http://dxdoi.org/10.1210/JC.2015-2284.

Fogel, S. M. and Smith, C. T. (2011) The function of the sleep spindle: a physiological index of intelligence and a mechanism for sleep-dependent memory consolidation. *Neuroscience and Biobehavioural Reviews*, **35** (5): 1154–1165.

Levine, D. (2012) Treating sleep improves psychiatric symptoms. *Scientific American* (November/December 2012), 14.

Lovato, N. and Lack, L. (2010) The effects of napping on cognitive functioning. *Progress in Brain Research*, **185**: 155–166.

Lu, J., Sherman, D., Devor, M., and Saper, C. B. (2006) A putative flip–flop switch for control of REM sleep. *Nature*, **441**: 589–594 (1 June 2006).

Prather, A. A., Janicki-Deverts, D., Hall, M. H., and Cohen, S. (2015) Behaviourally assessed sleep and susceptibility to the common cold. *Sleep*, **38** (9): 1353–1359.

Stickgold, R. and Walker, M. P. (2007). Sleep-dependent memory consolidation and reconsolidation. *Sleep Medicine*, **8** (4): 331–343.

Tononi, G. and Cirelli, C. (2006) Sleep function and synaptic homeostasis. *Sleep Medicine Reviews*, **10**: 49–62.

Tononi, G. and Cirelli, C. (2013) Perchance to prune. *Scientific American*, August 2013, 26–31.

Xie, L., Kang, H., Xu, Q., Chen, M. J., Liao, Y., Thiyagarajan, M., O'Donnell, J., Christensen, D. J., Nicholson, C., Iliff, J. J., Takano, T., Deane, R., and Nedergaard, M. (2013) Sleep drives metabolite clearance from the adult brain. *Science*, **342** (6156): 373–377 (18 October 2013).

Index

A1 allele (A1 receptor) 86, 141–142, 159
absences 265–267, 270, 280, 282
absorption (of drugs) 120–121
acetic acid 73
acetylcholine (ACh) 55, 72–73
acetylcholinesterase (AChE) 73, 319, 328
acetylcholinesterase inhibitors 328
acetyl-CoA 73, 319
ACPD receptor 66
acquired disorders 99
action potential 42–49
Adam principle 105
addiction to drugs (drug abuse) 138, 141–164
Addison's disease 81–83
Adenine 97, 205, 270, 298
adenosine receptors 161, 362–363
adenosine triphosphate (ATP) 41, 56, 147, 194, 301
adenylyl cyclase (AC) 56–57, 234
adrenal cortex 11, 33, 80–82, 84
adrenaline 57–58, 60, 83, 162, 174, 187
adrenal medulla 18, 59–60, 83, 172
adrenergic receptors 60
adrenocorticotropic hormone (ACTH) 11, 79, 82, 147, 173, 221, 243–245
adrenogenitalism 83–84
adrenogenital syndrome 82
affective disorder (Depression) 232–236
ageing brain 309–313
aggression 62, 84, 86–89
aggressive impulse personality disorder 89
agonist (drugs) 126–127
agouti-related protein (ARP) 190–191
akathisia 221
alanine 97
albumin (binding drugs in circulation) 121–122, 134–135
alcohol 88, 148, 157–160
alcohol dehydrogenase 159

alcohol withdrawal delirium 158
aldehyde dehydrogenase 159
aldosterone 81, 84
aliphatics 220–221
alleles 95–96, 109
allergic disorders 20
allosteric effect 54–55, 192
alpha-linolenic acid (ALA) 35
alpha-melanocyte stimulating hormone (α-MSH) 190–191
Alzheimer's disease (AD) 315–331
Alzheimer's disease drugs 328–331
Alzheimer's disease genetics 320–323
amine neurotransmitters 57
α-Amino-3-hydroxy-5-methyl-4-isoxazoleproprionate (AMPA) receptor 51, 65, 329–330
amitriptyline 252
amnesia 158, 308
amotivation 156
ampakines 329–330
amphetamines 150–153
amygdala 8–9, 85–86, 88, 90, 146–147, 169–172
amyloid β precursor protein (APP) 316
anandamide 155
androgens 81–82, 84, 86–87, 105
Angelman syndrome 113–114
anions 42
anorexia nervosa 190, 192–194
antagonist (drugs) 126–127
anterior cingulate circuit 19, 350
anticipation (in gene mutations) 99
anticonvulsants 119, 278–283
antidepressants 251–259
antidiuretic hormone (ADH) 11, 152, 344
antimanics (see mood stabilising drugs)
antimuscarinic drugs 294
antimuscarinic side effects 220–221, 253
anti-Parkinson drugs 293–295

antipsychotics 219–228
antisocial personality disorder (APD) 89
anxiety states (anxiety disorders) 183–186
anxiolytics 196–197
ApoE (apolipoprotein) genes 320–322
arachnoid mater 3
arcuate nucleus (of the hypothalamus) 69, 190–191
aspartate 67–68
Asperger's syndrome 339, 341–342
association areas 5–6
astrocytes 49–52
atonic 265
ATPase 260–261
attention deficit hyperactivity disorder (ADHD) 338–339
atypical antidepressants 253–255
atypical antipsychotics 223–227
autism Spectrum Disorder (ASD) 339–344
automatism 265
autonomic nervous system (ANS) 16–18
autosomal disorders 101–105
autosomal dominant nocturnal frontal lobe epilepsy (ADNFLE) 278
autosomes 94
autosomal recessive disorder 83, 301, 342
autoreceptors 49, 55, 60
AUTS genes (in autism) 340
avoidant personality disorder 195–196
axon 39–45
axoplasmic transportation 41–42

basal ganglia 9, 12–14
basal ganglia motor loop 10, 13
base sequence repeats (nucleotide repeats) 99
Batten's disease 311
behaviour 86–91
benign familial neonatal convulsions (BFNC) 270
benign occipital epilepsy 278
benserazide 294
benzodiazepines 196–197
beta-endorphins 148
Big Brain Theory 214
bioavailability (of drugs) 120–121, 125
biosimilar drugs 128
bipolar depression 232–236
blood-brain barrier 61, 321
body dysmorphic disorder (BDD) 349–350
body mass index (BMI) 194
borderline personality 196

brain 1–16
brain-derived neurotrophic factor (BDNF) 145, 173, 188
brain development 22–36
brain stem 15–16
broca's area 5, 29, 336–337
Brodmann numbers 4
bromo-benzodifuranil-isopropylamine (Bromo-DragonFly, BDF) 164
bromocriptine 126, 294
bulimia nervosa 190, 193
buspirone 197
butyrophenones 219, 220

cadherin 13 (*CDH13*) gene 87
caffeine 161–162
calcium (Ca) 35, 46–47, 51
calcium channel blockers 127, 151, 280–281
cannabidiol (CBD) 153–156, 164
cannabinoids 153–157
cannabinoid receptors 154
cannabis 153–157
Capgras syndrome 218
carbamazepine 260, 279–280, 282
carbidopa 294
carboxyl group 54–55
CASE de-escalation model (for aggression) 91
catecholamine-O-methyl transferase (*COMT*) gene 349
catecholamines 54, 83
catechol group 54–55
catenin delta-2 protein 112
cations 42, 44, 74, 259
caudate nucleus 12–13, 142, 180, 286–287, 289–290, 296
central nervous system (CNS) 23, 52
cerebellar vermis 176, 342
cerebellum 14–15
cerebrospinal fluid (CSF) 3–4
cerebrum (cerebral cortex) 2, 4–8
ceruloplasmin 302
channel blockers 127, 151, 279–281
channelopathies 272
childhood absence epilepsy (CAE) 278
childhood disintegrative disorder (CDD) 339, 342
chloride (Cl) 42, 48, 55
chlorpromazine 126, 137, 219–220
cholecystokinin (CCK) 68–69, 189, 216
cholesterol 33, 80–82, 245, 312
choline 72–73, 260, 319
choline acetyltransferase (ChAT) 72, 319

chromatin 96–97

chromosomes 94–97, 100–109, 323

cingulate gyrus (or cortex) 6–7, 19, 156, 178, 180, 207–208, 239

circadian rhythms 69, 233, 243, 248, 250, 260, 358

cleft lip and palate 105

clozapine 223–227

cocaine 149–151, 347

cocaine and amphetamine regulated transcript (CART) 190–191

cocaine psychosis 149, 151

cocainomania 149

communication disorders 333, 337–338

competitive antagonists 126, 136

compulsions 349

confusion 132–133, 315–316

congenital 18, 82, 269

congenital muscular dystrophies (CMD) 116

consciousness 5–7, 25–26, 265

convulsions 264–265

corpus callosum 7, 9, 85, 142, 180, 251, 273, 351

corpus striatum 13, 19, 178, 214–215, 286–290, 296

corticotrophin-releasing factor (CRF) 243

cortisol 79, 81–83, 173–174, 243, 245–247

Cotard's syndrome (or delusion) 218

cranial nerves 15, 17

craniofacial malformations (defects) 104–105, 115

cretinism 34, 80

Creuztfeldt-Jakob disease (CJD) 319

cri-du-chat syndrome 112

cryptopyrol 90

crystal methamphetamine 153

Cushing's syndrome 81

cyclic adenosine monophosphate (cAMP) 56–57, 144, 147, 233, 307

cyclic AMP-responsive element-binding protein (CREB) 147, 233, 307

cyclopia 105

cyclothymic disorder 233

cytochrome P-450 (CYP, P450) 123

cytokines 238, 245–247

cytosine 97, 110

cytoskeleton 41, 150, 319

Db gene 194

deafferentation 271, 273

deep brain stimulation 240, 351

default mode network (DMN) 7, 156

degenerative disorders 20, 286

déjà vu 276

deletions 99, 112, 291

delirium tremens (DT) 158

delta (δ) receptor 72, 145

delta-9-tetrahydrocannabinol (THC) 153, 156, 195

delusions 201, 212

dementia 306–328

dementia with cortical Lewy bodies (DCLB) 326–327

deoxyribonucleic acid (DNA) 77, 97

dependent personality 196

depersonalisation (out of body experience) 163, 182–183

depolarisation 43–44

depot drugs 121, 227–228

depression (affective disorder) 231–261

depression genetics 234, 237

derealisation syndrome 163

developmental disorders 339–345

diabetic risk (of antipsychotics) 227

diamorphine (heroin) 145

diazepam 129–130, 196–197, 282

dichorionic twins (in schizophrenia) 214

diffuse modulatory systems 19, 60–61, 224, 240–242, 349

diphenylbutylpiperidines 219, 222

DISC1 gene (in schizophrenia) 203, 205–206

dissociative disorders (dissociative states) 182

dizygotic (DZ) twins 89, 101, 202, 234, 237, 334, 340, 349

dominant genes 95–96, 320

dopa decarboxylase inhibitor 293

dopamine 57–59

dopamine agonists 294–295

dopamine hyperactivity 87

dopamine hypothesis (in schizophrenia) 214–215

dopamine receptors 58–59

doppelgangers 182

dorsolateral prefrontal circuit (cortex) 19, 31, 85, 189, 239, 323, 366

Down syndrome (Trisomy 21) 103–104, 325–326

dreams 364, 366–367

drug abuse 141–164

drug administration 121, 130–133

drug compliance 130–131, 133

drug interactions 134–137

duloxetine 255

dura mater 3

dynorphins 71–72

dysgraphia 336–337

dyslexia 333–336
dyspraxia 336–337
dysthymic disorder 233, 244
dystonia 110, 221, 299

eating disorders 190–195
Edwards syndrome (Trisomy 18) 102–103
ecstasy (MDMA) 151–153
Ekbom syndrome 218–219
electroencephalogram (EEG) 266–269
emotional memories 186–188
emotions response 168–172
endocannabinoids 155
endocrine glands 77
endogenous control (of behaviour) 31
endogenous opioids 70–72
endomorphines 71
β-endorphin (endorphins) 71
encephalin 71
enterohepatic cycle (of drug elimination)
    124–125
entorhinal cortex 208–209, 211–213, 216,
    306–308
epigenetics 112, 116, 323, 347
epilepsy 264–283
epileptogenic focus 270–273
ethosuximide 279–280, 282
Eve principle 105
exogenous control (of behaviour) 31
extended amygdala 146–147
extrapyramidal side effects (EPS, of
    antipsychotics) 19, 221

familial Alzheimer's disease (FAD) 315
F-BAR domain 24
fear 184–189
febrile convulsions 269, 277
fetal alcohol syndrome (FAS) 347–348
first pass metabolism (of drugs) 120–121
flashbacks 189–190
Florence Syndrome 179
fluoxetine 253–255
flupenthixol 222
follicle-stimulating hormone (FSH) 11
fragile X syndrome 110–111
free radicals 292–293, 311
Fregoli syndrome 218
frontal lobe 5
fusiform gyrus (in autism) 334, 342–343

GABA receptors 66–67
GABA transaminase (GABA-T) 51, 63, 280, 282

gamma-aminobutyric acid (GABA) 48, 63,
    65–67, 187, 240, 270, 281, 287
general adaptation syndrome (GAS, in stress)
    174–175
general anxiety disorder (GAD) 184
generalised epilepsy with febrile seizures plus
    (GEFS+) 278
generalised seizures 265–266
generalised tonic-clonic (Grand mal) seizure
    265, 273–275
genes (genetics) 94–116
genetic disorders 112–116
genotype 109
ghrelin 192
glial cells (neuroglia) 49
gliosis 50
globus pallidus 9, 12–13, 64, 146, 286–287,
    349–350
glucocorticoids 80
glucose transport molecules (GLUTs) 173, 216
glutamate (glutamic acid) 48–51, 63–66
glutamate receptors 65–66
glutamic acid decarboxylase (GAD) 51, 63, 281
glycine 66–67
glycogen synthase kinase 3 (GSK-3) 23, 234, 260
glymphatic system 356
Grave's disease 80
grey matter 2–3
growth hormone 11, 33, 70, 221, 243
guanine 97, 110, 205, 298
gyrus (gyri) 3, 310–311

half-life (of drugs) 123–124
hallucinations 162–164, 201, 212–213, 371–372
hallucinogenic drugs 162–164
hallucinogen persisting perception disorder
    (HPPD) 162
haloperidol 204, 220, 222, 224, 226–227
Hashimoto's encephalopathy 314
heroin (Diamorphine) 144–145
hippocampus 8–9, 30, 32, 38, 51, 60, 208–210
Hirano bodies 327
Histamine 73–75
histamine receptors 74–75
histrionic personality 196
homeostasis 78–79
homocysteine 313
homovanillic acid (HVA) 57, 215, 243
hormones 11–12, 77–83, 243
humour 177–178
huntingtin associated protein-1 (HAP-1) 298–299
huntingtin protein 297–301

Huntington's disease (HD) 295–301
Huntington's disease genetics 298
hydrocephalus 340
4-hydroxy-3-methoxymethamphetamine
  (HMMA) 151–152
5-hydroxytryptamine, 5-HT (Serotonin) 61–62,
  240, 364
hypsarrhythmia 277
hypermetamorphosis 186
hyperphosphorylation 319
hyperthyroidism 80
hypnotics 119, 148, 372–374
hypocretins (see orexins)
hypofrontality (in schizophrenia) 210–211
hypothalamo-pituitary-adrenal axis (HPA axis)
  79, 186, 243–244
hypothalamo-pituitary-thyroid axis (HPT axis)
  79, 243–244
hypothalamus 10–12
hypothyroidism (myxedema) 34, 80, 243

iatrogenic disorders 20
idiopathic disorders 20, 264
imipramine 252
immunity 244–248, 323–324
imprinting 112–115
infantile spasms 277
inflammation (in Alzheimer disease) 323
influenza virus (in schizophrenia) 216–217
inherited disorders 99–100
inhibitory metabotropic receptor 57
innate drives 87
insomnia 371–372
insular cortex 6
insulin 160, 174, 190, 194, 227, 312
intellectual disabilities 109–110, 112, 114–115,
  345–348
intelligence quotient (IQ) 108
interictal syndrome 276
interleukin-6 (Il-6) 152–153, 245, 324
intrathecal (administration of drugs) 121
iodine (I) 34, 79–80, 260
ionotropic receptors 55–56, 126
ions 42
iron (Fe) 35
irritable male syndrome 84

Jacksonian epilepsy 277
jamais vu 276
Jerusalem syndrome 178
Joubert syndrome 342

kainate (kainic acid, K) receptors 66
kappa (κ) receptor 71–72, 144, 175
karyotype 94–95, 101
K complexes 359–361
ketamine 163–164, 183, 259
α-ketoglutarate 63
K-hole effect 259
kinesin 41
Kleine Levin syndrome 371
Klinefelter's syndrome (XXY) 106–107
Kluver-Bucy syndrome 186
Korsakoff syndrome 158

L-AP4 receptor 66
Lafora disease (Lafora progressive myoclonic
  epilepsy) 270
large neutral amino acid transporter (LNAA) 61
lateralisation 29, 85, 213, 337
lateral orbitofrontal circuit 19
learned behaviour 86–87, 144, 188
learning 8–10, 27–30, 32, 34–35, 66
learning disorders 333–337
Leigh syndrome 291
Lennox-Gastaut syndrome 270, 279
Leptin 190–192
leptin receptors 190–191
levodopa (L-dopa) 293–294
Lewy bodies 289–290
limbic associated cortex (limbic cortex) 9, 32,
  170–171
limbic irritability 176
limbic system 8, 168–172
linolenic acid (LA) 35
lipofuscin 310–311
lipofuscinoses 311
lissencephalic disorders 115–116
lissencephaly genes 115
lithium 259–261
locus (of gene) 97–98
locus coeruleus 59, 171, 241–242, 345, 368
long-term memory 8, 30–31, 209, 307–309
long-term potential (LTP) 307–308, 329
love 178–179
lucid dreaming 366
lumbar puncture (LP) 4, 121, 128
luteinizing hormone (LH) 11
lysergic acid diethylamide (LSD) 90, 162

major affective disorder (MAFD) 234, 236
magnesium (Mg) 35, 66, 259
magnocellular layer (of thalamus) 335

major histocompatability complex (MHC) 205
mania 233–236
marijuana 195
mass psychogenic illness 188
medial forebrain bundle (MFB) 19, 141–143,
   145, 149
medial temporal epilepsy syndrome (limbic
   epilepsy) 276
medulla 15–16
melanin-concentrating hormone (MCH) 69
melanocortin-4 receptor (MC-4) 190
melatonin 250–251, 362–364, 372–373
memory 8–10, 29–31, 155, 158, 307–309
meninges 3, 18, 20, 121
mesocortical pathway (tract or system) 19, 58,
   137, 202, 214–215, 224–225, 364
mesolimbic pathway (tract or system) 19, 58,
   137, 202, 214–215, 224–225, 364
mesotelencephalic dopamine system 141, 146
metabolism (of drugs) 122–123
metabotropic receptors 55–56, 126, 174
methadone 144, 148–149
methamphetamine 153
methylation 115, 143, 323
3, 4-Methylenedioxymethamphetamine
   (Ecstasy) 151
met mouth 153
microcephaly 103–105, 110, 112, 345–346
microdeletions 115
microglia 52, 323–325, 343
midbrain 15–16, 24–25
mild cognitive impairment (MCI) 308, 315, 326
mild traumatic brain injury (MTBI) 314
Miller-Dieker syndrome (MDS) 115–116
mineralocorticoids 80–81
mirror neurons (in autism) 183, 343
mitochondria 39, 123, 270, 301
mixed bipolar 233
monoamine hypothesis (of depression) 57, 251
monoamine oxidase (MAO) 57, 251
monoamine oxidase B (MAO-B) 160, 294–295
monoamine oxidase inhibitors (MAOI) 252,
   255–257
monochorionic twins (in schizophrenia) 214
monosomies 101
monosomy (of 21) 102, 104
monotherapy 283
monozygotic (MZ) twins 89, 101, 202, 214, 234,
   237, 334, 340, 349
mood-stabilising drugs 259–261
morphine 144–146, 148

mosaic 101–103
motor cortex 5, 116, 208, 277
mu (μ) receptor 145, 147
murder 89–90
muscarinic (M) receptors 73
muscle tone 13–14
music 112, 178–182
music therapy 179
mutations 98–99
myelin 28, 40, 46
myelination 28, 52
myoclonic epilepsy and ragged red fibres
   (MERRF) 270–271
myoclonic seizures 265, 270–271
myxedema 80
myxedema madness 80

nabilone 156
narcissistic personality 196
narcolepsy 369, 371–373
near death experiences 183
negative symptoms (Type II, of schizophrenia)
   200–201
neural tube 22–23, 25–26
neurodevelopment 213, 328
neuroendocrine response 79, 169, 172–174, 192
neurofibrillary tangles (NFT) 315, 319–320
neuroglia (glial cells) 23, 49–52
neurokinin-1 (substance P) 69
neurokinin-2 (neurokinin A, substance K) 69
neurokinin (NK) receptors 69
neuroleptic malignant syndrome (NMS) 222
neuromelanin 289
neuromodulators 49
neuron 39–42
neuronal intranuclear inclusions (NII) 300
neuronal migration 24
neuropeptides 49, 191
neuropeptide Y (NPY) 69, 190–191
neurotransmission 42–46
neurotransmitters 49, 54–75
neurulation 22–23
nicotine 159–161
nicotinic (N) receptors 73
nightmares 366–367
nigrostriatal pathway (tract) 14, 19, 215, 224,
   289
N-methyl-d-aspartate (NMDA) receptor 66
N-methyl-4-phenyl-1,2,3,6-tetrahydropyridine
   (MPTP) 292
nodes of Ranvier 40, 45

non-rapid eye movement (NREM) sleep 358–361
non-syndromic (cleft lip and palate) 105
noradrenaline 59–60, 242
noradrenaline selective re-uptake inhibitors
    (NRIs) 255
nucleus accumbens 58–59, 141–146, 180, 215
nucleus of the solitary tract (NST) 191–192
nucleus reticularis pontis caudalis 171–172

obesity 194
OB gene 194
Obsessions 349
obsessive-compulsive disorder (OCD) 349–350
obsessive-compulsive personality 350
oestradiol 84
oestrogen 84
oligodendrocytes 52, 234, 357
omega-3 35–36
omega-6 35–36
opiate drugs 72, 144–145
opioid receptors 71–72, 147
optineurin (OPTN) 298–299
orbitofrontal cortex 9–10, 144, 168, 349–350
orexins (orexin A and B, hypocretins) 191
orthodromic impulse 271, 273
out of body experience (see depersonalisation)
oxidative stress 301, 319
oxytocin 12, 32, 90, 151, 188, 339, 344

panic attacks 183, 189, 197, 259
Panayiotopoulos syndrome 278
parahippocampal gyrus 168, 170, 208–209, 212,
    306
paranoia 154, 201
paranoid personality 219
parasympathetic nervous system 17–18, 69
parkinsonism 221
Parkinson's disease (PD) 288–293
Parkinson disease genetics 290–291
partial agonists 126–127
partial (focal) seizures 265–266
Patau syndrome (Trisomy 13) 102
penetrance (of genes) 95–96, 113, 270, 301
perforant pathway 208–210, 307
periaquaductal grey (PAG) 158
peripheral nervous system (PNS) 16, 23, 52, 105
personality disorders 177, 195, 197, 218–219
pervasive developmental disorder (not otherwise
    specified) (PDD-NOT) 339, 342
pethidine 144–145
pH 120, 134

pharmacodynamics 119, 125–127
pharmacogenetics 119, 138
pharmacokinetics 119–125
pharmacology 119–138
pharmacotherapeutics 119, 128–138
phencyclidine (PCP) 163
phenobarbital 279–280, 282
phenothiazines 219–222
phenotype 95–96, 109–110
phenylketonuria (PKU) 345–346
phenytoin 279, 282
phobias 183–188
phosphate (PO_4) 42, 319, 344
phosphodiesters (PDEs) 211
phosphomonoesters (PMEs) 211
phosphorylation-dephosphorylation cycle 319
phototherapy 350
Pick bodies 327
Pick disease 327–328
Pimozide 222, 228
pineal gland 250–251
pinealocytes 250
piperazines 220–221
piperidines 220–221
pituitary gland 10–12, 33, 58, 79, 82, 173, 221
planum (or planus) temporale 112, 182, 335–336
plaques (in Alzheimer disease) 315–319
plasticity 28
point mutations 98
polar temporal lobe 170
polygenic 99, 202, 216, 270
polymorphism 203–205
polypharmacy 132–134
positive symptoms (Type I, of schizophrenia)
    200–202, 205, 214–215, 219, 224
postpartum blues 249
postpartum depression (PPD) 249–250
postpartum psychosis 249
post-traumatic stress disorder (PTSD) 189–190
potassium (K) 35, 42–46
Prader–Willi syndrome 113–114
Predation 87
prefrontal cortex (or lobe) 7, 10, 19, 30–32
premenstrual syndrome 88
preschizophrenia 211–212
presenilin 316
prodrug 123, 163
progesterone 84, 249
prolactin 11, 58, 221, 224
prostaglandins 246, 324
protein kinase 56–57, 234, 299, 307

pseudohermaphroditism 82–83
psilocybin 163
psychic blindness 186
psychoimmunology 244
psychopath 89–91
putamen 9, 12–13, 142, 144, 146, 286, 289, 296, 351
pyridoxal phosphate (PLP) 63
pyridoxidine (vitamin B6) 63

raphe nuclei 61, 162, 240–241
rapid-cycling bipolar disorder 233
rapid eye movement (REM) sleep 183, 358–359
rapid tranquillisation 228
Rasmussen's encephalitis (RE) 266
reboxetine 255, 257
recessive genes 95–96
reflexes 16, 27
refractory phase 44–46
religious experiences 178
reminiscence bump 30
repolarisation 43–44
reserpine 251
resting membrane potential 42–43
reticular activating system (RAS) 16, 362
reticular formation (RF) 11, 16
Rett syndrome 340, 345
reversible monoamine oxidase inhibitors (RIMA) 256–257
Ritalin 339
Rolandic epilepsy (RE) 278

salience (salient) network 7, 341
saltatory action 46, 52
satiation (satiety centre) 11, 68
savantism (savants) 344
schizoaffectivedisorder 206, 218
schizoid/schizotypal personality 219
schizophrenia 200–219
schizophrenia genetics 202–206
seasonal affective disorder (SAD) 250
seizures (see epilepsy)
selective serotonin re-uptake inhibitor (SSRI) drugs 253–255
septo-hippocampal system 170–171
serotonergic toxicity (serotonin storm, hyperserotonaemia) 153, 258
serotonin (5-Hydroxytryptamine, 5-HT) 61–62, 240–242
serotonin and noradrenaline re-uptake inhibitors (SNRIs) 255, 257

serotonin receptors 62
serotonin syndrome (serotonin toxicity) 258
serotonin transporter (SERT) 195, 236, 240, 249
sex chromosomes (X and Y) 94–95, 105–106
sex-determining region Y (SRY) gene 105
sexual sadism 90
short-term memory 30, 307–308
Shy-Drager Syndrome (SDS) 291
sickness behaviour (sickness syndrome) 246
single nucleotide polymorphism (SNP) 205
sleep 355–374
sleep disorders 369–372
sleep medication 372–374
sleep spindles 359–360
sleep-wake cycle 11, 16, 358, 361
Smith-Magenis syndrome 116
smoking (affects on fetus) 347–348
social phobia 196
sodium (Na) 35, 42–46
sodium channel blockers 279
sodium valproate 279–280, 282–283
solvents 163–164
somatisation disorder 158
somatostatin 70
somnolence (hypersomnolence) 369
sonic hedgehog homolog (SHH) gene 105
SSRI discontinuation (withdrawal, cessation) syndrome 257
status epilepticus 275
stem cells 23, 331
Stendhal syndrome 178
steroids 77
Stockholm syndrome 177
stress (stressors) 172–177
stress and child abuse 176–177
stuttering (persistent developmental stuttering, PDS) 337–338
subcortical dementias 286
subgenual cingulate (Brodmann area 25) 239
substance P (neurokinin-1) 69
substantia nigra 12–14, 58, 143, 146, 155, 215, 287–290
substituted benzamide 222–223
subthalamus 12–14
suicide 226, 237–238
sulcus (sulci) 3, 310–311
sulpiride 222–223
superwoman syndrome (XXX) 106–107
suprachiasmic nucleus (SCN) 250, 363
Susac's syndrome 314
sympathetic nervous system 16–17, 83, 370

synapse 40, 46–48, 50, 307–308
synaptic homeostasis hypothesis (SHY) 356, 357
synaptic pruning 28, 30–32, 343, 357
synaptogenesis 28
syndromic (cleft lip and palate) 105
α-synuclein 290–292

tamoxifen 235–236
tardive dyskinesia 221
tau protein 314, 319–320, 329–330
Tay-Sachs disease 346
teenage brain 31–32, 150, 155
temporal lobe (psychomotor) epilepsy 183, 266, 276–277
teratogens (teratogenic) 18, 88, 217, 347–348
testosterone 33, 82–84, 86–90, 158–159, 195
tetracyclic antidepressants 252–253
thalamus 9–10, 13, 59, 212–213, 286–287, 289–290, 334, 360, 362
THC (delta-9-tetrahydrocannabinol) 153, 156, 195
therapeutic window 128–129, 137
thiamine (Vitamin B1) 34, 158, 373
thioxanthenes 219, 222
thought disorder 201, 210, 213
thymine 97, 205
thyroid gland 11, 33, 79–80, 260
thyroid hormone 11, 33–34, 79–80, 243, 260
thyroid-stimulating hormone (TSH) 11, 79–80
thyrotoxicosis 80
tic disorders 349, 351
Timothy syndrome 340
tolerance (to drugs) 138
Tourette's syndrome (TS) 350–351
toxic effects (of drugs; toxicology) 137, 238
Toxoplasma gondii 115, 217, 238
Traits 95–96
Translocations 99, 116, 202, 205
traumatic brain injury (TBI) 314
tricarboxylic acid (Krebs) cycle 51, 63
tricyclic antidepressants 148, 160, 252–253
tricyclic-related (see tetracyclic antidepressants)
triiodothyronine (T_3, see thyroid hormone)
trinucleotide repeat (see base sequence repeats)
trisomies 102–104
trisomy 8 (see Warkany syndrome) 102

trisomy 13 (see Patau syndrome)
trisomy 18 (see Edwards syndrome)
trisomy 21 (see Down syndrome)
trisomy X (see superwoman syndrome)
tryptophan 61–62, 241, 246
tryptophan hydroxylase (TRPH) 87, 151, 236
tuberoinfundibular pathway (tract) 214–215, 224
tumour necrosing factor (TNF) 193, 246, 324
Turner's syndrome (X) 107
twilight state 275
two-syndrome hypothesis (of schizophrenia) 202
tyromine 160, 256
tyrosine 57–58, 61, 345
tyrosine hydroxylase 57

ubiquitin 114, 291, 299, 300, 319
ultraviolet (UV) light (in schizophrenia) 216
unipolar depression 232–233, 236

vasoactive intestinal peptide (VIP) 69
venlafaxine 255, 257
ventral tegmental area (VTA) 7, 19, 57, 88, 141–146, 171–172, 215, 243
vigabatrin 279–280
vitamins 34
voltage-gated channels 43

Walker's lissencephaly 115
Walker-Warburg syndrome (WWS) 115–116
walking corpse syndrome (see Cotard's)
Warkany syndrome 2 (see trisomy 8)
Warrior gene 87
Wernicke's area 6, 29, 180, 335–336
Wernicke's encephalopathy 158
West syndrome 270
Williams syndrome 112
Wilson's disease 301–303
wnt pathway 205–206, 328

X chromosome 87, 105, 108–110, 112

Y chromosome 95, 105–106

zuclopenthixol 222